Prostaglandins and Reproduction

Prostaglandins and Reproduction

Edited by
S. M. M. Karim

Springer-Science+Business Media, B.V.

© 1975 Springer Science+Business Media Dordrecht
Originally published by MTP Press Ltd in 1975
Softcover reprint of the Hardcover 1st edition 1975

No part of this book may be reproduced
in any form without the permission from the publisher
except for the quotation of brief passages
for the purpose of review

ISBN 978-94-011-7169-4   ISBN 978-94-011-7167-0 (eBook)
DOI 10.107/978-94-011-7167-0

First published 1975

Contents

Advances in Prostaglandin Research

This book is one of three books on the Prostaglandins edited by Professor Karim which together are designed to represent a comprehensive, critical and entirely up to date review of prostaglandin research. The contents of the other two books in the series are shown below:

Prostaglandins: Physiological, Pharmacological and Pathological Aspects
Edited by S. M. M. Karim

Prostaglandins: Chemical and Biochemical Aspects
Edited by S. M. M. Karim

List of Contributors

Jean-Jacques Amy, M.D.
Research Associate,
Department of Obstetrics,
State University of Ghent,
Ghent, Belgium.

Mike Cooper, Ph.D.
Pharmaceuticals Division,
Imperial Chemical Industries Ltd.,
Mereside Alderley Park,
Macclesfield, Cheshire.

Anthony P. F. Flint, Ph.D.
Research Fellow,
Nuffield Department of Obstetrics and Gynaecology,
University of Oxford,
Oxford.

Keith Hillier, Ph.D.
Research Fellow,
Nuffield Department of Obstetrics and Gynaecology,
University of Oxford, Oxford.
Department of Physiology and Biochemistry,
University of Southampton,
Southampton.

Sultan M. M. Karim, Ph.D., D.Sc.
Research Professor of Obstetrics and Gynaecology,
University of Singapore,
Kandang Kerbau Hospital,
Singapore, Republic of Singapore.

Kenneth T. Kirton, Ph.D.
Research Section Head,
Fertility Research,
The Upjohn Company,
Kalamazoo, Michigan, U.S.A.

Anant P. Labhsetwar, Ph.D.
Adjunct Associate Professor,
Division of Biology,
Kansas State University,
Manhattan, Kansas, U.S.A.

Bhashini Rao, Ph.D.
Research Fellow,
Department of Obstetrics and Gynaecology,
University of Singapore,
Kandang Kerbau Hospital,
Singapore, Republic of Singapore.

Michel Thiery, M.D., Ph.D.
Professor and Chairman,
Department of Obstetrics,
State University of Ghent,
Ghent, Belgium.

Arthur L. Walpole, Ph.D.
Pharmaceuticals Division,
Imperial Chemical Industries Ltd.,
Mereside Alderley Park,
Macclesfield, Cheshire.

Preface

This is the first in a series of three books on advances in prostaglandin research. In recent years there has been an unparalleled interest in these compounds and as a result a vast amount of research data has accumulated since the publication of my earlier book in 1972. At that time it was possible to present a fairly comprehensive review of the various aspects of prostaglandins research in one volume. This is no longer possible, and the contents are divided into three volumes: the present volume dealing with prostaglandins and reproduction and two further volumes to be published shortly dealing with other areas of prostaglandin research.

The authorship represents international scientists consisting of physiologists, pharmacologists, reproductive biologists, veterinary scientists and obstetrician gynaecologists actively engaged in different areas of prostaglandins research. Certain areas not covered in my 1972 book are included, i.e. effects of prostaglandins on the reproductive systems of the laboratory animals, (sheep and goat) and practical applications in animal husbandry. An attempt has been made to provide a total coverage of current advances relating to prostaglandins and reproduction. For the sake of completeness and continuity, material covered in my 1972 book is either briefly summarised or reference made to that edition.

The need for rapid publication in a fast expanding field is obvious. Attempts have been made to cover work published until the end of 1974 (although some omissions are inevitable) and publication date set for autumn 1975. This has only been possible as a result of the co-operation of the contributors in submitting their manuscripts on time and the efforts of the publishers in bringing out the book within a few months of receiving the manuscripts.

Tables and figures previously published are in general acknowledged by a reference in the legends and I am grateful to the respective authors, editors and publishers for their permission.

My thanks are due to my various colleagues, particularly Mr P. G. Adaikan, Drs Keith Hillier, Bhashini Rao, John Salmon and R. L. Tambyraja for discussion and advice on the subject matter of some of the chapters and to Miss Lo Pia Yong and Miss Leong Yun Kiew for cross-checking the journal references and proof reading. I am also grateful to Professor S. S. Ratnam, Head of the Department of Obstetrics and Gynaecology, University of

Singapore for his support and encouragement. I should also like to thank Miss Lily Koh for expert secretarial assistance.

Singapore, March 1975   Sultan M. M. Karim

1
General Introduction and Comments

S. M. M. KARIM and B. RAO

1.1 INTRODUCTION

The last decade has been the most prolific and stimulating period in the area of prostaglandin research. The flood of information that has come out of laboratories around the world is quite staggering (Figure 1.1). This book in itself is a witness to the vast amount of information that has accumulated in the area of reproduction alone. Such an interest in the field is exciting and augurs well for further development. However, this very fact also makes the task of the reviewer difficult.

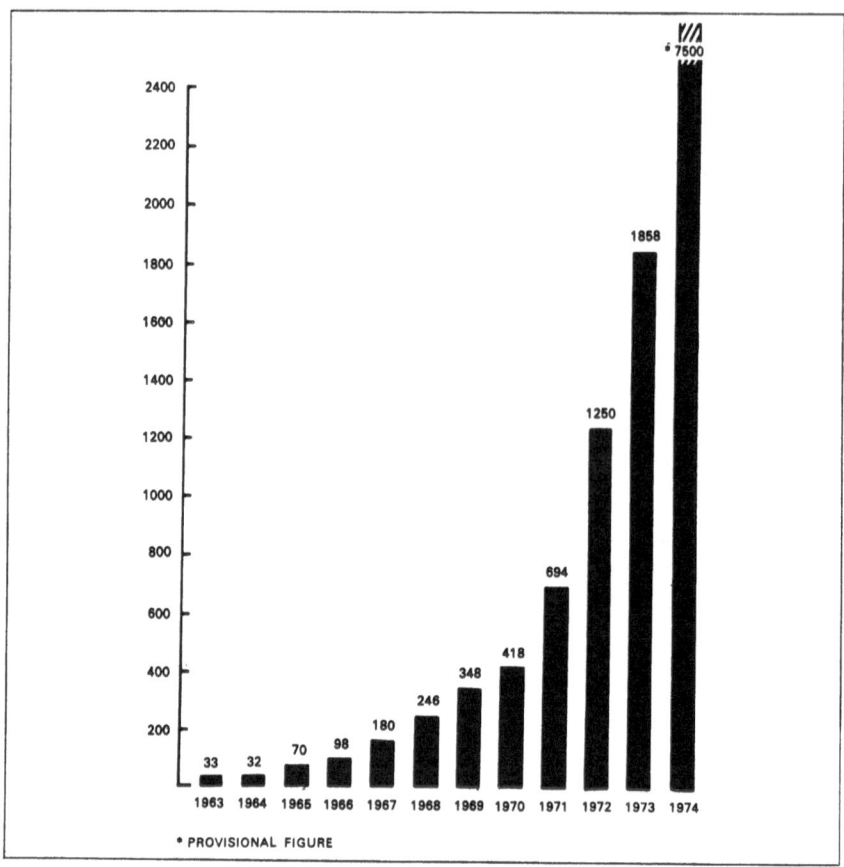

Figure 1.1   Cumulative growth of the literature in prostaglandins, 1930–1974

The increase in research activity in the field unfortunately does not seem to have brought with it a proportionate increase in the basic understanding of either the role of prostaglandins in normal reproductive processes or the basic mechanisms of their pharmacological action. Nevertheless, it has become quite evident that prostaglandins hold a key position in the common pathway through which hormones and drugs exert control over different aspects of reproduction. If the present interest in the field continues one could, with a degree of confidence, predict that what may seem at the present time to be disparate pieces of information may in fact turn out to be integral parts of the same jigsaw puzzle. Meanwhile any attempt to bring together information obtained from different experimental models (often contradictory) and to seek some common basis must therefore seem premature. And yet it is important, at different stages of development of a field, not only to look for possible generalisations but also to a certain extent indulge in speculations since meaningful generalisation and speculation play an important role in stimulating new thoughts and in pointing to new directions. In any attempt of this kind it is difficult for the authors to completely avoid personal views and prejudices.

This chapter aims at presenting to the reader a brief overall review of historical development and the state of knowledge of the role of prostaglandins in different aspects of reproduction. Instead of merely cataloguing numerous publications an attempt is made to interpret what seems to be significant and point to the gaps in our knowledge. It is hoped that this will stimulate further research in the field.

1.2 HISTORICAL

The biological activity of seminal fluid and prostate gland extracts has been recognised for many years. Thus in ancient China seminal fluid from young adults was considered to be of therapeutic value in patients with gastric ulceration (Chau, 1972). Amongst some North African tribes oral ingestion of the father's semen is used to initiate labour when this is delayed (Harley, 1941). Pharmacological activity of prostate was first demonstrated by Japelli and Scafa (1906) who observed a rise in blood pressure of the dog upon injecting extracts of bull and dog prostate glands. In contrast aqueous extracts of human prostate gland produced a fall in blood pressure in the dog (Battez and Boulet, 1913). Kurzrok and Lieb (1930) found that fresh human semen altered the motility of the human uterus *in vitro*. A few years later Von Euler (1934, 1935) and Goldblatt (1933, 1935) independently observed the smooth muscle stimulating activity of extracts of human seminal fluid. It was Von Euler (1936) who firmly established that the pharmacological effect of the active principle in the human seminal fluid extracts was due to a completely new substance and called it prostaglandin in the belief that it was secreted by the prostate gland. Although this assumption proved incorrect when Eliasson (1959) showed that human seminal prostaglandins originate from the seminal vesicles the name prostaglandin had become firmly established. Von Euler's studies also showed that the biological activity of the seminal fluid extract was associated with a fraction containing lipid soluble acids. Similar activity was also present in the seminal fluid of the monkey, sheep, goat and extracts of sheep seminal vesicles.

1.3 PURIFICATION, ISOLATION AND CHEMICAL STRUCTURES OF PROSTAGLANDINS

After a gap of several years the work on the identification of prostaglandins was commenced in 1949 by Bergström who confirmed Von Euler's findings that the biological activity of human seminal fluid extract was due to a new group of highly active lipid soluble unsaturated hydroxy fatty acids. Bergström also recognised that seminal fluid extract contained more than one prostaglandin. The isolation in pure crystalline form from sheep vesicular glands of the first two prostaglandins—now called prostaglandin E_1 (PGE$_1$ and prostaglandin $F_{1\alpha}$ (PGF$_{1\alpha}$) was reported by Bergström and Sjövall in 1957. Several related prostaglandins have since been isolated from human seminal plasma and from sheep vesicular glands and their chemical structures elucidated (see Bergström, Carlson and Weeks, 1968). The chemical structure of naturally occurring prostaglandins, their metabolites and their nomenclature have been previously discussed by Schneider (1972) and only a brief summary will be given here.

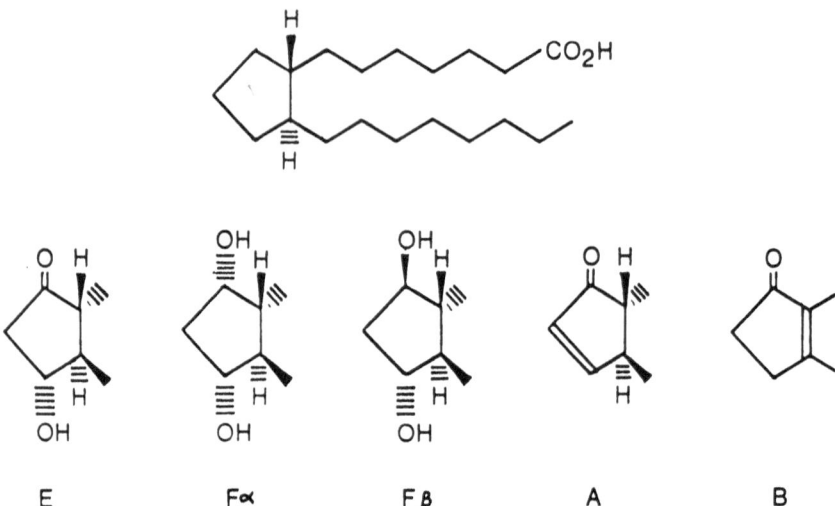

Figure 1.2 Prostanoic acid (Top) and structural differences (Bottom) between prostaglandins of the E, F, A and B series

Chemically all prostaglandins are 20-carbon hydroxy fatty acids with a cyclopentane ring and two side-chains and are derivatives of prostanoic acid (Figure 1.2). They are divided into four groups designated by the letters E, F, A and B corresponding to differences in the five-membered cyclopentane ring (Figure 1.2). The naturally occurring prostaglandin of the E and F groups (i.e. E_1, E_2, E_3, $F_{1\alpha}$, $F_{2\alpha}$ and $F_{3\alpha}$) are referred to as primary prostaglandins because other prostaglandins are derived from these compounds. All primary prostaglandins have an OH group in the 15 position and contain a 13, 14-*trans* double bond. The subscript number after the letter denotes the degree of unsaturation in the side chains of the prostaglandin molecule. Thus, PGE$_1$, PGF$_{1\alpha}$, A$_1$, B$_1$ have only one pair of double bonds; E$_2$, F$_{2\alpha}$, A$_2$ and B$_2$ have two pairs of double bonds. F$_{1\beta}$ and F$_{2\beta}$ are isomeric alcohols obtained by chemical reduction of E prostaglandins. Only the α-isomers occur naturally.

In addition to the thirteen naturally occurring prostaglandins originally reported present in the semen, Taylor and Kelly (1974) have shown that fresh human semen also contains 19-hydroxylated PGE$_1$ and PGE$_2$ (Figure 1.3). Intermediate groups of prostaglandins (intermediate between Es and Bs) of a generally unstable nature have also been identified.

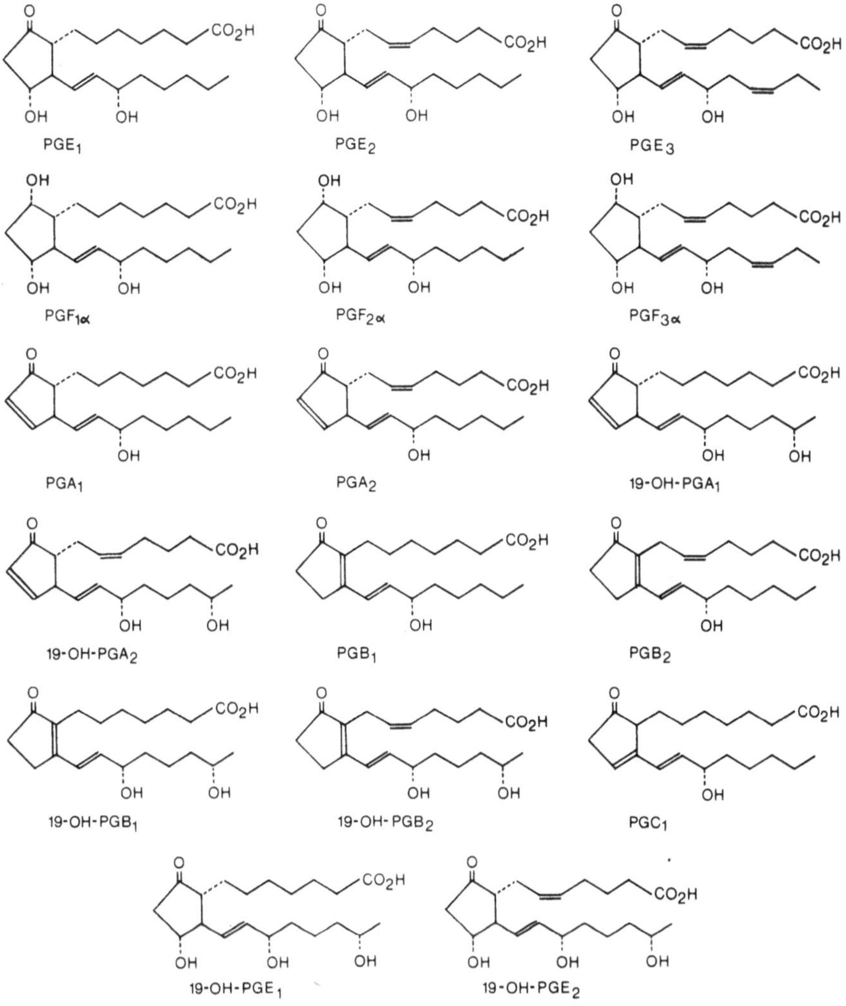

Figure 1.3 Chemical structures of naturally occurring prostaglandins

1.4 BIOSYNTHESIS AND SYNTHESIS

The precursors for the biosynthesis of prostaglandins are three unsaturated acids, e.g. 8,11,14-Eicosatetranoic acid (di-homo-γ-linoleic acid), 5,8,11, 14-Eicosatetraenoic acid (arachidonic acid) and 5,8,11,14,17-Eicosapentaneoic acid. These precursor acids are derived from the essential fatty acid—linoleic acid. Natural synthesis of prostaglandins from their fatty acid precursors is under the control of a microsomal synthetase system (prostaglandin synthetase). The pathways are outlined in Figure 1.4. Prostaglandin synthetase activity has been demonstrated in a large number of organs and this activity is inhibited by non-steroidal anti-inflammatory drugs such as aspirin, indomethacin and fenamates. Several different routes of total synthesis

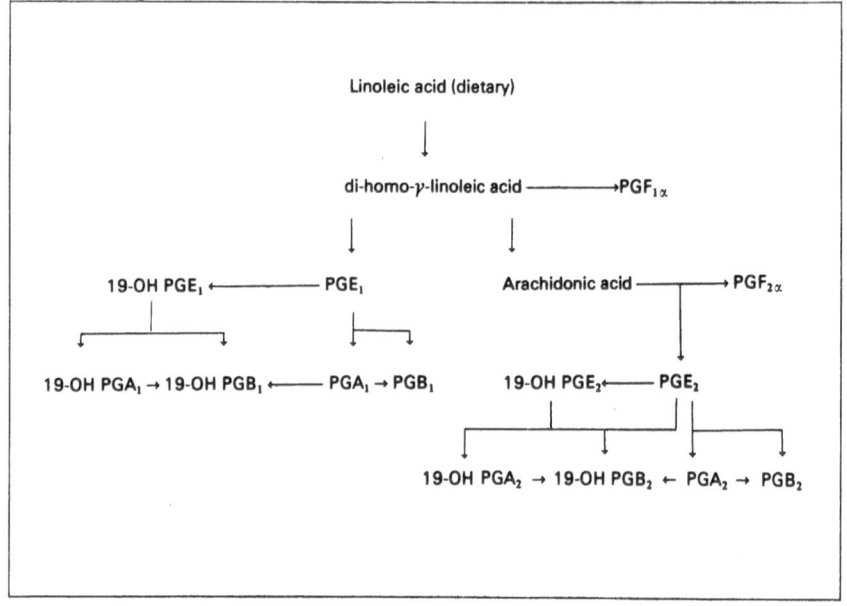

Figure 1.4   Outline of prostaglandin biosynthesis from linoleic acid

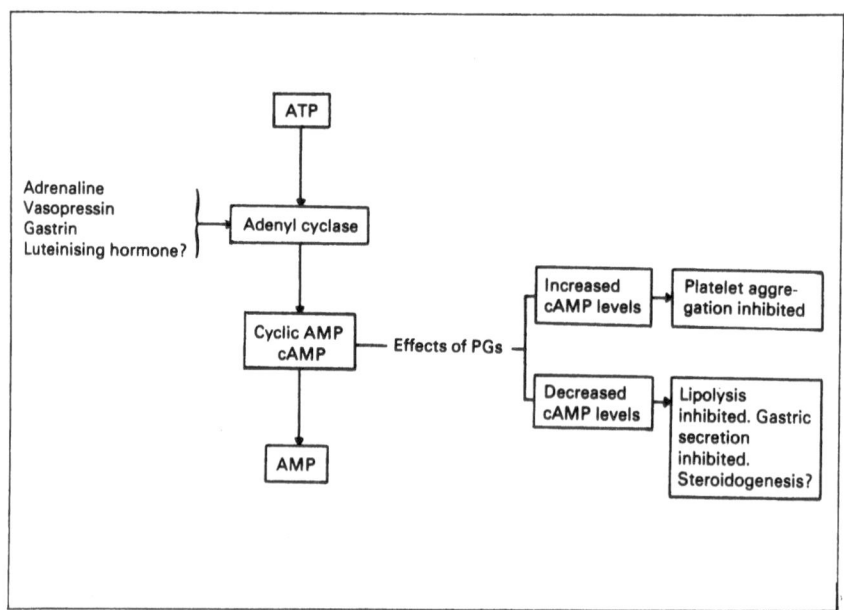

Figure 1.5   Schematic representation of prostaglandins with cyclic AMP system

Table 1.1 Occurrence of prostaglandins in human tissues and fluids

Source	Prostaglandins	References
Seminal fluid	E_1, E_2, E_3, $F_{1\alpha}$, $F_{2\alpha}$ A_1, A_2, B_1, B_2, 19-hydroxy A_1, 19-hydroxy A_2, 19-hydroxy B_1, 19-hydroxy B_2, 19-hydroxy E_1, 19-hydroxy E_2	Chapter 2
Menstrual fluid Endometrium	E_2, $F_{2\alpha}$	Chapter 2
Amniotic fluid during pregnancy and labour	E_1, E_2, $F_{1\alpha}$, $F_{2\alpha}$	Chapter 2
Maternal blood during gestation and labour	$F_{2\alpha}$, E_2	Chapter 2
Decidua	$F_{2\alpha}$, E_2	Chapter 2
Fallopian tube	$F_{2\alpha}$, E_2	Chapter 2
Umbilical and placental blood vessels	E, F	Chapter 2
Umbilical cord blood	$F_{2\alpha}$	
Aqueous humour	E_2	Wyllie and Wyllie (1971); Podos et al. (1972); Eakins et al. (1973)
Blood (normal)	$F_{2\alpha}$, E, A, F	Unger et al. (1971); William (1971); Jubiz et al. (1972); Wolfe et al. (1972); Jaffe et al. (1973); Hennam et al. (1974); Pletka and Hickler (1974)
Urine	$F_{1\alpha}$, $F_{2\alpha}$, E_1, E_2	Frölich et al. (1973)
Gastric juice and gastric mucosa	E_2	Bennett et al. (1968, 1970, 1973); Peskar et al. (1974)
Eccrine sweat	E_2	Frewin et al. (1973); Förström et al. (1974)
Kidney	A, E	Vance (1973)
Skin perfusate (normal)	E_1, E_2, $F_{1\alpha}$, $F_{2\alpha}$	Greaves et al. (1971)
Lung	E_2, $F_{2\alpha}$	Änggard (1965); Karim et al. (1967)
Thymus	E_1,	
Thyroid	E_2, $F_{2\alpha}$,	
Vagus nerve	E_2, $F_{2\alpha}$,	Karim et al. (1967)
Cervical sympathetic nerve	E_2, $F_{2\alpha}$,	
Bronchi	E_2, $F_{2\alpha}$,	
Cardiac muscle	E_2	
Gingival tissue	E_2	Goodson et al. (1974)
Cells in tissue culture: epidermal, fibroblasts	E	Jaffe et al. (1973); Förström et al. (1974b)
Cerebrospinal fluid	$F_{2\alpha}$	La Torre et al. (1974)

of prostaglandins have been worked out and most of the presently used prostaglandins are prepared by total synthesis.

The Gorgonian plexaura homomalla is the richest natural source of prostaglandins. This Caribbean coral contains 15-epi-PGA$_2$ and its diester in amounts of 0.2 and 1.3% respective of the dried cortex. The coral prostaglandins have been used as intermediates to prepare biologically active natural prostaglandins and their synthetic analogues (Weinshenker and Andersen, 1973; Schneider, 1975).

1.5 DISTRIBUTION OF PROSTAGLANDINS

Prostaglandins are widely distributed in mammalian tissues, although with considerable qualitative, quantitative and species variation (Table 1.1). Their possible occurrence in tissues of lower animals and in plants is being investigated. Since the most abundant free fatty acid in the body is arachidonic acid, the majority of tissues contain either PGE$_2$ or PGF$_{2\alpha}$ or both. Unlike many other biologically active substances prostaglandins are formed immediately prior to release and are not stored in the body. Biosynthesis and release of prostaglandins from tissues occur so readily in response to a variety of physiological and pathological stimuli that it would appear that any distortion of cell membrane is an adequate trigger mechanism. The ease with which prostaglandins are biosynthesised implies that prostaglandin concentration values reported for many tissues do not accurately reflect the true endogenous concentration. Experimentally induced release may indicate accelerated biosynthesis rather than activation of release mechanism.

1.6 PHARMACOLOGICAL ACTIONS OF PROSTAGLANDINS

The various biological actions of prostaglandins on the tissues of male and female reproductive systems are discussed in detail in the chapters that follow. Beyond this, prostaglandins have a wide range of pharmacological actions. This is illustrated in Table 1.2 which lists in a general way some of the many actions of prostaglandins. Generally but not invariably the individual prostaglandins of a group have the same biological action on any one system but can differ quantitatively. However, the same prostaglandins may have qualitatively dissimilar effects upon different tissues and likewise prostaglandins from separate groups may have dissimilar actions. Thus PGE$_1$ relaxes the umbilical blood vessels *in vitro* whereas PGE$_2$ has a stimulant action. Prostaglandins E$_1$ and E$_2$ are bronchodilators whereas PGF$_{1\alpha}$ and F$_{2\alpha}$ induce bronchoconstriction. The prostaglandin type, the tissue, or species can determine the pharmacological or physiological effect.

Certain target organs are keenly sensitive to the prostaglandins. For instance, although over 90% of PGE and PGF compounds are metabolised during one circulation through the lungs and liver only minute doses are required to selectively stimulate human uterine muscle *in vivo*. While the actions of the prostaglandins are limited by their rapid inactivation, it has recently been shown that certain of their breakdown products which are more

Table 1.2 A generalised account of some of the actions of prostaglandins

Effect	Prostaglandins	General reference
Central nervous system	E, F	Horton (1972); Coceani and Pace —Asciak (1975)
Meiosis, intraocular pressure	E	Eakins (1973, 1975)
Bronchodilatation and bronchoconstriction	E, F	Cuthbert (1973); Smith (1975)
Cardiovascular effects	E, A, F	Nakano (1973); Karim and Somers (1972); Malik and McGiff (1975)
Gastrointestinal motility and secretion	E, F	Bennett (1972, 1975); Waller (1973)
Pancreatic function	E	Wilson (1974)
Natriuresis, diuresis, redistribution of blood supply Renal blood flow	E, A	Lee (1973); Malik and McGiff (1975); McGiff (1975)
Inhibition of platelet adhesiveness and aggregation	E	Mody (1972); Willis and Weiss (1973); Howie (1975)
Inflammatory processes	E, F	Vane (1973); Søndergaard (1973); Greaves (1975)
Endocrine involvement Cyclic AMP effects	E, F	Hittlemann and Butcher (1973); Kuehl et al. (1975)
Autonomic neurotransmission	E, F	Hedqvist (1973, 1975)
Lipid metabolism	E	Paoletti and Puglisi (1973)

All 1975 references quoted in this table refer to the two other volumes in this series

resistant to metabolism, can be biologically active. This may explain in part why pharmacological effects persist for a longer period than would be expected. It is known that the lung metabolises prostaglandins of the A and B series to a lesser extent than prostaglandin of the E or F series and the former are more likely to act as circulating hormones. It is probable that the E and F series are only physiologically important as local hormones.

To alter the duration of action and potency of the prostaglandins, chemical structural modifications have been effected to protect groups sensitive to enzymatic inactivation by the lungs. This has resulted in 15-methyl and 16, 16-dimethyl derivatives which have enhanced actions and on certain systems increased selectivity (Chapters 2–8).

Pharmacological and physiological investigations of the prostaglandins have been considerably aided by the use of inhibitors of their synthesis and receptor interaction. Compounds structurely related to the prostaglandins and certain non-steroidal anti-inflammatory drugs like aspirin, indomethacin and fenamates are effective inhibitors of synthetase activity (Vane, 1973; Lands and Rome, 1975). The interaction of prostaglandins at receptor level can be blocked by compounds such as polyphloretin phosphate and some dibenzoxapenine derivatives (Eakins and Sanner, 1972; Sanner, 1974; Sanner and Eakins, 1975). There are reasons to suspect that the prostaglandins may be linked to the physiology of many bodily functions and to disorders of these functions. Disturbed production of prostaglandins might contribute to

Table 1.3 Pathological conditions which cause changes in the release of prostaglandins (From Nakano (1973a), by courtesy of *Residents and Staff Physician*)

System	Increase	Decrease
General	Malignant tumours, sepsis, fever, trauma, burn, shock	EFA deficiency Malnutrition Aspirin and idomethacin
Central nervous system	Fever (thermoregulatory centre in hypothalamus) Subarachnoid haemorrhage Cerebral embolism, haemorrhage and trauma	
Cardiovascular system	Pulmonary hypertension Circulatory failure	
Respiratory system	Bronchial asthma (PGF$_{2\alpha}$) Anaphylactic bronchospasm Pulmonary embolism Aspiration, pneumonia	
Gastrointestinal system	Diarrhoea due to infections (cholera) Gastritis. Intestinal obstruction	Gastric hyperacidity? Peptic ulcer? Constipation?
Renal system	Essential hypertension Renovascular hypertension Renal ischaemia	
Haematological system	Thromboembolism (PGE$_2$) Sickle-cell crisis Polycythemia. Leucocytosis	
Reproductive system	Habitual and threatened abortion. Dysmenorrhoea. Endometriosis? Labour. Intrauterine devices	Uterine inertia Male sterility? Hysterectomy (Pseudopregnancy)
Endocrine system and metabolism	Endocrine disorders (Hyperfunctions) Obesity	Endocrine disorders (Hypofunctions)
Musculoskeletal and skin system	Arthritis. Inflammation Allergy	Dermatitis due to EFA Deficiency
Eye	Glaucoma. Eye injury Uveitis	
Tooth	Gingivitis. Periodontal abscess	

symptomatology associated with some pathological conditions (Table 1.3) and administration of prostaglandins or inhibitors of prostaglandin synthesis or action may limit the symptoms.

One unifying hypothesis for many of the diverse actions of prostaglandin is their ability to modify the production of cyclic adenosine monophosphate (cyclic AMP). Two types of effects have been observed (Figure 1.5). As an example cyclic AMP enhances lipolysis and gastric secretion and in these systems PGEs both inhibit adenyl cyclase conversion to cyclic AMP and also inhibit lipolytic and gastric secretory activities. In the platelet aggregation system, increased cyclic AMP production inhibits the aggregation of platelets and prostaglandin E$_1$ enhances the formation of cyclic AMP and also inhibits platelet aggregation (Hittleman and Butcher, 1973; Kuehl, 1975) (Table 1.4).

Table 1.4   Cyclic AMP-mediated biological actions of PGE₁ (From Nakano (1973a), by courtesy of *Residents and Staff Physician*)

Tissue	Species	Responses
Stimulatory effects		
Heart	Guinea-pig	Positive inotropic and chronotropic actions
Lung and Diaphragm	Rat	Bronchodilatation
Aorta	Rat	Vasodilation
Kidney	Dog, rat	Inhibition of sodium and water reabsorption
Bone	Rat	Bone resorption (calcitonin effect)
Leukocyte	Human	Emigration and lysosomal membrane stabilisation
Erythrocyte*	Human	Fragility, erythropoiesis
Platelet	Rat, human, rabbit	Inhibition of aggregation
Anterior pituitary	Rat	Stimulation of ACTH, TSH, growth hormone, LH secretion
Corpus luteum*	Bovine	Progesterone secretion
Thyroid*	Dog, rat	Thyroxin secretion
Adrenals	Rat	Corticosterone secretion
*PGE₂		
Inhibitory effects		
Renal tubules medulla	Rabbit Hamster	Inhibition of water transport
Bladder	Toad	Inhibition of water transport
Stomach	Dog	Inhibition of gastric secretion
Adipose tissue	Rat and human	Inhibition of lipolysis
Cerebellum	Cat	Inhibition of action potential discharge

1.7 PROSTAGLANDINS AND REPRODUCTION

The various pharmacological actions and physiological roles of prostaglandins in relation to reproduction in different laboratory animals, subhuman primates and human are discussed in detail in Chapters 2–8.

In the male, prostaglandins are implicated in the processes of erection, ejaculation, sperm motility and morphology. In the female on the other hand, enough evidence has accumulated to suggest that prostaglandins are involved in menstruation, spontaneous abortion and labour, ovulation and luteolysis.

1.7.1 Male

Human seminal fluid is the richest known mammalian source of prostaglandins. Fifteen different prostaglandins belonging to four groups (PGA, PGB, PGE and PGF) are present. Together they amount to 300 μg ml^{-1} of semen. The level of prostaglandin in the seminal fluid can be reduced by prostaglandin synthetase inhibitors such as aspirin. Seminal vesicles have been shown to be the major source of prostaglandins present in the seminal fluid but it is quite possible that other glandular systems contributing to the ejaculate may also synthesise some prostaglandins (Chapter 2). It is also not clear whether spermatozoa itself contains any prostaglandins. Very little is known about the distribution of prostaglandins in the semen of laboratory animals.

The physiological significance of the presence of prostaglandins in the seminal fluid is not clear. Being potent inhibitors of lipolysis they may act as membrane stabilising agents by preventing lipid peroxidation damage to the sperm membranes. Seminal prostaglandin may also be of importance in the transport of the spermatozoa in the female reproductive tract.

Although prostaglandins have been shown to relax or stimulate the smooth muscle of the human penis, clearly much more work is needed in this area to test the suggestion that prostaglandins may be involved in erection or ejaculation (Chapter 2).

Attempts have been made to establish a correlation between the prostaglandin content of seminal fluid and male fertility. There is some evidence to show that semen sample from men in infertile marriages contained less PGE compounds compared with samples from men with recently documented fertility (Chapter 2). However it has not been possible to show any correlation between prostaglandin content of seminal fluid and the number or degree of motility of the spermatozoa—two important requirements for fertility. This lack of effect on motility or number does not, however, rule out the possibility of other biochemical and morphological changes in the spermatozoa which can go undetected under light microscopy. Such changes may influence the fertilising ability of the spermatozoa. It would be very useful to explore the effect of prostaglandins on the spermatozoa at the ultrastructural and biochemical level.

1.7.2 Female

The possibility that prostaglandins might be used pharmacologically for fertility control has acted as a great stimulus to research on the role of prostaglandins in female reproduction. Various aspects of female reproduction such as sperm transport, tubal and ovarian contractility, luteolysis, menstruation, abortion, parturition and closure of umbilical blood vessels after birth have been studied.

1.7.3 Ovulation

The fact that prostaglandins are present in the ovary has been known for a long time but their precise distribution with respect to various ovarian compartments (corpus luteum, follicle and interstitium) remains to be elucidated. Recent investigations from a number of laboratories have indicated that prostaglandins play a significant role in the process of ovulation both in the primates and subprimates. In the human most of the research has concentrated on the effect of prostaglandins on ovarian contractility. This may indirectly influence the rupture of the follicle (Chapter 2).

The most interesting points to have emerged from the *in vivo* and *in vitro* studies are:

1. Both PGF and PGE are synthesised in the follicle. As ovulation approaches the ratio of PGF to PGE in the follicle increases (Chapter 5).
2. Indomethacin, an inhibitor of prostaglandin synthesis, prevents ovulation if injected intravenously or directly into the follicle. The indomethacin block can be reversed by administration of increasing doses of luteinising hormone (LH) or prostaglandins (Chapters 5 and 6).
3. Ovulation can also be blocked by intrafollicular injection of antisera to prostaglandins.
4. Follicles in which ovulation is blocked by indomethacin go through luteinisation without any impairment of their hormonal pattern. Thus cycles treated with indomethacin, though infertile, appear to be normal in duration and hormonal secretion. This result in itself is of particular interest since it points to the fact that follicle rupture and luteinisation are two independent events with different control mechanisms. While follicular prostaglandins are important in the physiology of ovulation they seem to have no effect on luteinisation of granulosa cells (Chapter 6).

The mode of action of prostaglandins in facilitating follicular rupture is still unclear. Prostaglandins could trigger follicular rupture by altering vascular permeability or by affecting contractile activity of the ovary. The fact that $PGF_{2\alpha}$ stimulates ovarian contractions and that there is a greater increase of PGF as compared to PGE during ovulation suggests that prostaglandins of the F, rather than that of E series may play a more important role in the process of ovulation. The significance of the presence of PGE in the follicular fluid is still not clear. There are indications that in the rhesus monkey granulosa cell cultures, prostaglandins E_1 and E_2 stimulate progesterone synthesis and morphological luteinisation of the granulosa cells (Chapter 5).

1.7.4 Sperm transport

It has been suggested that prostaglandins can influence sperm transport by altering uterine motility. Very little concrete evidence is available for this suggestion. The demonstration that $PGF_{2\alpha}$ increases sperm penetration and drive of the spermatozoa through the cervical mucus is an exciting one (Chapter 2). It is not known whether other naturally occurring prostaglandins share this property of $PGF_{2\alpha}$. It is conceivable that the relationship between the deficiency of prostaglandins in seminal fluid and male infertility is due to a decrease in the sperm penetration and drive through cervical mucus.

It could be interesting to investigate whether cervical mucus contain any prostaglandin metabolising enzymes and whether female infertility, or the mechanism of action of oral contraceptives is due to alterations in the concentration of these enzymes.

1.7.5 Tubal motility or egg transport

The possible role of prostaglandins in the passage of the ovum through fallopian tubes is suggested by studies using two different experimental approaches:

1. Effect of prostaglandins on tubal motility both *in vivo* and *in vitro*.
2. Effect of prostaglandins on egg transport.

Although it seems reasonable to believe that tubal motility can influence egg transport there is as yet no direct experimental evidence to support this belief. The effects of prostaglandins on tubal motility have been studied in the human, monkey, sheep and rabbit.

Human fallopian tubes have been shown to contain $PGF_{2\alpha}$ and PGE_1. *In vivo* tubal motility seems to vary with the phase of the menstrual cycle. Furthermore, $PGF_{2\alpha}$ has a stimulatory effect, while PGE_2 produces inhibition of tubal motility. Results from *in vitro* experiments suggest that the response of the fallopian tube is dependent not only on the type of the prostaglandin used but also on the anatomical position of the segment of the tube studied. The physiological implication of these findings is not clear (Chapter 2).

Variation of tubal motility with the phase of menstrual cycle has also been shown to be true in the rhesus monkey. Prostaglandin E_2 and E_1 depressed spontaneous motility while $PGF_{2\alpha}$ had a stimulating effect. These contrasting effects of PGF and PGE have been confirmed both in the sheep and in the rabbit (Chapters 6 and 7).

Experiments on the transport of ovum through the fallopian tube have been carried out mainly in the laboratory animals. Results are often contradictory. In the rabbit $PGF_{2\alpha}$ has been shown to accelerate the passage of the eggs through the fallopian tube while PGE_2 was ineffective. In the hamster, on the other hand, prostaglandins have no effect on egg transport. Clearly more information is required before one can define the role of different prostaglandins in egg transport.

1.7.6 Luteolysis

The importance of corpus luteum in the normal menstrual cycle and in maintaining early pregnancy is well-established. If a way could be found to inhibit corpus luteum function after fertilisation and/or implantation of the ovum, then a postcoital contraceptive to be taken once a month by the woman could be developed. One of the obstacles in understanding the role of prostaglandin in the physiology of luteolysis is the variation amongst species. Yet from the vast amount of data collected it is possible to extract some similarities.

1. In animals where the process of luteal maintenance and regression depends upon the presence of the uterus, prostaglandins are effective in causing luteal regression both in the pregnant and in the non-pregnant cycle. The sheep and the rabbit are typical examples of this group (Chapters 6 and 7).
2. Primates belong to the second group where luteolysis in the normal cycle is not controlled by the uterus. Administration of prostaglandin

$F_{2\alpha}$ in the non-pregnant monkey has little effect on the hormone levels in the early luteal phase and in the late luteal phase very high doses are required to cause luteolysis or to shorten the length of the menstrual cycle. Moreover administration of prostaglandin $F_{2\alpha}$ antiserum or inhibitors of prostaglandin synthesis are without any effect on the corpus luteum function or cycle length. These studies indicate that the primate corpus luteum of the normal menstrual cycle is not as vulnerable to prostaglandin-induced luteolysis as the corpus luteum of the sheep or many laboratory animals. However, in humans and monkeys during early pregnancy, administration of $PGF_{2\alpha}$ is followed by a decrease in plasma progesterone levels. The decrease in steroid level is associated with the onset of vaginal bleeding. It is debatable whether this drop in progesterone level reflects a direct effect of $PGF_{2\alpha}$ on the corpus luteum or whether it is the result of an indirect luteolytic effect brought about by the removal of the possible luteotrophic support of the conceptus, the latter being dislodged by the direct uterine stimulant effect of prostaglandins (Chapter 5).

In the human, several studies have been carried out to assess the effects of prostaglandins on the corpus luteum of the normal cycle. Prostaglandins have been administered either intravenously or intravaginally. Overall results are equivocal. But if one were to make a generalisation, it would be that exogenous prostaglandins when given intravenously or intravaginally are not luteolytic in the non-pregnant cycle. In very early pregnancy when corpus luteum is the major source of progesterone and its functional integrity is essential for the maintenance of pregnancy, a marked depression in progesterone level is observed after prostaglandin administration. Again as in the sub-human primates it can be argued that this decline in progesterone level does not represent a true luteolytic effect but is due to the demise of the corpus luteum function indirectly by removal of its trophic support. At this stage, when so little information is available on the nature of either the 'trophic support' or the 'natural luteolysin' in the primates, it is difficult to distinguish between direct and indirect luteolysis (Chapters 2 and 3).

The mechanisms by which prostaglandins cause luteolysis are unclear. Altered gonadotrophin secretion, vascular insult, antagonism to luteotrophins at the ovarian level and direct effect on the lutein cells are some of the mechanisms suggested. There is not enough evidence, at this stage, to accept any of these mechanisms completely. An appreciation of the complexity of the problem leads to the realisation that there will be no single answer to the problem of luteolysis. Rather, it should be viewed as an expression of a series of related events in which more than one mechanism may be involved.

1.7.7 Umbilical cord and placenta

It has been shown that the blood vessels of the full-term human umbilical cord and the large surface vessels of the placenta contain prostaglandins Es and Fs. They are not present in blood vessels from early pregnancy. They do however appear during spontaneous abortion. These observations have led to the suggestion that prostaglandins play an important role in the spontaneous closure of the umbilical blood vessels that occurs at birth. Prostaglandins have also been implicated in the regulation of fetal and placental circulation. Recently it has been shown that prostaglandins A_2 and B_2 are several times more potent than prostaglandins E_2, $F_{2\alpha}$ and $F_{1\alpha}$ in constricting the umbilical blood vessels. The possible presence of A and B prostaglandins in the umbilical blood and blood vessels has so far not been investigated (Chapter 2).

1.8 CLINICAL APPLICATIONS OF PROSTAGLANDINS

Practical applications of prostaglandins in the area of reproduction are discussed in detail in Chapters 3, 4 and 8 (Table 1.5). In addition prostaglandins promise to be of therapeutic value in several other areas (Karim and Hillier, 1974). The investigation of the physiological roles of prostaglandins in reproduction has proved of benefit in two ways. Firstly, by using exogenous prostaglandins it has been possible to mimic some of these processes, i.e. induction of menstruation, abortion and labour. Secondly, the use of prostaglandin synthesis inhibitors or receptor antagonists has a promise of practical applications. In some laboratory animals ovulation blockade with prostaglandin synthetase inhibitors has already been demonstrated. Such an effect in the human could form the basis of a once-a-month contraceptive. Prevention of premature labour by inhibiting prostaglandin synthesis in the human female has already been demonstrated. The implication of the last finding is far reaching and there is a growing conviction that one of the physiological stimuli for uterine contractions during labour is a prostaglandin.

In terms of practical applications, major advances have been made in developing the use of prostaglandins for the termination of pregnancy at almost any

Table 1.5 Established and potential clinical applications of prostaglandins and prostaglandin synthesis inhibitors in relation to human reproduction

Prostaglandins
Induction and acceleration of labour at term
Induction of labour in case of intrauterine fetal death
Induction of labour in case of anencephalic pregnancy
Cervical ripening at term
Termination of first and second trimester pregnancy
Termination of molar pregnancy
Termination of pregnancy in case of missed abortion
Menstrual induction
Preoperative cervical dilatation in the first trimester of pregnancy
Preoperative cervical dilatation in non-pregnant women
Management of 3rd stage of labour and prevention of postpartum haemorrhage
Treatment of male infertility

Prostaglandin synthesis inhibitors
Prevention of premature labour
Prevention of spontaneous abortion
Treatment of dysmennorhea
Ovulation block
Male contraception

stage of gestation. The failure to demonstrate a direct luteolytic effect of prostaglandins during very early human pregnancy has been a disappointment since such an effect could form the basis for an ideal method of fertility control by causing luteolysis and thus terminating pregnancy as soon as it is established. However, the fact that pregnancy can be terminated with intra-uterine administration of prostaglandins (possibly through uterine stimulation) during the first two weeks following a missed menstruation is encouraging. The route of drug administration not lending itself to self-treatment and the high incidence of gastrointestinal side-effects are at present limiting factors for widespread use of prostaglandins for menstrual induction. There are indications that these disadvantages will be overcome by employing one of the many synthetic analogues of prostaglandins now being evaluated.

The first ever clinical application of a prostaglandin was for the induction of labour at term (1968). The vast amount of clinical data accumulated in the past six years is discussed in Chapters 3–4. Until recently oxytocin has been the only drug available for the induction of labour at term. Several decades of experience has made it a safe and useful drug for the purpose. However it falls short by a considerable margin of being an ideal drug for the induction of labour. Controlled clinical trials have established that $PGF_{2\alpha}$ is as efficacious as oxytocin. However Liggins (1974) has suggested that the action of prostaglandin on the pregnant uterus is far more complex than that of oxytocin and that comparison based on their administration by identical techniques may do scant justice to the prostaglandins. 'Although prostaglandins, may, like oxytocin, fall short of the ideal, it is becoming apparent from preliminary work that prostaglandins have attributes for induction of labour that will ultimately rank them far superior to oxytocin'. In certain areas prostaglandins have already been shown to be superior to oxytocin. They clearly emerge as the agents of choice for induction of labour in pregnancies complicated by intrauterine fetal death or gross fetal malformation. Because of the ability of prostaglandins to stimulate the uterus at any stage of pregnancy, they are very effective when induction of labour is indicated before term. A major advantage of prostaglandins over oxytocin is the ability to stimulate the pregnant uterus at term when administered by mouth. Oral PGE_2 is as efficacious as intravenous oxytocin for the induction of labour, providing an advantage of simplicity.

It also needs to be emphasised that most studies of induction of labour with prostaglandins have utilised $PGF_{2\alpha}$. There are reasons to believe that PGE_2 may be superior to $PGF_{2\alpha}$ for this purpose.

Prostaglandins may also be the physiological substance involved in cervical ripening, enhanced sensitivity to oxytocin and eventually typical uterine activity associated with normal labour. If such proves to be the case, the full potential of prostaglandins in the induction of labour will be realised only by methods of administration that give these more subtle effects time to develop. It may be possible eventually to induce labour safely, even in out-patients by insertion into the vagina of a device liberating enough prostaglandin to start labour after a latent period of 48 hours or so, during which time the uterus becomes prepared to effect delivery efficiently and safely (Liggins, 1974).

The hypotensive property of PGA compounds may prove useful for the induction of labour in hypertensive patients since these prostaglandins are also able to stimulate the pregnant human uterus. The possible use of prostaglandins in the management of the postpartum period also remains unexplored. Some synthetic analogues of prostaglandins are able to produce sustained contractions of the uterus—a property which is essential for preventing postpartum haemorrhage.

In the area of second trimester pregnancy termination prostaglandins have received an unqualified acceptance. Pregnancy termination at this period of gestation requires a combination of uterine stimulation and cervical dilatation. It is often assumed that the latter will automatically follow the former. This does not seem to be the case because oxytocin in massive doses is able to produce high intensity, high frequency contractions of the uterus during second trimester of pregnancy, yet fail to dilate the cervix. Prostaglandins E_2 and $F_{2\alpha}$ in contrast produce uterine contractions and cervical dilatation. The latter effect may be the result of reduction in steroid hormone levels (particularly progesterone) brought about by prostaglandins (see Chapters 2 and 4). Earlier studies demonstrating the efficacy of prostaglandins for second trimester pregnancy termination were carried out with intravenous infusions of the compounds. In view of the wide range of pharmacological actions of prostaglandins, it was not surprising that the procedure was associated with gastrointestinal and other side-effects. These have been virtually eliminated by utilising the local routes, i.e. intra-amniotic and extra-amniotic. By applying the drugs directly to the target organ the efficacy is considerably increased. Further progress in the area in terms of increased efficacy and safety and reduced side-effects have come with the use of synthetic analogues of prostaglandins. It is hoped that with an appropriate prostaglandin analogue second trimester pregnancy termination will be possible by routes which do not invade the uterus. It is estimated that during the first full year of commercial availability of prostaglandins in the USA 25% of all second trimester pregnancies were terminated with prostaglandins. The figure is thought to be higher in the United Kingdom.

Although prostaglandins given by various routes are able to terminate pregnancy in the first trimester, the procedure does not compare favourably with the vacuum aspiration method. The latter is simple and less time consuming and can also be carried out on an outpatient basis. However, in a proportion of women it is necessary to mechanically dilate the cervix prior to the evacuation of the uterus. There is growing evidence that this leads to an increased incidence of spontaneous second trimester abortion or prematurity in subsequent pregnancy. Prostaglandin analogues (particularly 15-methyl-PGE_2 or 15-methyl-$PGF_{2\alpha}$) given as a single extra-amniotic dose a few hours prior to uterine evacuation have been found to be effective in dilating the cervix. It is assumed that cervical dilatation with prostaglandin does not lead to incompetent cervix since it occurs gradually.

The possible use of prostaglandins for the dilatation of the non-pregnant human cervix also remains unexplored.

References

Änggard, E. (1965). The isolation and determination of prostaglandins in lungs of sheep, guinea pig, monkey and man. *Biochem. Pharmacol.*, 14, 1507–1516

Battez, G. and Boulet, L. (1913). Action de l'extrait de prostate humaine sur la vessie et sur la pression arterielle. *C. R. Seanc. Soc. Biol.*, **74**, 8–9

Bennett, A., Murray, J. G. and Wyllie, J. H. (1968). Prostaglandins and gastric secretion in man. *Brit. J. Pharmacol.*, **32**, 339–349

Bennett, A. and Fleshler, B. (1970). Prostaglandins and gastro-intestinal tract. *Gastroenterology*, **59**, 790–800

Bennett, A. (1972). Effects of prostaglandins on the gastrointestinal tract. In: *The Prostaglandins: Progress in Research*, 205–221 (S. M. M. Karim, editor) (Lancaster: M.T.P.)

Bennett, A., Stamford, I. F. and Unger, W. G. (1973). PGE_2 and gastric acid secretion in man. *Adv. Biosciences*, **9**, 265–269

Bergström, S. (1949). Prostaglandins Kemi. *Nord. Med.*, **42**, 1465–1466

Bergström, S. and Sjövall, J. (1957). The isolation of prostaglandin. *Acta Chem. Scand.*, **11**, 1086

Bergström, S., Carlson, L. A. and Weeks, J. R. (1968). The Prostaglandins: A family of biologically active lipids. *Pharmacol. Rev.*, **20**, 1–48

Chau Eric (1972). *The Dragon and the Golden Phoenix* (Translation: New York, 1972)

Cuthbert, M. W. (1973). Prostaglandins and Respiratory smooth muscle. In: *The Prostaglandins*, 253–286 (M. F. Cuthbert, editor) (London: Heinemann)

Eakins, K. E. and Sanner, J. H. (1972). Prostaglandin antagonists. In: *The Prostaglandins: Progress in Research*, 263–292 (S. M. M. Karim, editor) (Lancaster: M.T.P.)

Eakins, K. E. (1973). Ocular effects. In: *The Prostaglandins*, 214–238 (P. W. Ramwell, editor) (N.Y., London: Plenum Press)

Eakins, K. E., Whitelocke, R. A. F., Perkins, E. S., Bennett, A. and Unger, W. G. (1973). Inflammation in rabbits and man. *Adv. Biosciences*, **9**, 427–433

Eliasson, R. (1959). Studies on prostaglandin. Occurrence, formation and biological actions. *Acta Physiol. Scand.*, **46, Suppl. 158**, 1–73

Förström, L., Goldyne, M. E. and Winkelmann, R. K. (1974a). Prostaglandin activity in human eccrine sweat. *Prostaglandins*, **7**, 459–464

Förström, L., Goldyne, M. E. and Winkelmann, R. K. (1974b). Prostaglandin production by human epidermal cells *in vitro*: A model for studying pharmacologic inhibition of prostaglandin synthesis. *Prostaglandins*, **8**, 107–115

Frewin, D. B., Eakins, K. E. and Downey, J. A. (1973). Prostaglandin-like activity in human eccrine sweat. *Aust. J. Exp. Biol. Med. Sci.*, **51**, 701–702

Frölich, J. C., Sweatman, B. J., Carr, K., Splawinski, J., Watson, J. T., Änggard, E. and Oates, J. A. (1973). Occurrence of prostaglandin in urine. *Adv. Biosciences*, **9**, 321–330

Goldblatt, M. W. (1933). A depressor substance in seminal fluid. *J. Soc. Chem. Ind. (London)*, **52**, 1056–1057

Goldblatt, M. W. (1935). Properties of human seminal plasma. *J. Physiol. (London)*, **84**, 208–218

Goodson, J. M., Dewhirst, F. E. and Brunetti, A. (1974). Prostaglandin E_2 levels in human peridontal disease. *Prostaglandins*, **6**, 81–85

Greaves, M. W., Søndergaard, J. and McDonald-Gibson, W., (1971). Recovery of prostaglandins in human cutaneous inflammation. *Brit. Med. J.*, **2**, 258–260

Harley, G. W. (1941). *Native African Medicine with Special Reference to its Practice in the Mano tribe of Liberia*, 237–238 (Cambridge, Mass.: Harvard University Press)

Hedqvist, P. (1973). Autonomic Neurotransmission. In: *The Prostaglandins*, Vol. 1, 101–131 (P. W. Ramwell, editor) (N.Y., London: Plenum Press)

Hennam, J. F., Johnson, D. A., Newton, J. R. and Collins, W. P. (1974). Radioimmunoassay of prostaglandin $F_{2\alpha}$ in peripheral venous plasma from men and women. *Prostaglandins*, **5**, 531–542

Hittelman, K. J. and Butcher, R. W. (1973). Cyclic AMP and the mechanism of action of the prostaglandins. In: *The Prostaglandins*, 151–166 (M. F. Cuthbert, editor) (London: Heinemann)

Horton, E. W. (1972). Prostaglandins. *Monogr. Endocrinol.*, **7**, 1–197 (Berlin: Springer-Verlag)

Jaffe, B. M., Behrman, H. R. and Parker, C. W. (1973). Radioimmunoassay measurement of prostaglandin E, A and F in human plasma. *J. Clin. Invest.*, **52**, 398–405

Jaffe, B. M., Philpott, G. W., Hamprecht, B. and Parker, C. W. (1973). Prostaglandin production by cells *in vitro*. *Adv. Biosciences*, **9**, 179–182

Japelli, G. and Scafa, G. M. (1906). Sur les effets des injections intraveineuses d'extrait prostatique de chien. *Arch. Ital. Bio.*, **45**, 165–182

Jubiz, W., Frailey, J., Child, C. and Bartholomew, K. (1972). Physiologic role of prosta-glandins of the E (PGE), F (PGF) and AB (PGAB) groups. Estimation by radioimmunoassay in unextracted human plasma. *Prostaglandins*, 2, 471–483

Karim, S. M. M., Sandler, M. and Williams, E. D. (1967). Distribution of prostaglandins in human tissues. *Brit. J. Pharmacol. Chemother.*, 31, 340–344

Karim, S. M. M. and Somers, K. (1972). Cardiovascular and renal effects of prostaglandins. In: *The Prostaglandins: Progress in Research*, 165–202 (S. M. M. Karim, editor) (Lancaster: M.T.P.)

Karim, S. M. M. and Hillier, K. (1974). Prostaglandins—Pharmacology and clinical applications. *Drugs*, 8, 176–207

Kuehl, F. (1975). Prostaglandins and cyclic AMP. In: *Prostaglandins: Progress in Research*, Vol. II (S. M. M. Karim, editor) (Lancaster: M.T.P.) (to be published in July 1975)

Kuzrok, R. and Lieb, C. C. (1930). Biochemical studies of human semen. II. Action of semen on the human uterus. *Proc. Soc. Exp. Biol. Med.*, 28, 268–272

La Torre, E., Patrono, C., Fortuna, A. and Grossi-Belloni, D. (1974). Role of prostaglandin $F_{2\alpha}$ in human cerebral vasospasm. *J. Neurosurg.*, 41, 293

Lands, W. E. M. and Rome, L. (1975). Prostaglandin synthetase inhibitors. In: *Prostaglandins: Progress in Research*, Vol. II (S. M. M. Karim, editor) (Lancaster: M.T.P.) (to be published in July 1975)

Lee, J. B. (1973). Renal homeostasis and the hypertensive state: A unifying hypothesis. In: *The Prostaglandins*, Vol. I, 133–188 (P. W. Ramwell, editor) (N.Y., London: Plenum Press)

Liggits, G. C. (1974). Prostaglandins: current therapeutic status in obstetrics. *Drugs*, 8, 161–163

Mody, N. J. (1972). Effects of prostaglandins on platelet function. In: *The Prostaglandins: Progress in Research*, 239–262 (S. M. M. Karim, editor) (Lancaster: M.T.P.)

Nakano, J. (1973). Cardiovascular Actions. In: *The Prostaglandins*, Vol. If 239–316 (P. W. Ramwell, editor) (N.Y., London: Plenum Press)

Nakano, J. (1973a). The Prostaglandins: Their effect on 14 clinical conditions. *Residents and Staff Physician*, 19, 93–106

Paoletti, R. and Puglisi, L. (1973). Lipid Metabolism. In: *The Prostaglandins*, Vol. I, 317–326 (P. W. Ramwell, editor) (N.Y., London: Plenum Press)

Peskar, B. M., Holland, A. and Peskar, B. A. (1974). Quantitative determination of prosta-glandins in human gastric juice by radioimmunoassay. *Clin. Chim. Acta*, 55, 21–27

Pletka, P. and Hickler, R. B. (1974). Blood prostaglandin A (PGA) levels in normal human subjects. *Prostaglandins*, 7, 107–115

Podos, S. M., Jaffe, B. M. and Becker, B. (1972). Prostaglandins and glaucoma. *Brit. Med. J.*, 4, 232

Sanner, J. H. (1974). Substances that inhibit the actions of prostaglandins. *Arch. Int. Med.*, 133, 133–146

Sanner, J. H. and Eakins, K. E. (1975). Prostaglandin antagonists. In: *The Prostaglandins: Progress in Research*, Vol. II (S. M. M. Karim, editor) (Lancaster: M.T.P.) (to be published in July 1975)

Schneider, W. P. (1972). The chemistry of the prostaglandins. In: *Prostaglandins: Progress in Research*, 293–319 (S. M. M. Karim, editor) (Lancaster: M.T.P.)

Schneider, W. P. (1975). The chemistry of the prostaglandins. In: *Prostaglandins: Progress in Research*, Vol. II (S. M. M. Karim, editor) (Lancaster: M.T.P.) (to be published in July 1975)

Smith, A. P. (1972). Effects of prostaglandins on respiratory system. In: *The Prostaglandins: Progress in Research*, 223–238 (S. M. M. Karim, editor) (Lancaster: M.T.P.)

Söndergaard, J. (1973). Skin. In: *The Prostaglandins*, Vol. I, 189–202 (P. W. Ramwell, editor) (N.Y., London: Plenum Press)

Taylor, P. L. and Kelly, R. W. (1974). 19-hydroxylated prostaglandins as the major prostaglan-dins in human semen. *Nature (London)*, 250, 665–667

Unger, W. G., Stamford, I. F. and Bennett, A. (1971). Extraction of prostaglandins from human blood. *Nature (London)*, 233, 336–337

Vance, V. K. (1973). Quoted by James, B. L. in Cardiovascular renal effects of prostaglandins. *Arch. Int. Med.*, 133, 56

Vane, J. R. (1973). Inhibition of prostaglandin biosynthesis as the mechanism of action of aspirin-like drugs. *Adv. Biosciences*, 9, 395–411

Von Euler, U. S. (1934). Zur Kenntnis der pharmakologischen Wirkung von nativsekreten und extrakten mánnlicher accessorischer Geschlechtsdrüsen. *Arch. Exp. Pathol. Pharmak.*, **175**, 78–84

Von Euler, U. S. (1935). A depressor substance in the vesicular gland. *J. Physiol. (London)*, **84**, 21P

Von Euler, U. S. (1936). On the specific vasodilating and plain muscle stimulating substances from accessory glands in man and certain animals (prostaglandin and vesiglandin) *J. Physiol. (London)*, **88**, 213–234

Waller, S. (1973). Prostaglandins and the gastrointestinal tract. *Gut*, **14**, 402–417

Weinshenker, N. M. and Andersen, N. H. (1973). Chemistry. In: *The Prostaglandins*, Vol. I, 5–82 (P. W. Ramwell, editor) (London: Plenum Press)

William, E. A. (1971). The extraction of PGE_1 from human plasma. *Life Sci.*, **10**, Part I, 1181–1191

Willis, A. L. and Weiss, H. J. (1973). A congenital defect in platelet prostaglandins production associated with impaired hemostasis in storage pool disease. *Prostaglandins*, **4**, 783–794

Wilson, D. E. (1974). Prostaglandins. Their actions on the gastrointestinal tract. *Arch. Int. Med.*, **133**, 112–118

Wolfe, L., Mamer, O. and Rostworowski, K. (1972). Prostaglandin levels in human body fluids. *Clin. Res.*, **20**, 925

Wyllie, A. M. and Wyllie, J. H. (1971). Prostaglandins and glaucoma. *Brit. Med. J.*, **3**, 615–617

2
Physiological Roles and Pharmacological Actions of Prostaglandins in Relation to Human Reproduction

S. M. M. KARIM and K. HILLIER

2.1 INTRODUCTION

The physiological involvement of prostaglandins in various reproductive processes and modification or simulation of these processes by exogenous

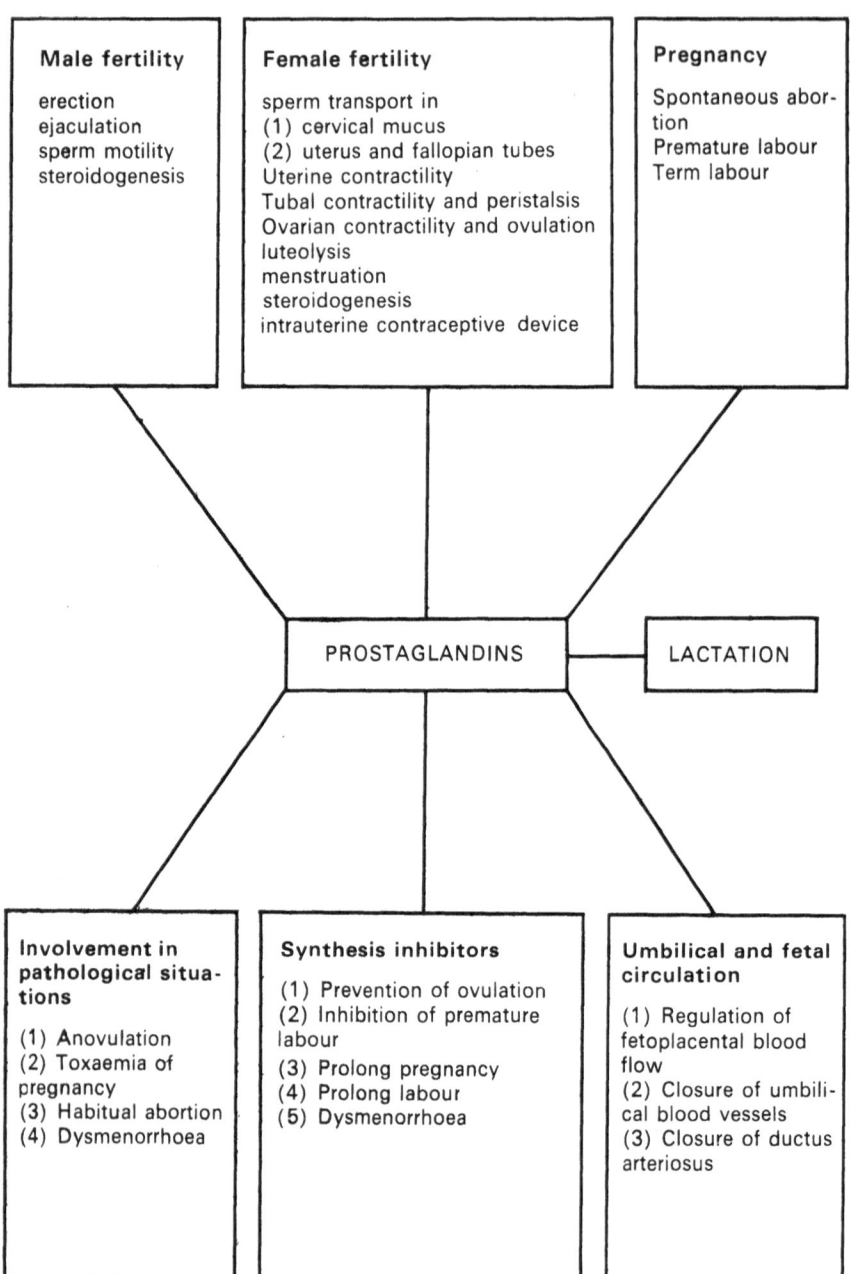

Figure 2.1 Prostaglandin and their inhibitors: Modulation and mediation of reproductive process

prostaglandins form a major area of research (Figure 2.1). Since the publication of the first volume in this series (Karim, 1972a), a vast amount of data has accumulated as a result of research carried out in many laboratories. The purpose of the present chapter is to discuss new information with due reference to or brief summary of data covered in the previous volume. The chapter is restricted to human studies although occasional reference to investigations in sub-human primates and laboratory animals is made. The latter are dealt with in detail in Chapters 5, 6 and 7.

2.2 MALE REPRODUCTION

In the male, prostaglandins are implicated in the processes of erection, ejaculation, sperm motility and morphology, testicular and penile contractions and in steroidogenesis. Prostaglandins thus could have an influence on male potency and fertility.

2.2.1 Seminal fluid prostaglandins

Human seminal fluid is the richest known mammalian source of prostaglandins. Thirteen different prostaglandins belonging to four groups (PGA, PGB, PGE and PGF) are present in total amounts of around 300 μg ml^{-1} (Table 2.1 for references). It has been reported that 19-hydroxy derivatives of prostaglandins A and B are present in the human semen at an average concentration of 40 μg ml^{-1} (Hamberg and Samuelsson, 1966; Bygdeman et al., 1970). Using a new approach for the measurement of E prostaglandins (which involves protecting the unstable β-ketol system by oximation in the fresh unextracted semen), Taylor and Kelly (1974) found very low levels of 19-hydroxy PGA and PGB compounds. Instead they identified 19-hydroxy PGE$_1$ and 19-hydroxy PGE$_2$ at an average total concentration of 100 μg ml^{-1}.

Taylor and Kelly (1974) suggested that the 19-OH prostaglandins have probably been missed before because they are converted to A series if left in semen (almost all 19-OH prostaglandins E had disappeared in a semen sample

Table 2.1   Concentration of prostaglandins in human seminal fluid. (From Bygdeman et al. 1966; Bygdeman and Samuelsson, 1966, 1967; Hamberg and Samuelsson, 1966; Taylor and Kelly, 1974)

Prostaglandin	Concentration $\mu g\,ml^{-1}$ semen
PGE$_1$	25
PGE$_2$	23
PGE$_3$	5.5
PGF$_{1\alpha}$	3.6
PGF$_{2\alpha}$	4.4
PGA$_1$, PGA$_2$, PGB$_1$, PGB$_2$	200
19-OH PGA$_1$; 19-OH PGA$_2$ 19-OH PGB$_1$; 19-OH PGB$_2$	50
19-OH PGE$_1$; 19-OH PGE$_2$	100*

left at 37 °C for 60 hours) and they are more difficult to extract from semen than the hydroxylated A and B compounds. The physiological significance of these new findings is at present not clear.

In view of their presence in large amounts in the seminal fluid it has been assumed that prostaglandins have special functions, presumably connected with reproduction. Because these substances also have effects on the female reproductive system it is likely that reproductive processes in both the donor and the recipient are affected. Studies by Eliasson (1959) have provided evidence that seminal fluid prostaglandins originate from the seminal vesicles and not the prostate as was originally assumed. The method of prostaglandin assay employed by Eliasson, however, does not permit the definite conclusion that all prostaglandin present in the semen originates only from the seminal vesicles. Other glandular systems contributing to the ejaculate may also provide some prostaglandins, although the testes do not secrete prostaglandins Es, As and 19-OH As because the amounts of these compounds in semen are not reduced after vasectomy (Brummer, 1973a).

2.2.2 Erection and ejaculation

In man, it has been postulated that seminal prostaglandins through their smooth muscle stimulating and vasodilator actions could act as a stimulus for the emptying of the genital glands. It has also been suggested that prostaglandins may contribute to the maintenance of peristalsis involved in ejaculation (Goldblatt, 1935; Euler, 1936). In spite of the gap of almost 40 years since this suggestion was made, the effect of prostaglandins on the male accessory genital glands remains unexplored. Virtually nothing is known of their effects on the smooth muscle of the human seminal vesicles, testicular capsule and other parts of the male reproductive system.

In the rabbit, prostaglandins affect the contraction of the testicular capsule and have an effect on testicular blood flow. Hargrove *et al.* (1971) and Ellis *et al.* (1972) have shown that PGE_1 decreases the resting tone and frequency of spontaneous rhythmic contractions of the rabbit testicular capsule. $PGF_{1\alpha}$ on the other hand increases the tone and frequency of contraction and stimulates the inactive capsule. No data from human studies are available and whether the observed effect of prostaglandin on testicular capsule contractions has physiological implication in ejaculation is not known. Strips of corpus cavernosa muscle from the human penis *in vitro* exhibit spontaneous activity which may be due to a release of prostaglandins. Aspirin and indomethacin (which are known to inhibit prostaglandin synthesis) added to the perfused strip (10 μg ml^{-1} upwards) produced a dose dependent inhibition of spontaneous activity and reduction in the resting tone of the muscle (Karim and Adaikan, 1975) (Figure 2.2).

Prostaglandin E_1 added to spontaneously contracting strips of cavernosa muscle caused a reduction in frequency of spontaneous contractions and resting tone. PGE_2 produced a similar effect at low dose but had a stimulant action with higher doses. All other prostaglandins (A_1, A_2, B_1, B_2 and $F_{2\alpha}$) tested increased the tone and frequency of contractions of the penile muscle; PGA_2 being the most potent compound (Figure 2.3, Table 2.2). The

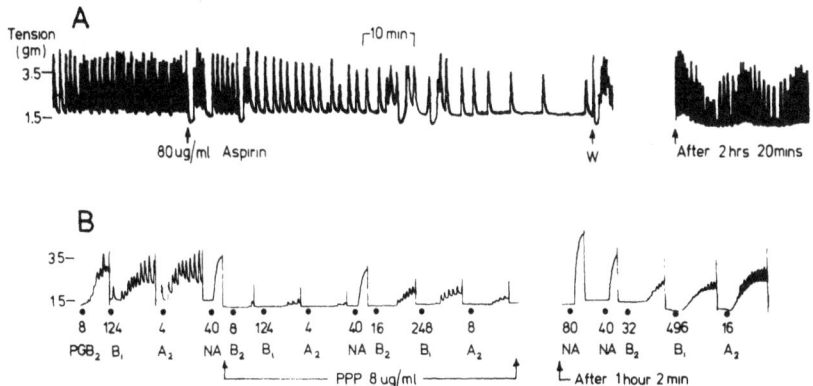

Figure 2.2 Isometric recording of longitudinal strips of the corpus cavernosa muscle of human penis *in vitro*. Krebs Hensleit solution, 37 °C bubbled with 95% oxygen, 5% CO_2.
Upper section A. Effect of 80 μg ml^{-1} (bath volume) aspirin.
Wash at W.
Lower section B. Polyphloretin phosphate (PPP 8 μg ml^{-1}) added one minute before PGB$_2$, PGB$_1$ and PGA$_2$ inhibited responsiveness without significantly reducing the noradrenaline induced contraction (doses ng ml^{-1}). One hour of repeated washing to remove PPP resulted in partial recovery of prostaglandin induced contractility. (From Karim and Adaikan, 1975, in press)

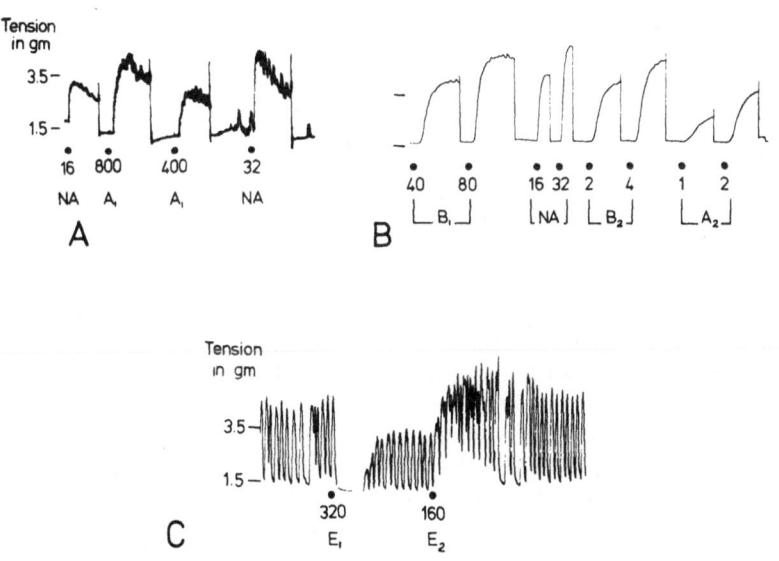

Figure 2.3 Isometric recording of longitudinal strips of the corpus cavernosa muscle of human penis *in vitro*. Krebs Hensleit solution, 37 ° C bubbled with 95% oxygen, 5% CO_2. Sections A, B and C from different penes. Doses ng ml^{-1} bath fluid. Effect of noradrenaline (NA), prostaglandin A$_1$ (A$_1$), prostaglandin A$_2$ (A$_2$), prostaglandin B$_1$ (B$_1$), prostaglandin E$_1$ (E$_1$) and prostaglandin E$_2$ (E$_2$). (From Karim and Adaikan, 1975, in press)

Table 2.2 Stimulant effect of various prostaglandins on corpus cavernosa muscle from human penis *in vitro*, relative to noradrenaline (assigned a potency of 1) (From Karim and Adaikan, 1975, in press)

Prostaglandin	Mean potency (noradrenaline $\equiv 1) \pm SD$	Range	Threshold dose range $ng\ ml^{-1}$	No. of experiments
A_2	8.21(± 1.41)	3.88–14.8	1–32	7
B_2	6.58(± 0.92)	5.24–9.33	8–40	4
A_1	0.04(± 0.01)	0.02–0.09	100–500	4
B_1	0.61(± 0.18)	0.2 –1.07	10–80	5
$F_{2\alpha}$	0.31(± 0.08)	0.15–0.46	30–160	4

stimulant action of prostaglandins was abolished by polyphloretin phosphate (PPP, a prostaglandin receptor blocking drug) without significantly altering responses to adrenaline and noradrenaline. A combination of prostaglandins induced smooth muscle stimulation and vasodilatation in the penis may be important in the physiology of erection and ejaculation (Karim and Adaikan, 1975).

2.2.3 Male fertility and infertility

Results of several investigations have shown that there is no correlation between the prostaglandin content of seminal fluid and the number and degree of motility of spermatozoa, nor does addition of prostaglandin E_1 to sperms affect their motility or metabolism (Eliasson, 1959). However, there are indications of a correlation between the amounts of E prostaglandins and male infertility. Bygdeman *et al.* (1970) found that semen samples from men in infertile marriages contained less PGE compounds compared with samples from men with recently documented fertility. If this is of physiological significance, the lack of any effect on sperm count and motility suggests that prostaglandins are of importance in fertility after semen is deposited into the vagina (see effect on cervical mucus, Section 2.3.1).

Collier and Flower (1971) have shown that in normal therapeutic doses soluble aspirin given for seven days reduces both E and F prostaglandins in the semen of healthy males. Horton *et al.* (1973) studied the effects of high doses of aspirin (3.6 and 7.2 g/day) in man given in divided doses for three days. During treatment with aspirin in two subjects the levels of prostaglandin E fell by 52% and 60% respectively at the 3.6 g/day dose level and 78 and 82% respectively at the 7.2 g/day level. The reduction was maximal after 48 hours treatment and although at 72 hours the concentrations had risen slightly, they were still lower than pretreatment values. A return to basal levels occurred within 48 hours of cessation of aspirin ingestion. Aspirin also lowered the amounts of 19-hydroxy PGA and B and PGF compounds. No information is available from the above publications as to whether aspirin and reduced levels of prostaglandins had any effect on subsequent sperm count, motility or on erection and ejaculation.

2.3 FEMALE REPRODUCTION

Prostaglandins may affect fertility after deposition in the vagina by an action on cervical mucus, vaginal secretion or by affecting sperm transport in the uterus and fallopian tubes. In addition to prostaglandins present in seminal fluid, the tissues and fluids of the female genital tract also contain prostaglandins which could be of physiological significance (Ogra *et al.*, 1974).

2.3.1 Sperm transport in cervical mucus

The ability of cervical mucus and the uterotubal junction to act as barriers to sperm transport is well recognised. Eskin and Azarbal (1973) and Eskin *et al.* (1973) have studied the effect of prostaglandin $F_{2\alpha}$ and PGE_2 *in vitro* on sperm motility, sperm penetration and drive of the spermatozoa through the

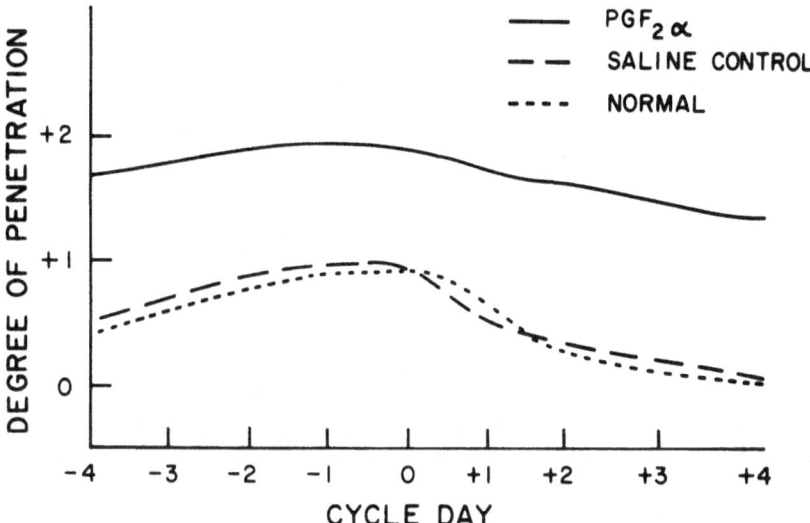

Figure 2.4 Degree of spermatozoa penetration through cervical mucus incubated at 37 °C for one hour. Scores assigned arbitrarily were (0)—no penetration; (1)—average penetration; (2)—exceptionally effective penetration. The latter score indicated that the spermatozoa had reached the distal edge of the mucus specimen. The figure shows the average daily score. (From Eskin *et al.*, 1973, by courtesy of *Obstetrics and Gynecology*)

cervical mucus during the periovular period in normally cycling women. Prostaglandin $F_{2\alpha}$ added to the mucus specimens (250 ng ml^{-1}) and incubated at 37 °C for one hour produced a significant increase in all parameters studied and the effect was greatest in samples obtained 24 hours prior to ovulation (Figures 2.4 and 2.5). PGE_2 had little effect. The authors suggest that $PGF_{2\alpha}$ could be of value in infertility problems resulting from (a) incompatibility between spermatozoa and mucus, (b) idiopathic hostility of cervical mucus, (c) reduced penetration characteristics of spermatozoa, and (d) reduced number of spermatozoa.

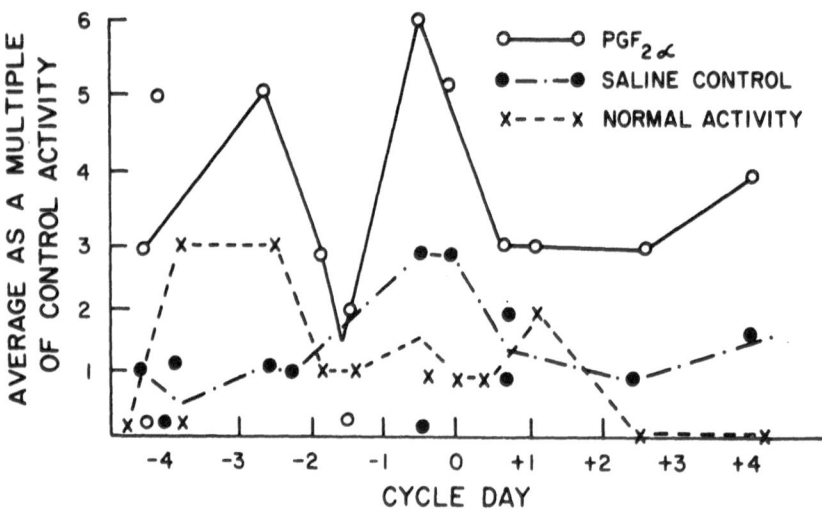

Figure 2.5 Spermatozoa motility (using a high power lens) expressed as multiples of the activity seen in the original specimen before being used in the experiment. Spermatozoa and mucus were incubated at 37 °C for one hour before assessment. (From Eskin *et al.*, 1973, by courtesy of *Obstetrics and Gynaecology*)

2.3.2 Sperm transport in uterus and fallopian tubes

In addition to prostaglandins aiding sperm transport by affecting the cervical mucus, they may also help in the passive migration of sperm by altering the motility of the uterus and fallopian tubes. It has been suggested that seminal fluid prostaglandins by alternately stimulating and inhibiting uterine motility could aid sperm migration from the vagina into the uterine cavity and to the fallopian tube. The subject has been discussed in detail previously (Karim, 1972b).

2.3.3 Ovulation—tubal and ovarian contractility

The effects of prostaglandins on oviduct contractility have been extensively studied in animals and are discussed in Chapter 5. Sandberg *et al.* (1963, 1964, 1965) showed that the response of the human fallopian tubes *in vitro* to prostaglandins was dependent upon the prostaglandin used and the anatomical position of the segment of the tube studied. Independent of the phase of the menstrual cycle, E prostaglandins caused a contraction of the proximal quarter of the fallopian tube but relaxed the strips from the distal three-quarters of the tube whereas PGF compounds produced contractions of all segments. Although the above findings have been basically confirmed *in vivo*, the physiological implications are not clear. Sandberg *et al.* (1964, 1965) have postulated that the predominance of E prostaglandins in the semen may result in contraction of the proximal section and relaxation of the rest of the fallopian tube. Such an effect could result in suction allowing the entrance of the ovum into the tube and its retention in the middle part of the oviduct until fertilisation.

Coutinho (1971, 1974) and Coutinho and Maia (1971) have most widely studied the responsiveness of the human fallopian tube and ovary in *vivo* to prostaglandins, gonadotrophins, steroid hormones, adrenergic drugs and oxytocin. The motility and mutual functioning of these organs physiologically may be dependent upon interplay between many hormonal factors and may play an important part in the release, transport and fertilisation of the ovum.

The motility of the fallopian tube *in vivo* recorded directly with indwelling catheters is dependent upon the phase of the menstrual cycle (Coutinho, 1971). The phasic appearance of tubal motility interspersed with a more quiescent pattern occurred at roughly one hour intervals in the follicular phase, whereas overall motility was less in the luteal phase but low amplitude bursts of activity occurred more frequently. The asynchronous nature of the bursts of activity in contralateral tubes (Coutinho, 1971; Sico-Blanco *et al.*, 1971) suggested local control independent of uterine activity. The isthmus was also observed to contract asynchronously to the ampulla.

Coutinho and Maia (1971) studied the effect of prostaglandins upon tubal and ovarian contractility. Four patients were infertile because of tubal occlusion and four required tubal ligation having no tubal pathology. Direct pressure recordings were made via indwelling tubal and ovarian stromal catheters. 100 μg PGE_2 or $PGF_{2\alpha}$ intravenously both stimulated uterine contractility but concomitantly the amplitude of tubal contractions was inhibited by PGE_2 whereas $PGF_{2\alpha}$ increased resting tone and frequency of contraction (Figure 2.6). Direct intratubal application of 0.5 μg E_2 or 0.1 μg $PGF_{2\alpha}$ had a similar effects. When injected together these drugs were mutually antagonistic. The duration of the response to a single injection of $PGF_{2\alpha}$ was more

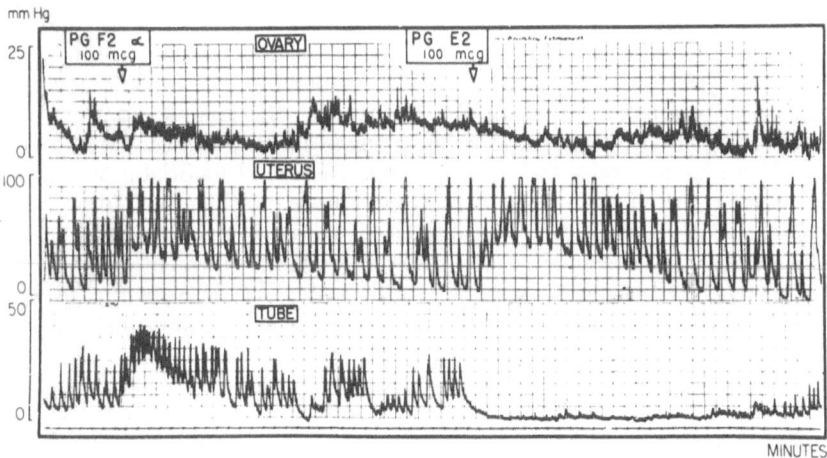

Figure 2.6 The response of the human ovary, uterus and fallopian tubes to prostaglandins $F_{2\alpha}$ and E_2 *in vivo*. At the arrow 100 μg of either $PGF_{2\alpha}$ or PGE_2 was injected intravenously. Note the stimulatory response of the ovary, tube and uterus to $PGF_{2\alpha}$. The uterus is stimulated by PGE_2 but the fallopian tube is caused to relax completely; the ovaries are little affected. (From Coutinho and Maia, 1971, by courtesy of *Fertility and Sterility*)

than 30 min whereas PGE_2 induced suppression lasting only 5–10 min. Prostaglandin $F_{2\alpha}$ intravenously (100 μg) also had a marked stimulant effect upon intraovarian pressure whereas the same dose of PGE_2 had little effect. Coutinho and Maia (1971) suggest that PGE_2 may have a physiological effect aiding sperm penetration into the tube by contracting the uterus and relaxing the isthmus, while $PGF_{2\alpha}$ may be important in expelling the ovum. These tenuous findings require much further proof and investigation. Of equal importance was the finding that intravenous HCG (3000 U) results in a large increase in intraovarian pressure about ten minutes after its injection.

The response was seen only at the preovulatory and ovulatory phase and probably required oestrogen priming. LHRH caused a similar response.

In human ovarian tissue *in vitro* HCG administration has been shown to increase the content of $PGF_{2\alpha}$ (Armstrong, unpublished) which may explain the contractile effect of the former and the latency of response. The postulate may be made that prostaglandins are involved with gonadotrophins in ovarian contractility to facilitate follicular rupture and ovum expulsion. An increased pressure within both tubes and ovary is also seen with exogenous oxytocin, vasopressin and adregenic stimulants. These effects may also be modulated by steroid hormone balance as oestrogen enhances and progesterone diminishes ovarian contractility.

Indirect and non-invasive techniques using the tubal insufflation test of Rubin corroborate Coutinho's (1971) findings. Using this test Eliasson and Posse (1965) showed that total seminal fluid prostaglandin extract increased the resistance to gas flow (a reflection of tubal contractility) in four of seven infertile patients studied. Embrey and Hillier (unpublished observations) have shown in three patients that PGE_2 intravenously (20 μg) inhibits tubal motility and $PGF_{2\alpha}$ (100 μg) enhances tubal contractility. In one additional case PGE_2 (40 μg) was without effect. The duration of action of PGE_2 was 1–2 min while the $PGF_{2\alpha}$ effect lasted for over six minutes.

Zetler and Wiechell (1969) have identified PGE_1 and $PGF_{2\alpha}$ in the ampulla but not the isthmus of the tube. Using immunofluorescence techniques Ogra *et al.* (1974) showed that $PGF_{2\alpha}$ was localised in the human oviductal mucosal surface before ovulation but in the oviductal lamina propria after ovulation. No $PGF_{2\alpha}$ was found in the postpartum or postmenopausal oviduct. These findings raise the possibility that passage of fimbrial prostaglandins to the ovary might occur; alternatively release of follicular fluid prostaglandins at rupture might affect tubal motility.

Insufficient data are at present available to relate the effects of prostaglandins on tubal and ovarian contractility to the phase of the menstrual cycle, and the possibility of assigning a physiological role must await further experimentation.

2.3.4 Menstruation and luteolysis

Prostaglandins E_2 and $F_{2\alpha}$ are present in human menstrual fluid and in endometrial curettings obtained during the proliferative and secretory phase of the menstrual cycle. Prostaglandin-like activity in peripheral blood obtained during menstruation has also been reported (Pickles, 1957, 1967; Clithero and Pickles, 1961; Clithero, 1961; Eglinton *et al.*, 1963; Pickles and Hall, 1963; Pickles and Ward, 1965).

Attempts have been made to correlate the levels of prostaglandins in the endometrium and in peripheral circulation with luteolysis and onset of menstruation. Downie *et al.* (1974) measured endometrial prostaglandins at different stages of the menstrual cycle. PGE_2 and $PGF_{2\alpha}$ increase progressively in the luteal phase of the cycle (Figure 2.7). The ratio of $PGF_{2\alpha}$:PGE_2 increased from 0.6 in the early proliferative phase to 1.5–1.7 around ovulation, it peaked in the mid-luteal phase at 3.2 and dropped to 1.4 at menstruation.

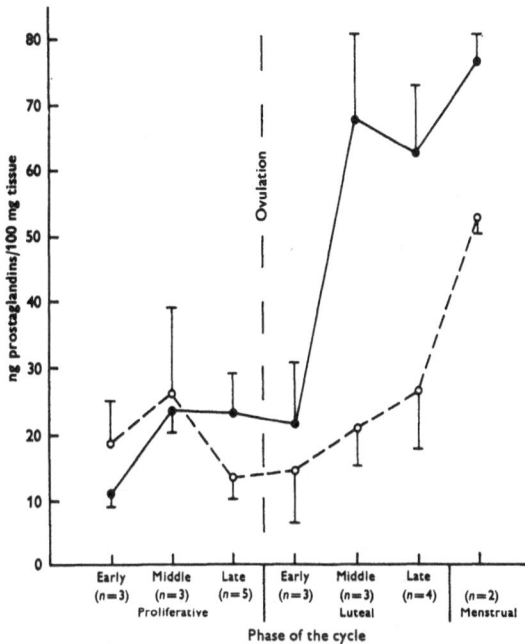

Figure 2.7 Levels of prostaglandin $F_{2\alpha}$ ($PGF_{2\alpha}$ •—•) and prostaglandin E_2 (PGE_2 o---o) in the human endometrium during the menstrual cycle (*n* = number of separate determinations in each group). (From Downie *et al.*, 1974, by courtesy of *J. Physiol.*)

They suggest from this study that the synthesis of PGE_2 and $PGF_{2\alpha}$ from their common precursor (arachidonic acid) can be preferentially directed; also that peak concentrations are present when oestrogen and progesterone are present together at high levels. The elevated concentration of prostaglandins in the presence of low premenstrual amounts of progesterone may account for the greater degree of uterine activity at that time. The physiological significance of these changes is at present obscure but could be associated with the increasing number of lysosomes in endometrial cells as the menstrual cycle progresses (Henzl *et al.*, 1972). According to Bitensky and Cohen (1965) the lysosomes also increase in fragility towards menstruation. These factors would predispose to increased prostaglandin synthesis.

Several investigators have measured levels of prostaglandins in peripheral blood during different stages of the menstrual cycle. The results are listed below:

1. plasma: Luteal phase concentrations 200–300 pg ml^{-1}
Caldwell *et al.*, 1971
2. plasma: Two peaks of activity rising from 80–100 pg ml^{-1} PGFs to 250–300 pg ml^{-1} at days 8–10 and 22–24
(van Orden and Farley, 1973)
3. serum: Different volunteers at varying times of the cycle 500–2500 pg ml^{-1} PGFs. No discernible pattern (Kirton *et al.*, 1972)
4. plasma: F$_{1\alpha}$ wide daily fluctuations tending to be higher in follicular phase. PGF$_{2\alpha}$ relatively constant mid-cycle levels with a significant luteal phase increase. No concentrations given
(Patrona *et al.*, 1974, abstract)
5. plasma: No alteration in PGF concentrations through the cycle or with
 or dysmenorrhoea. Range 100–3500 pg ml^{-1}
 serum (Wilks *et al.*, 1973)
6. plasma: Concentrations of 23.8±11.9 pg ml^{-1} at unspecified times in menstrual cycle
(Hennam *et al.*, 1974)
7. plasma: 6.38±2.7 pg ml^{-1} in follicular phase and 5.7±2.3 pg ml^{-1} in luteal phase
(Dray and Charbonnel, 1973)

The short halflife of the prostaglandins has led to suggestions that a more accurate reflection of prostaglandin synthesis would obtain from the measurement of metabolites. Thus Levine and Gutierrez-Cernosek (1973) measured serum levels of 13,14-dihydro-15-keto-PGF$_{2\alpha}$ levels in four women through the menstrual cycle, two of whom were taking a combined contraceptive. Variable patterns apparently unrelated to ovulation or to contraceptive practice were noted. In three a downward trend from approximately 500–12 000 pg ml^{-1} to 2000–7000 pg ml^{-1} throughout the cycle occurred whereas in the fourth patient concentrations increased from 500 pg ml^{-1} to a maximum of 26 000 pg ml^{-1}. Thus far the variety and lack of agreement between the reported levels of prostaglandins in the non-pregnant female make any clear interpretation impossible. It is probable that artificially high levels produced by non-prostaglandin interference with assay systems would mask any changes that might occur. Only the concentrations reported by Dray and Charbonnel (1973) and Hennam *et al.* (1974) closely approach the physiological levels estimated by GLC-mass spectrometry. It remains to be seen whether any alteration in peripheral plasma prostaglandins will be detected at different times in the menstrual cycle using these sensitive techniques more extensively.

2.3.5 Luteolysis studies in non-pregnant women

The factors controlling the integrity and demise of the corpus luteum are of great importance in the understanding of the physiology of the menstrual cycle and maintenance of early human pregnancy. Unlike most endocrine

Table 2.3 The effect of prostaglandins on peripheral progesterone levels in the non-pregnant female

Drug	Dose μg min⁻¹	Time (hours)	Route	N	Stage of cycle	Progesterone concentration	Reference
$F_{2\alpha}$	12.5–250	4–8	i.v.	4	late luteal	decline	Hillier et al. (1972)
$F_{2\alpha}$				3	early luteal	no change	Hillier et al. (1972)
$F_{2\alpha}$	75mg kg⁻¹min⁻¹	3.5–6	i.v.	7	mid-luteal	decline 4/7	Coudert et al. (1974)
$F_{2\alpha}$	100	8	i.v.	3	luteal	no change	Jewelwicz et al. (1972)
$F_{2\alpha}$	50	8	i.v.	13	luteal	transient decline	Wentz and Jones (1973)
$F_{2\alpha}$	25–46	8–14	i.v.	6	luteal	no change	Lemaire and Shapiro (1972)
$F_{2\alpha}$	4	4	i.v.	1	luteal	no change	Lehmann et al. (1972)
$F_{2\alpha}$	83	5	i.v.	1	luteal	marked decline	Lehmann et al. (1972)
$F_{2\alpha}$	8–100	8	i.v.	6	early luteal	slight transient decline	Wiqvist et al. (1971)
E_2	5–15	8×2–3 days	i.v.	7	luteal	no change	Henzl et al. (1973)
$F_{2\alpha}$	50–100 mg total dose	2×24 hour interval	i.vag.	7	late luteal	slight transient decline 5/7	Bolognese and Corson (1973)
$F_{2\alpha}$	25–75 mg total	over 24 hours	i.vag.	3	mid-luteal	no change	Okamura et al. (1974)
$F_{2\alpha}$	25–75 mg total	over 24 hours	i.vag.	3	mid-luteal	17_α–OH progesterone no change	Okamura et al. (1974)
$F_{2\alpha}$	100 mg total	over 24–48 hours	i.vag.	10	mid-luteal	no change	Tom et al. (1972)

organs the corpus luteum has a limited life span. In the absence of fertilisation and implantation it reaches a maximum level of steroid secretion and then regresses; in the primate menstruation follows. If fertilisation and implantation take place then the life span of the corpus luteum is extended and progesterone production which is essential for early pregnancy maintenance continues. There is evidence that in subprimates $PGF_{2\alpha}$ (and possibly other PGs and precursors) may be responsible for causing regression of the corpus luteum (see Chapters 5 and 7); such evidence in the human and subhuman primate is lacking. Exogenous administration of prostaglandins $F_{2\alpha}$ in subprimates results in premature demise of the corpus luteum; similar effect in the human could form the basis of pre- or postimplantation contraception by ensuring low levels of progesterone incompatible with implantation and the maintenance of early pregnancy. Experiments in humans to assess whether prostaglandin can pharmacologically induce luteolysis have basically taken two forms; (a) short term administration in the luteal phase of menstrual cycle and (b) during early pregnancy at the time when pregnancy maintenance depends upon a functional corpus luteum.

Several groups have carried out studies to assess experimentally whether prostaglandins administered during the luteal phase of the cycle would interfere with corpus luteum function. In most of the studies the drugs have been given acutely by intravenous infusion although the intravaginal route has also been explored. The objective of these experiments has been to assess the effects of high doses of prostaglandins upon corpus luteum function. Overall results are equivocal (Table 2.3). Hillier *et al.* (1972) reported a reduction in progesterone output with very little effect on oestrogens on infusing 12.5–250 μg min^{-1} $PGF_{2\alpha}$ in four subjects in the late luteal phase of the menstrual cycle (Figure 2.8) but no effect was observed in three patients in the early luteal

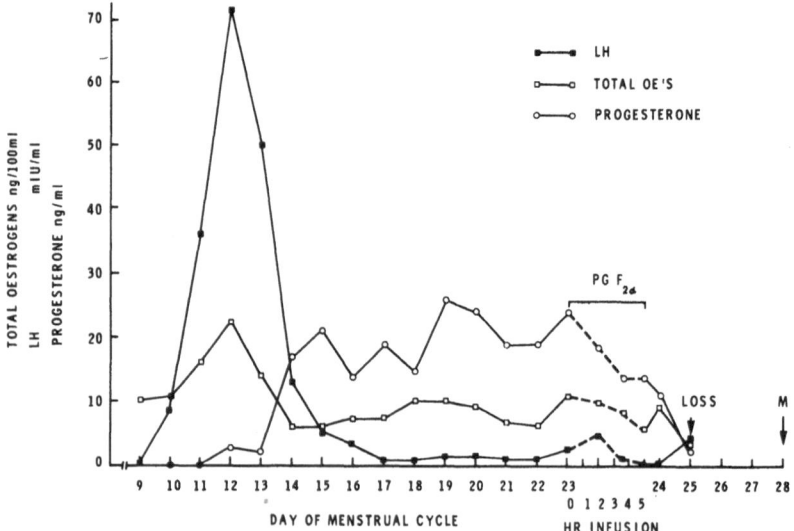

Figure 2.8 $PGF_{2\alpha}$ and luteolysis in the human. Effect of $PGF_{2\alpha}$ 12.5–250 μg min^{-1} infused for five hours in the late luteal phase on peripheral progesterone, total oestrogens and gonadotrophins. (From Hillier *et al.*, 1972, by courtesy of *Brit. Med. J.*)

phase of the cycle. Vaginal spotting occurred following prostaglandin infusion which lasted until the expected day of menstruation. The menstrual cycle length was not shortened.

A transient fall in progesterone concentration of 23–70% was observed by Wentz and Jones (1973) with intravenous infusion of 50 μg min^{-1} PGE$_{2\alpha}$ for eight hours in nine patients in the luteal phase of the menstrual cycle (Figure 2.9). In contrast to the observation of Hillier et al. (1972) they also observed

PROSTAGLANDIN F$_{2\alpha}$ INFUSION

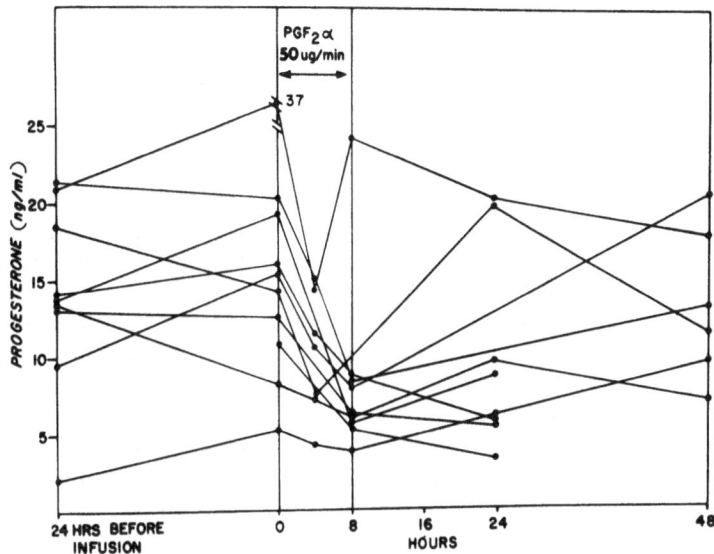

Figure 2.9   PGF$_{2\alpha}$ and luteolysis in human. The effect of 50 μg min^{-1} intravenous PGF$_{2\alpha}$ infused for eight hours on progesterone concentration in non-pregnant volunteers on days 3–12 from the LH surge. (From Wentz and Jones, 1973, by courtesy of *Obstet. Gynecol. (N.Y.)*)

a reduction in plasma progesterone levels when 50 μg min^{-1} PGF$_{2\alpha}$ was infused before progesterone level had reached its peak in the early luteal phase. They also observed an overall shortening of the luteal phase length in ten out of thirteen patients given PGF$_{2\alpha}$.

Three studies utilising the vaginal route of administration have been reported. Luteolysis was not induced (Table 2.3).

It is not possible at present to state the reasons for discrepancies in results of all the above investigators. Individual volunteer variation may account for some differences as may differences in administered dosage and blood sampling frequencies. It is not known whether the uterine, tubal and ovarian contractility that must result from the prostaglandin administered would in any way contribute to the demise of the corpus luteum but this is a distinct possibility. It may be concluded that PGF$_{2\alpha}$ and PGE$_2$ administered systemically (and vaginally) are not (or are only weakly) luteolytic. However, a number of points should be borne in mind; naturally occurring prostaglandins E$_2$ and F$_{2\alpha}$ are rapidly broken down in the lung and liver and only a small amount may reach the corpus luteum. The experimental conditions could well be insufficient for functional luteolysis to be induced. These arguments must remain academic until results of prostaglandin administrations for several days are available. The pre-existing hormone balance may affect the response of the corpus luteum to prostaglandins (Shaikh, 1972). Treatment with oestrogens and prostaglandins in the monkey results in regression of the corpus luteum whereas prostaglandins alone are effective only when very large doses are used (Kirton, 1973). This approach will no doubt be tried in humans.

The effects of prostaglandins upon steroidogenesis *in vitro* in the human ovary has only recently been investigated. Human corpora lutea slices from the luteal phase of the menstrual cycle and at 12–20 weeks of pregnancy were incubated with acetate-1-^{14}C for three hours. The effect of 10 μg ml^{-1} PGF$_{2\alpha}$ was to increase the progesterone and 20α-OH progesterone content of the tissue and generally to increase the incorporation of radioactive acetate into progesterone and 20α-OH progesterone (Puri et al., 1973). Contrary to these results Archer and Petrilli (1973), using corpora lutea of mid-pregnancy incubated for three hours, found that PGF$_{2\alpha}$ and PGE$_1$ (50 μg ml^{-1}) reduced the incorporation of acetate-1-^{14}C into progesterone while only marginally reducing the tissue content of progesterone. The latter finding (which at first sight does not support the data obtained from incorporation of labelled acetate) may be due to the fact that the conversion of cholesterol to progesterone is not affected by prostaglandins and a finite and as yet unknown time is necessary to exhaust this pool.

Patwardhan and Lanthier (1974) incubated human single follicles or corpus luteum for three hours using pregnenelone-7(N)-^{3}H as substrate for follicular incubates or sodium acetate-1-^{14}C or progesterone-4-^{14}C as substrate for corpus luteum incubates. Prostaglandin E$_2$ (10 μg ml^{-1}) in 0.1 ml ethanol was added to the incubates with suitable controls. PGE$_2$ increased the progesterone content and incorporation of acetate-^{14}C label into progesterone (Table 2.4). In one experiment only where PGF$_{2\alpha}$ was used no effect was noted.

Table 2.4   **PGE$_2$ (10 μg ml^{-1}) effect on progesterone content and incorporation of sodium acetate-1-^{14}C into progesterone and digitoninprecipitate sterols (DPS) in human corpora lutea incubated** *in vitro* (From Patwardhan and Lanthier, 1974)

	Progesterone content μg g^{-1}		Acetate-^{14}C incorporation into progesterone dpm g^{-1} DPS			
	Control	PGE$_2$	Control	PGE$_2$	Control	PGE$_2$
1	50.1	106	11 943	35 089	57 064	124 170
2	40.5	62.1	27 823	53 169	144 650	201 700

In addition to this effect PGE$_2$ also stimulated the utilisation of progesterone-4-^{14}C to form 17-OH progesterone, androstenedione, testosterone and oestradiol-17β in corpus luteum tissue. Marsh and Lamaire (1974) have also shown similar effects indicating stimulation of progesterone biosynthesis and *de novo* synthesis from acetate-^{14}C by prostaglandins. In contrast to the increased progesterone in corpora lutea invoked by PGE_2, it inhibited the utilisation of pregnenelone-7(N)-^{3}H by follicles to form progesterone, 17-OH progesterone, androstendione and dehydroepiandosterone (Table 2.5). Therefore, as previously suspected, prostaglandins may have different effects upon steroidogenesis in different compartments of the human ovary. Both *in vitro* and *in vivo* investigations of steroidogenic influences of prostaglandins are in their infancy; further work should clarify some of the apparent paradoxes and gaps in our knowledge.

Table 2.5 Pregnenolone-7(N)-^{3}H metabolism by isolated follicles from human ovaries. Conversion of substrate per 100 mg of tissue expressed as percentage of control (From Patwardhan and Lanthier, 1974)

Metabolite	Control (%)	Prostaglandin E_2 (10 μg ml^{-1})	
		1	2
Progesterone	100	55	70.7
17-hydroxy progesterone	100	45.7	57.1
Androstenedione	100	47.9	38.3
Dehydroepiondesterone	100	—	43.7

Powell *et al.* (1974) have shown the presence of a discrete receptor for $PGF_{2\alpha}$ in human corpora lutea. Minced corpora lutea were homogenised and centrifuged at 600 g for 10 min. The supernatant was recentrifuged at 100 000 g for 60 min and in the presence of indomethacin, ^{3}H-PGF$_{2\alpha}$ was added with or without 3 μg unlabelled $PGF_{2\alpha}$ and incubated for 90 min at 10 °C. Bound and free $PGF_{2\alpha}$ were separated and two populations of receptors identified, one with high affinity (Kd 55 nM) with a receptor site concentration of 0.05 pmol/mg protein, and one with a low affinity (Kd 500 nM) with receptor site concentration of 0.08 pmol/mg protein. The presence of specific receptor sites gives credence to a specific corpora luteal controlling function of the prostaglandins.

Investigations in lower animals have suggested that prostaglandins may be involved in gonadotrophin secretion at the pituitary and hypothalamic levels (Labhsetwar, 1973) (see Chapter 6). Patrona and Serra (1974) have assessed the pituitary response to LHRH (20 or 50 μg single intravenous injection) in man prior to and following indomethacin (50 mg daily for four days or 100 mg daily for three days). No modification of the LH release was effected by indomethacin treatment. This indicates that the prostaglandins do not mediate LHRH induced LH release. It is apparent, however, that prostaglandin synthetases in different organs have varying sensitivities to inhibitors and further investigation is required before one can be certain that pituitary and hypothalamic synthetases were inhibited at the dose levels used. No direct effect of prostaglandins infusion upon LH levels in the luteal phase has been reported in non-pregnant females (Hillier *et al.*, 1972; Wentz and Jones, 1973).

Dhont *et al.* (1974) and Vanderheyden *et al.* (1974) showed that PGE_2 and $PGF_{2\alpha}$ enhanced cortisol secretion and human growth hormone but did not alter LH, FSH, prolactin or TSH in postmenopausal women. Following dexamethasone pretreatment PGE_2 failed to increase cortisol secretion, therefore failing to over-ride the negative feedback exerted by dexamethasone on the secretion of ACTH. This suggests that the effect of prostaglandins upon cortisol secretion is at the hypothalamus or higher CNS centres.

2.3.6 Luteolysis and abortion in early pregnancy

Until approximately the seventh week of pregnancy (calculated from last menstrual period) maintenance of pregnancy is dependent upon a functional corpus luteum (see Csapo et al., 1972 for references). This is based on evidence that luteectomy during this period results in a reduction in peripheral plasma progesterone followed by abortion. Contribution of progesterone by the placenta may also be essential for the maintenance of early pregnancy. In a case of tubal pregnancy complete removal of the conceptus sac in addition to luteectomy evoked a reduction in plasma progesterone concentration more readily than luteectomy alone (Csapo et al., 1974). Placental tissue obtained from early pregnancy termination (up to seven weeks from LMP) contains progesterone and is able to synthesise this hormone in vitro (Rao and Karim, 1975).

Because of the established luteolytic effect of some prostaglandins in animals (both during non-pregnant cycle and in pregnancy) there has been a great deal of interest in studying the effects of these compounds in humans during the period when pregnancy maintenance is dependent upon the functional integrity of the corpus luteum. There is a general agreement that with appropriate doses of various prostaglandins it is possible to terminate early human pregnancy (during the first two weeks of delayed menstruation). The procedure is usually described as menstrual induction or menstrual regulation as the induced abortion resembles menstrual loss. The results of such clinical studies are described in Chapter 3. In the present section the possible mechanisms by which prostaglandins might cause termination of early pregnancy are discussed. Several possibilities are considered.

1. The prostaglandins have a direct luteolytic effect in early pregnancy.
2. That termination of pregnancy is unrelated to luteolytic factors but is the result of intense myometrial activity dislodging and expelling the embryo.
3. That interruption of pregnancy is due to an indirect luteolytic effect brought about by the removal of the possible luteotrophic support of the conceptus as a result of direct action of prostaglandins.
4. That progesterone and other hormone production by the early placenta may also be essential for the maintenance of early pregnancy and prostaglandins directly interfere with this balance.

These mechanisms are in many ways inter-related and it is impossible at present to categorically state which of the four is responsible for the early termination of pregnancy. A reduction in plasma progesterone could result through all four mechanisms operating individually or together. From clinical studies reported so far it is evident that consistent and high efficacy in terms of pregnancy termination with an acceptable rate of unwanted side-effects is achieved only when prostaglandins are given by the intrauterine route and results obtained by this route alone are discussed.

Table 2.6   Progesterone and oestradiol-17 levels before and after the intrauterine injection of 5 mg PGF$_{2\alpha}$ (From Csapo, 1974)

	Progesterone ng ml^{-1}				*Oestradiol-17β ng ml^{-1}*			
Hour	0	3	6	24	0	3	6	24
Mean	19.7	16.08	13.17	10.69	0.47	0.32	0.28	0.27
± SE	± 2.17	± 2.44	± 2.09	± 1.88	± 0.66	± 0.04	± 0.03	± 0.03

Only two out of 22 patients were curetted, probably unnecessarily. The 44% progesterone withdrawal is significant ($p < 0.5$)

Csapo (1974) reported a reduction in progesterone and oestradiol-17β during the first 24 hours following a single intrauterine dose of 5 mg PGF$_{2\alpha}$ (Table 2.6). His hypothesis (quoted from Csapo, 1974) on the mechanism of menstrual induction of prostaglandins (and also for the mechanism of prostaglandin induced abortion at other periods of gestation) involves the following events:

1. vasoconstriction in the uterine microcirculation
2. sustained uterine contracture
3. suppression of the endocrine function of the conceptus
4. withdrawal of placental and luteal progesterone
5. decrease in excitability threshold of the myometrium
6. conversion of the refractory uterus to a reactive organ
7. evolution of advanced cyclic intrauterine pressure
8. clinical progress of cervical dilatation
9. expulsion of uterine contents
10. restoration of non-pregnant state and normal menstrual cycle.

The postconceptional role for prostaglandins as envisaged by Csapo (1974) involves their oxytocic potency and also their ability to 'convert' the progesterone dominated uterus into 'a spontaneously active and pharmacologically reactive organ'. He suggests that this is brought about by compromising the endocrine function of the feto–placental unit and is in part a result of vasoconstriction induced by prostaglandins.

The overwhelming impact of massive doses of prostaglandins administered by Karim (1973), Csapo (1974) and Ylikorkala et al. (1974) rapidly brings about this change in hormonal balance and effectively ensures a state of non-pregnancy. However, the efficacy of smaller doses of prostaglandins employed by other investigators suggests more subtle effects.

In a recent study Hillier et al. (1975) have studied the effect of small doses of PGE$_2$ in 16 women during pregnancy (delay in menstruation of up to 21 days). Twelve patients were given single intrauterine dose of 0.5 mg and four received 0.1 mg. Pregnancy test became negative in all within 7–38 days following treatment. All developed uterine contractions and attendant cramps.

In most patients peripheral blood samples were taken at 4–6 hourly intervals during the first 24 hours following prostaglandin administration. Subsequently blood samples were taken at periodic intervals for at least one month. The effects on the hormonal profile were variable but generally a reduction was seen in the first 24 hours following prostaglandin administration. By analysis

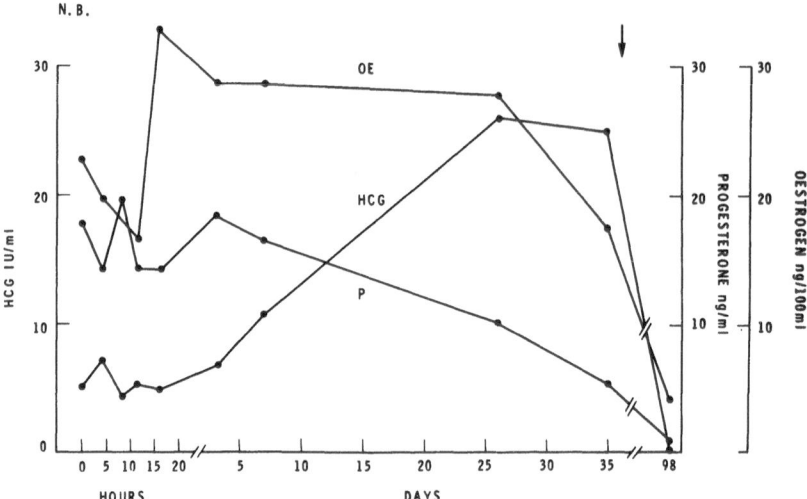

Figure 2.10 Intrauterine prostaglandin E₂ (0.1 mg) after nine days delay in expected menstruation. The effect on peripheral progesterone (P), oestrogen (OE) and gonadotrophin (HCG). Bleeding commenced on day 36 following treatment (indicated by arrow). (From Hillier *et al.*, 1975)

of steroids, gonadotrophins and clinical observation, abortion occurred from 24 hours to 36 days after treatment; a total of six patients aborted within 24 hours and 19 within seven days. Figure 2.10 shows the steroid profile in a patient with delayed abortion. The patient (nine days delay in menstruation) was treated with 0.1 mg PGE₂, showed little change (during first 24 hours) in progesterone or HCG but oestrogen level was elevated compared with preinjection values after a transient decline. During the subsequent 35 days the progesterone and oestrogen levels fell while HCG continued to rise. Bleeding commenced 36 days after treatment.

In general removal of the support of HCG was roughly paralleled by changes in progesterone and oestrogen concentration. However, the observation (albeit in one case in this small series) that HCG could be maintained while progesterone and oestrogens decline suggests the possibility of direct luteolysis. Measurements of 17α-hydroxy progesterone should clarify this.

Complete comparison of this study with that of Karim (1973), Mocsary and Csapo (1973), Csapo (1974) and Ylikorkala *et al.* (1974) is difficult because of differences in dosage of drug administered and the slightly earlier gestational stage of other investigators' patients. Overall, similar success rates were obtained and although diagnosis of the precise time of early abortion is difficult this appears to differ between series. Karim (1973), Mocsary and Csapo (1973) and Ylikorkala *et al.* (1974) generally observed bleeding within a few hours of drug administration although a delay of six days was noted in one patient in the latter study.

In the study of Hillier *et al.* (1975) bleeding started within 24 hours in none of four patients treated with 0.1 mg PGE₂ and in seven out of 12 patients treated with 0.5 mg PGE₂. This may well represent less uterine activity produced by smaller administered doses, but without analysis of individual uterine pressure records this must remain a tenuous point. By analysis of steroid and gonadotrophin hormones abortion was assessed as occurring from 24 hours to up to as long as 36 days after treatment (Figure 2.10). It is doubtful that initiation of bleeding can be taken as the unqualified time of abortion as it may be merely traumatic and has been noted following prostaglandins in non-pregnant volunteers.

The results of this study with small doses of prostaglandins (Hillier *et al.*, 1975) do not deny the hypothesis of Csapo (1974) but indicate that changes other than falling concentrations of oestradiol-17β and progesterone levels can occur. Progressive changes can proceed in the absence of contractility although the irreversible change may have been effected by uterine stimulation. It would be of value to study the abortifacient effectiveness and hormone profile of other oxytocics at this stage of gestation. Increased oestrogen output that occurred in some patients has been noted following prostaglandin infusion in animals (see Chapter 7).

It should be noted that the intravenous administration of $PGF_{2\alpha}$ in high doses in the luteal phase in non-pregnant patients causes a transient decline in progesterone levels (Hillier *et al.*, 1972; Wentz and Jones, 1973) or no change. The marked depression of progesterone observed by Csapo (1974) and Hillier *et al.* (1975) which can occur following prostaglandin administration in very early pregnancy may not be due to a greater sensitivity of the corpus luteum to prostaglandin at that time but that an indirect effect of compromised fetus and placenta may be the prime abortifacient mechanism.

2.3.7 Mechanism of prostaglandin-induced abortion and labour

The mechanism of action of prostaglandins in terminating pregnancy after it is no longer dependent upon a functional corpus luteum (beyond seven weeks from the LMP) has been investigated by several groups. Two possible mechanisms exist:

1. A direct myometrial stimulant action.
2. Inhibition of steroid and gonadotrophin production by the feto–placental unit.

That prostaglandins have a direct myometrial stimulant action both *in vitro* and *in vivo* has been recognised for several years. In mid-pregnancy it is also likely that as a result of myometrial stimulation (and other effects) the production of steroid hormones by the feto–placental unit is impaired, contributing to subsequent enhanced myometrial activity and termination of pregnancy. The mechanism of action of prostaglandins in inducing abortion as proposed by Csapo (1974) involves immediate induced contraction followed by progesterone withdrawal; the regulatory imbalance converts the refractory uterus to a reactive organ. (See page 44).

Csapo's hypothesis necessarily implies that prostaglandins are initially able to stimulate the myometrium tetanically but progesterone withdrawal is necessary for the development of cyclic (high frequency, high amplitude) uterine activity. Although reduction in plasma progesterone with prostaglandin treatment has been reported by several investigators, it is not possible to categorically state that evolution of cyclic activity follows progesterone withdrawal in

Simultaneous shortening and stretch in the myometrial cells
↓
Vasoconstriction? Direct myometrial activity
↓
Sustained contracture with low level cyclic activity
↓
Decrease in uterine blood flow
↓
Suppression of the endocrine function of the feto-placental unit
↓
Decrease in luteotrophin support and luteolysis (when applicable)
↓
Decrease in progesterone and oestradiol-17β levels
↓
Decrease in threshold: increase in endogenous PG synthesis
↓
Evolution of uterine activity and reactivity
↓
Promotion of this evolution process by exogenous stimulation
↓
High level cyclic IUP and progress in cervical dilatation
↓
Abortion and delivery

every case. As short a period as 30–60 min after prostaglandin administration in many patients some degree of cyclic intrauterine activity is present without significant reduction in progesterone levels. It is however possible that progesterone reduction will enhance subsequent uterine activity.

During $PGF_{2\alpha}$ induced labour Lemaire *et al.* (1972) noted a significant fall in progesterone and a marked increase in oestriol levels both of which were of greater magnitude than in oxytocin induced patients. It is suggested that prostaglandin may bring about the effect upon oestrogen production via the stimulation of adenyl cyclase, that has been observed in placental homogenates by Satoh and Ryan (1972).

Evidence that the prostaglandins can alter the placental production of oestrogens is derived from the investigations of Alsat and Cedard (1973) using whole human term placenta perfused *in vitro*. They showed that the output of oestrogens in the perfusion fluid while infusing testosterone was greatly increased by the addition to the perfusion fluid of 3×10^{-6} M $PGF_{2\alpha}$, PGE_2 or pge$_1$. The increase was of long duration and had a dose–response relationship since 8×10^{-6} M $PGF_{2\alpha}$ had a greater effect than 3×10^{-6} M $PGF_{2\alpha}$ (Figure 2.11).

In the mid-trimester the reduction in steroid hormones correlates with the time to abortion (Craft *et al.*, 1973a; Csapo, 1973; Tyack *et al.*, 1974) but is contrary to the findings of Wiqvist *et al.*, (1971) and Speroff *et al.* (1972), who noted that progesterone values did not decline overall in patients induced with intra-amniotic $PGF_{2\alpha}$ until abortion occurred. However, Speroff *et al.* (1972) did note a reduction in oestrogens, particularly oestriol. Symonds

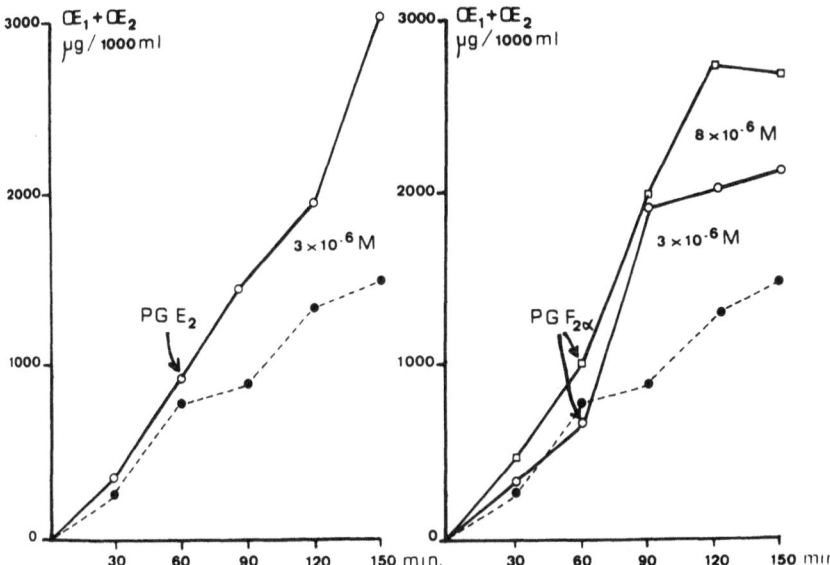

Figure 2.11 The action of prostaglandins PGE_2 and $PGF_{2\alpha}$, on the quantity of oestrogens (oestrone and oestradiol) in the placental perfusion fluid following addition of 10 mg of testosterone. Solid line with addition of prostaglandin and dotted line without addition. (From Alsat and Cedard, 1973, by courtesy of *Prostaglandins*)

et al. (1972) in a similar study showed that in three of seven patients studied there was a reduction in plasma steroid hormones within six hours of intra-amniotic $PGF_{2\alpha}$ injection. The discrepancy in the results from different centres is probably due to the fact that samples were taken infrequently or were not taken sufficiently close to the time of abortion to observe a delayed decline. Speroff *et al.* (1972) sampled blood serially during the abortion process but the final sample taken was in some cases many hours from the actual time of abortion. Souka and Hillier (unpublished data) have observed that the reduction in progesterone does not necessarily occur until fairly close to the time of abortion and this can be overlooked with infrequent sampling at this time (see also Chapter 3). These findings would not support Csapo's hypothesis.

Great variability in the reduction in progesterone concentrations occurs prior to abortion (Tyack *et al.*, 1974); the ratio of the concentration at delivery to that prior to onset of treatment in ten patients treated with intra-amniotic $F_{2\alpha}$ was 0.225–0.834 (mean 0.557). It is therefore evident that abortion can take place with only a modest decrease in progesterone occurring.

In a study using hypertonic saline to induce abortion (Tyack *et al.*, 1973) two of nineteen patients studied had no reduction in progesterone at the time of successful abortion. In these two abortion was not delayed. The mean reduction in progesterone at abortion was 53.6% of control concentrations. It should be noted that Gustavii and Green (1972) showed that amniotic fluid prostaglandins can be elevated in hypertonic saline induced abortion and may be the mediators of the uterine responsiveness in this situation.

In explaining the onset and progress of term labour the unifying hypothesis of Csapo (1974) appeared to be inconsistent with findings that progesterone concentrations do not alter prior to parturition. However, recent findings (Csapo et al., 1971; Turnbull et al., 1974) suggest that a reduction in progesterone does occur prior to onset of labour. The latter study also showed a significant concomitant rise in oestrogens. According to Csapo et al. (1971) a slight or even insignificant decrease in progesterone during labour is, however, sufficient to cause the evolution of uterine activity as sufficient uterine stretch is present which can promote myometrial activity at high levels of progesterone. Lemaire et al. (1972) have also indicated a greater reduction in progesterone and elevation in oestrogens in $PGF_{2\alpha}$ induced labour compared with oxytocin (Section 2.3.7).

2.3.8 Physiological role of prostaglandins in labour

Evidence implicating prostaglandins in the physiology of labour has been based on the following observations:

- (a) Presence of prostaglandins in maternal blood obtained during labour.
- (b) Presence in intrauterine tissues and fluids.
- (c) The ability of prostaglandins to stimulate pregnant human uterus.
- (d) Delay in onset of labour and prolongation of active labour by prostaglandin antagonists and synthesis inhibitors.

(a) Prostaglandins in maternal circulation

Assessment of the role of prostaglandins in the physiology of labour has thus far relied heavily upon their quantification in biological fluids; their measurement in plasma or serum is technically difficult and levels reported previously are significantly higher than those presently being measured. It is important to interpret data with the knowledge that all methods of analysis including biological assay, radioimmunoassay and gas liquid chromatography/mass spectrometry have given in many cases widely different blood prostaglandin levels. It is also important that different investigators have used serum or plasma for estimation of prostaglandin levels and there is now no doubt that human serum (if the blood is allowed to clot at room temperature or 37 °C but not at 4 °C) contains very much higher levels of prostaglandins than plasma (Challis and Tulchinsky, 1974). It is also true that the manner of plasma collection can affect its prostaglandin content. It has been suggested that E prostaglandins can be generated in plasma on storage (Jubiz and Frailey, 1974). Plasma collected and centrifuged at room temperature has a higher prostaglandin content than if collected into iced tubes centrifuged at 4 °C and deep frozen. For the plasma level to be considered a reflection of endogenous production it should not be allowed to regain room temperature before extraction.

Concentrations of PGF in serum through gestation estimated by radioimmunoassay after dialysis purification showed a peak at 17–20 weeks of pregnancy (mean 800 pg ml^{-1}) with lower levels at other stages of gestation (Gutierrez-Cernosek et al., 1972). However, Brummer (1972, 1973b), using a less specific antisera and no column chromatographic step, reported the opposite in that early and late pregnancy serum concentrations were around 500–600 pg ml^{-1} whereas at 17–20 weeks they were 100–400 pg ml^{-1}. Caldwell *et al.* (1971) measured 600–900 pg ml^{-1} PGF in plasma during the first trimester of pregnancy rising to 1200–2000 pg ml^{-1} in labour to 3000–5000 pg ml^{-1} at delivery. This confirmed the original work of Karim (1968) who published the first observations on the increasing concentrations of PGF in plasma during labour, rising to a mean concentration of 8000 pg ml^{-1} as estimated by biossay.

Jubiz *et al.* (1972) have carried out prostaglandin estimations in a number of biological situations on unextracted human plasma. In the normal male (590 ± 330 pg ml^{-1}) and female (930 ± 500 pg ml^{-1}) good agreement was seen between estimates of PGE$_2$ in extracted or unextracted plasma. However, in pregnancy the unextracted plasma concentration was 140 ± 170 pg ml^{-1} and extracted 820 ± 500 pg ml^{-1} and in woman on the contraceptive pill 140 ± 170 pg ml^{-1} in unextracted plasma compared with 2000 ± 3100 pg ml^{-1} after extraction. Considerable variation in levels throughout the day and through the menstrual cycle was noted in PGE levels, but generally they were higher in the luteal phase. The methodology used and variation in results obtained make interpretation difficult.

Hertelendy *et al.* (1973) estimated PGE levels in chromatographed peripheral plasma or serum during labour. The levels in non-pregnant and pregnant groups were approximately 300 pg ml^{-1} which rose to 1428 ± 440 pg ml^{-1} at 6–9 cm cervical dilation.

Highest levels were observed in plasma or serum or cord blood (1870 ± 255 pg ml^{-1}) after spontaneous and (2246 ± 1150 pg ml^{-1}) after PGE$_2$ induced labour. Hertelendy *et al.* (1973) found no difference in the PGE content of serum and plasma. This is contrary to the findings of Challis *et al.* (1974) who have consistently estimated higher levels in serum. Craft *et al.* (1973b) have estimated PGF levels in maternal serum immediately prior to and following delivery, in umbilical artery and vein, maternal femoral artery and uterine vein. Umbilical artery and vein samples were also taken at elective Caesarean section within a week of term. The mean ± SEM concentrations (pg ml^{-1}) in maternal, fetal arterial and fetal vein levels following labour were respectively 497 ± 52, 905 ± 103 and 915 ± 110. At elective Caesarean section the concentrations in maternal femoral artery, uterine vein, umbilical artery and umbilical vein were 725 ± 103, 739 ± 131, 1079 ± 205 and 974 ± 133 pg ml^{-1}. The umbilical artery and vein differences were statistically significant ($p < 0.2$). Hillier *et al.* (1974) reported concentrations of between 260–1400 pg ml^{-1} in peripheral plasma during labour. There was no increase with the progression of labour.

It is now appreciated that all the preceding results may incorrectly reflect the circulating prostaglandin concentrations *in vivo* because:

(a) Samples were incorrectly collected at a time when there was not prior knowledge that conditions of temperature and clotting processes may artificially increase prostaglandin levels in samples.

(b) Non-specific antisera, the absence of chromatographic purification and non-specific 'blank' values may also contribute to falsely high levels which may mask subtle changes in concentration. The previous results of plasma levels of natural prostaglandins generally have been so variable between investigations so as to make impossible any overall interpretation of the results.

Using sophisticated gas chromatography and mass spectrometic methods during the second trimester of pregnancy Wolfe and Pace-Asciak (1972) reported plasma concentration of 400 ± 270 pg ml^{-1} PGF$_{2\alpha}$ (1974) and levels of 150 pg ml^{-1} have been reported by Green et al., at 16–24 weeks gestation. Hennam et al. (1974) estimated 23.8 ± 11.9 pg ml^{-1} PGF$_{2\alpha}$ in non-chromatographed venous plasma from non-pregnant women. During the first, second and third trimesters they detected 29.6 ± 4.1, 20.4 ± 4.7 and 26.7 ± 7.6 pg ml^{-1} respectively. During labour the levels rose to 33.1 ± 11.6 pg ml^{-1}. The second trimester concentrations were significantly lower than in samples taken at other times during pregnancy. Challis et al. (1974) collected samples into chilled heparinised tubes and centrifuged at 4 °C. Estimates were made following column chromatography. They found as did Sharma et al. (1973) that a peak of PGF$_{2\alpha}$ occurs 45–60 s following a contraction. Umbilical artery and vein plasma had a significantly higher PGF concentration during labour than when obtained from patients not in active labour at Caesarean section (Table 2.7).

Table 2.7 The concentration of PGF in the maternal peripheral vein and umbilical cord plasma of women at term (From Challis et al., 1974)

	No.	PGF pg ml^{-1} $\pm$ SEM		
		Peripheral vein	Umbilical artery	Umbilical vein
I Elective CS	4	34 ± 20	180 ± 69[a]	130 ± 36[c]
II Oxytocin-induced	6	66 ± 24	430 ± 127	616 ± 163[d]
III Spontaneous	9	8 ± 29	537 ± 85[b]	636 ± 118[e]

Group II and III vaginal delivery
b was significantly greater than a $p < .05$

d was significantly greater than c $p < .05$
e was significantly greater than c $p < .02$

These results are in contrast to Craft et al.'s (1973b) study using serum without column chromatography. The latter could show no difference between umbilical artery or vein samples from spontaneous labour compared with Caesarean section. Also concentrations were higher than measured by Challis et al. (1974). However, both investigators agreed that umbilical artery concentrations were higher than vein at the time of Caesarean section but not during induced or spontaneous labour.

Sharma et al. (1973) found that a peak of PGF appeared in plasma 15–45s after the peak of a uterine contraction in the first stage of labour (Figure 2.12). Samples were not extracted and were not collected into tubes at 4 °C. Concentrations in the range of 75 pg ml^{-1}–1190 pg ml^{-1} were noted. (It was not possible to determine whether the prostaglandin levels were causally related to the uterine contractions.) This work confirmed the results of Karim (1968) but the absolute levels measured were lower in the study of Sharma et al. (1973). Conclusion drawn from the measurement of prostaglandins in plasma must be made with utmost caution. Using only those estimates giving lower more accurate levels:

(a) increase in concentrations during labour has been shown by Karim

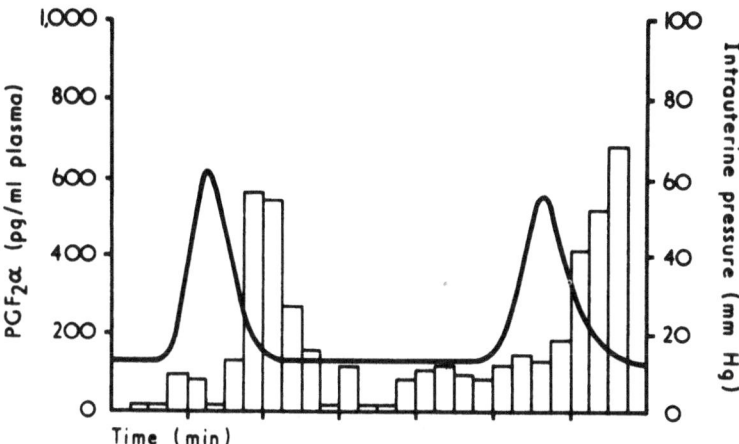

Figure 2.12   Prostaglandin $F_{2\alpha}$ concentrations in peripheral venous plasma (histogram) in relation to uterine contractions (tocograph tracing). Continuous sampling of blood was made with 15 s aliquots. (From Sharma *et al.*, 1973, by courtesy of *Brit. Med. J.*)

    (1968), Challis *et al.* (1974) and Hennam *et al.* (1974), but not by Gréen *et al.* (1974),

(b) concentrations may increase in relation to contractions (Karim, 1968; Sharma *et al.*, 1973; Challis *et al.*, 1974) although Gréen *et al.* (1974) failed to show this,

(c) concentrations are significantly higher in umbilical cord blood than peripheral blood (Challis *et al.*, 1974),

(d) no increase in peripheral plasma prostaglandin levels before labour was noted (Hennam *et al.*, 1974),

(e) no significant difference in plasma $PGF_{2\alpha}$ levels was noted between oxytocin induced and spontaneous labour (Challis *et al.*, 1974).

(b) Prostaglandins in intrauterine tissues and fluid

The low circulating levels of the natural prostaglandins and the ability of many tissues to rapidly synthesise and metabolise them has led investigators to look at the involvement of prostaglandins in reproductive processes in a purely local capacity. The uterine milieu has been the subject of much examination in the human. Because of its accessibility and the possibility of obtaining frequent samples, the amniotic fluid has been studied with the hope that it may reflect the uterine involvement of the prostaglandins.

    The amniotic fluid does not metabolise prostaglandins readily (Keirse *et al.*, 1974a). When large amounts of prostaglandins are injected into amniotic fluid they disappear (presumably by diffusion or active transport) relatively slowly. Figure 2.13 shows that following an injection of 15–25 mg $PGF_{2\alpha}$ the concentration had diminished to half the peak value attained within 3–5 hours (Hillier and Dilley, 1974). This agrees with similar findings by Pace-Asciak *et al.* (1972).

    However, the rapid fluctuations in amniotic fluid concentrations that have been noted in the second stage of labour (Hillier *et al.*, 1974) suggest that rapid endogenous changes can occur.

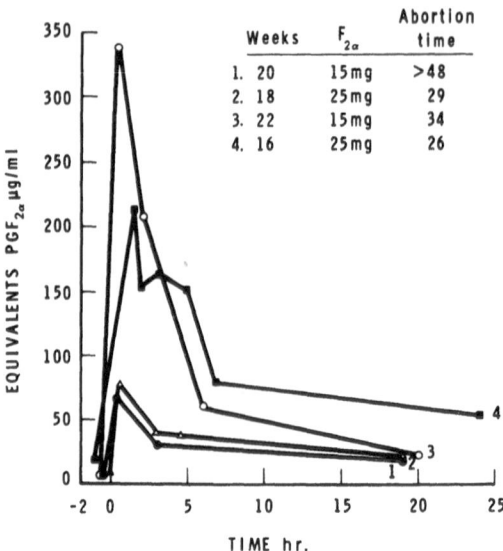

Figure 2.13 Disappearance of $PGF_{2\alpha}$ from amniotic fluid after injection of 15–25 mg $PGF_{2\alpha}$ at 18–26 weeks gestation. (From Hillier and Dilley, 1974, by courtesy of *Prostaglandins*)

Prostaglandins were first identified in amniotic fluid by Karim (1966) and Karim and Devlin (1967). With the methods available they showed that high levels (up to 20 000 pg ml⁻¹ $PGF_{2\alpha}$ and 500 pg ml⁻¹ PGE_2) appeared in amniotic fluid only during active labour. At elective Caesarean section and before the onset of spontaneous labour the concentrations were low. This elevation during labour was not confined to term pregnancy because amniotic fluid obtained during or following spontaneous abortion but not hysterectomy or termination hysterectomy was first shown by Karim and Hillier (1970) to contain high concentrations of PGE_2 and $PGF_{2\alpha}$. These results were used in part as evidence by Karim (1972a) in postulating an involvement of prostaglandins in the processes of spontaneous labour and abortion. Karim and Devlin (1967) also showed that the decidua contained relatively high contrations of prostaglandins during labour and suggested that this may be their source. Since that time several studies have confirmed and extended these findings both qualitatively and quantitatively. Hibbard *et al.* (1974) and Salmon and Amy (1973) have shown an increase in amniotic fluid PGF concentrations in late pregnancy and labour. With an assay that did not involve chromatographic separation of prostaglandins Hibbard *et al.* (1974) found less than 75 pg ml⁻¹ PGF before 36 weeks of gestation; after this time but before the onset of labour a progressive rise with advancing gestation occurred generally to higher than 300 pg ml⁻¹. Further increases were noted in the first stages of labour. Hillier (unpublished data) has shown that PGF concentrations in amniotic fluid, estimated by radioimmunoassay following column chromatography, are significantly higher at 36–40 weeks gestation (396 ± 58.2 SEM) compared with 47.5 ± 5.7 pg ml^{-1} in the mid-trimester. Salmon and Amy (1973) assayed prostaglandins in unextracted amniotic fluid using a double antibody technique. Concentrations measured at 16 weeks gestation were in the region of 400 pg ml^{-1} compared with about 40–75 pg ml^{-1} estimated by other investigators. They noted a rise in prostaglandins after 35–36 weeks of pregnancy, which agrees qualitatively with the findings of Sharma *et al.* (1973) although measured concentrations in the former investigations were generally higher. A further increase in liquor PGF concentration occurred during labour, rising most steeply after 5–6 cm cervical dilatation.

Keirse and Turnbull (1973) measured E prostaglandins in late pregnancy and labour using a gas liquid chromatographic technique. Before the onset of labour, concentrations were below 500 pg ml^{-1} but in labour a progressive increase in PGE concentration was noted reaching from 1200–17 000 pg ml^{-1}.

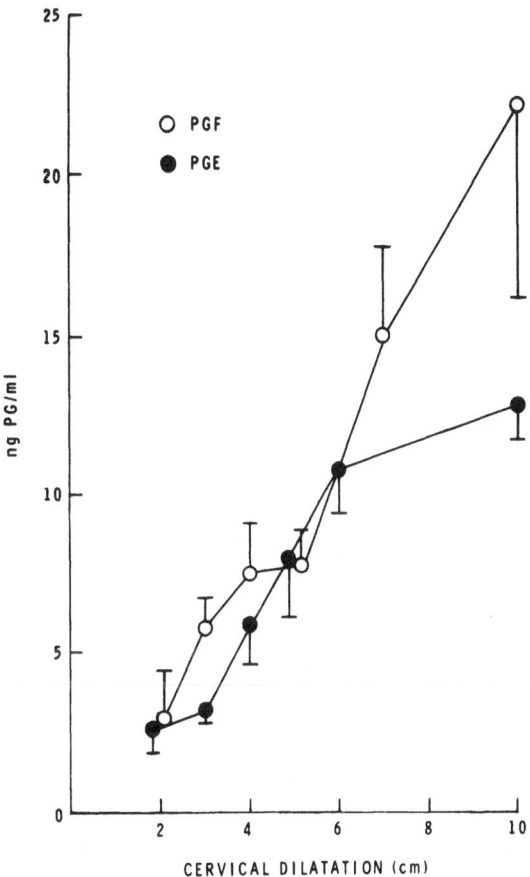

Figure 2.14 Comparison of PGE$_2$ and PGF$_{2\alpha}$ content of amniotic fluid during spontaneous labour, plotted against cervical dilatation. Values are ng ml^{-1} mean ($\pm$ SEM) of at least three determinations in each case. PGF$_{2\alpha}$ estimation by radio-immunoassay and PGE$_2$ by gas liquid chromatography. (From Keirse *et al.*, 1974, by courtesy of *J. Obstet. Gynaecol. Brit. Cwlth.*)

Keirse *et al.* (1974a) showed that concentration of PGF at term before the onset of labour was significantly higher (1655 ± 210) than in the mid-trimester
(650 ± 130 pg ml⁻¹). These levels are considerably higher than estimated by
Hillier *et al.* (1974) and Sharma *et al.* (1973). Keirse *et al.* (1974a) also found
an increase during labour of both PGE_2 and $PGF_{2\alpha}$ and levels were almost
identical (Figure 2.14). The concentrations measured in the acceleratory
phase of labour accord reasonably well with those of Hillier *et al.* (1974) and
Salmon and Amy (1973).

The studies already mentioned have utilised separate single amniotic fluid
samples from different patients. Because of interpatient variability that can
occur, Hillier *et al.* (1974) obtained serial liquor samples from patients in
spontaneous or induced labour. Generally this was performed after amniotomy by passing a transcervical catheter, but in four patients in spontaneous
labour a transabdominal catheter was inserted. Figures 2.15 and 2.16 show
results obtained in individual patients. During either spontaneous (Figure
2.15) or induced labour (Figure 2.16) there was a progressive but

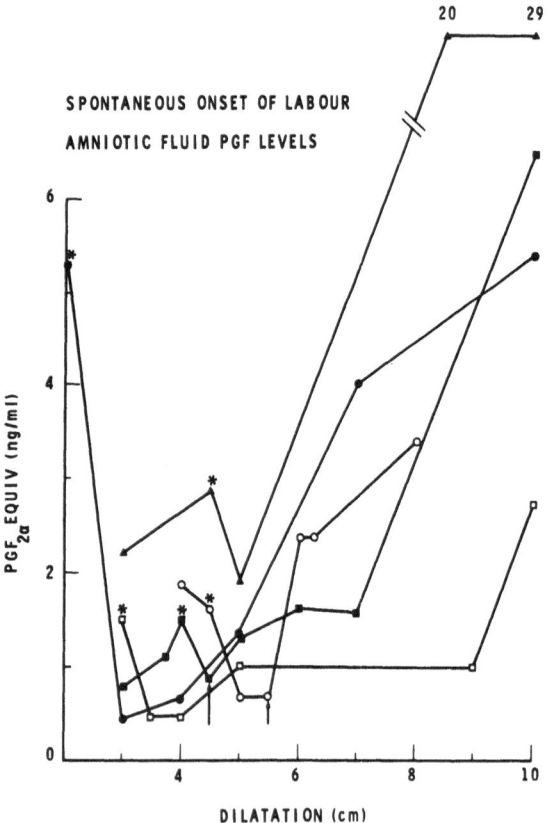

Figure 2.15 Amniotic fluid concentrations of $PGF_{2\alpha}$ equiv ml⁻¹ in individual
patients throughout labour (spontaneous onset of labour); * indicates amniotomy. The arrows
indicate addition of oxytocin in two patients for augmentation of labour. (From Hillier *et al.*,
1974, by courtesy of *J. Obstet. Gynaecol. Brit. Cwlth.*)

OXYTOCIN INDUCED LABOUR - AMNIOTIC FLUID PGF LEVELS

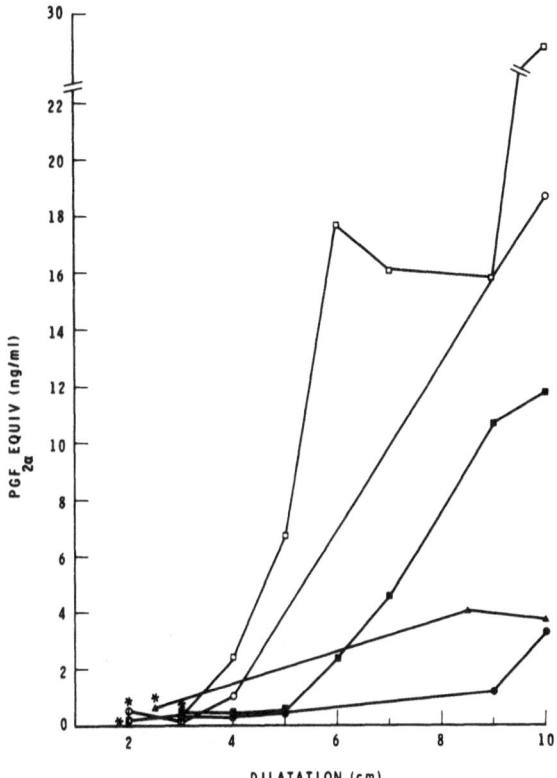

Figure 2.16   Amniotic fluid concentrations of $PGF_{2\alpha}$ equiv ml^{-1} in individual patients throughout labour (oxytocin induced labour). Oxytocin was administered immediately after amniotomy indicated by *. (From Hillier *et al.*, 1974, by courtesy of *J. Obstet. Gynaecol. Brit. Cwlth.*)

very variable increase in PGF concentration. The increase in the induced groups appeared to relate only to the acceleratory phase of labour. Significant changes in prostaglandin concentrations were not observed before this phase (Figure 2.16). It is also noteworthy that the concentrations in patients in early spontaneous labour were higher than those in early induced labour at a time when contractility in the latter patients was equivalent or greater than in the spontaneously labouring group. Samples from patients with transabdominal catheters before and after artificial rupture of membranes indicated a transient fall in concentration following amniotomy.

Increasing amounts of prostaglandins in amniotic fluid in the latter weeks of pregnancy seem to parallel the increasing amounts of oestrogens and decreasing progesterone detected in plasma at the same time. These increases clearly precede the identifiable onset of labour but it is not known whether the increased myometrial contractility known to occur after the 35th week of gestation (Theobald *et al.*, 1968) can cause or is a consequence of increased prostaglandin concentrations. An hormonal involvement in the control of prostaglandin production may be necessary. Liggins *et al.* (1972) and Currie *et al.* (1973) have shown that uterine PGF production near term in sheep, parallels the increase in oestrogen production and coincident reduction in progesterone levels.

The prostaglandin increase in amniotic fluid after 35–36 weeks of gestation in the human may well depend upon changes in oestradiol and progesterone which have been shown to occur (Turnbull *et al.*, 1974). In the very early stages of labour there appear to be subtle differences in the concentration of amniotic fluid prostaglandin dependent upon whether the labour is spontaneous in onset or induced. The higher levels of prostaglandins present in spontaneous labour may indicate an endogenous involvement in uterine contractility. Where exogenous oxytocics are used it is not until the acceleratory phase of labour that a spontaneous or endogenous component becomes apparent and prostaglandin concentrations rise.

It has been intimated that prostaglandins may be released by vaginal and cervical distension and stretch. In sheep the circulating prostaglandin F levels are elevated by vaginal distension and infused oxytocin (see Chapter 7). The mechanism of this phenomenon has not yet been clarified. In humans the elevated amniotic fluid concentrations during labour may be due to progressive cervical and vaginal dilatation and distension. Experiments carried out to investigate this in humans have so far given equivocal results. If manipulation does elevate prostaglandin concentrations it is possible that the fall noted following artificial rupture of membranes may be due to prior stimulation creating an artificially high concentration. The plasma levels of prostaglandins during vaginal examination in humans have not been measured.

It is possible that the endometrium, decidua, amniotic membranes, umbili-

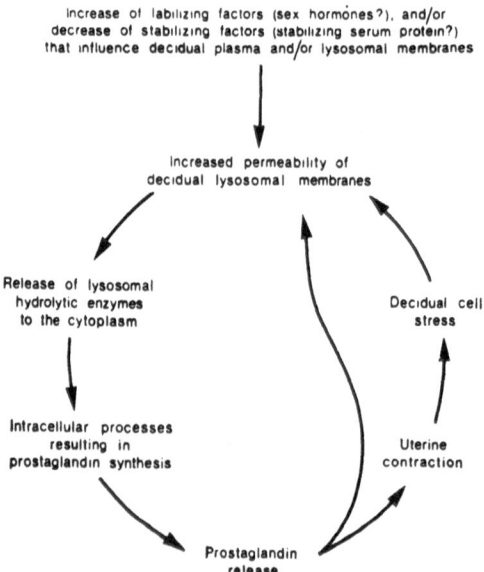

Figure 2.17 Hypothetical model for the mechanism initiating uterine contractions. (From Gustavii, 1972, by courtesy of *Lancet*)

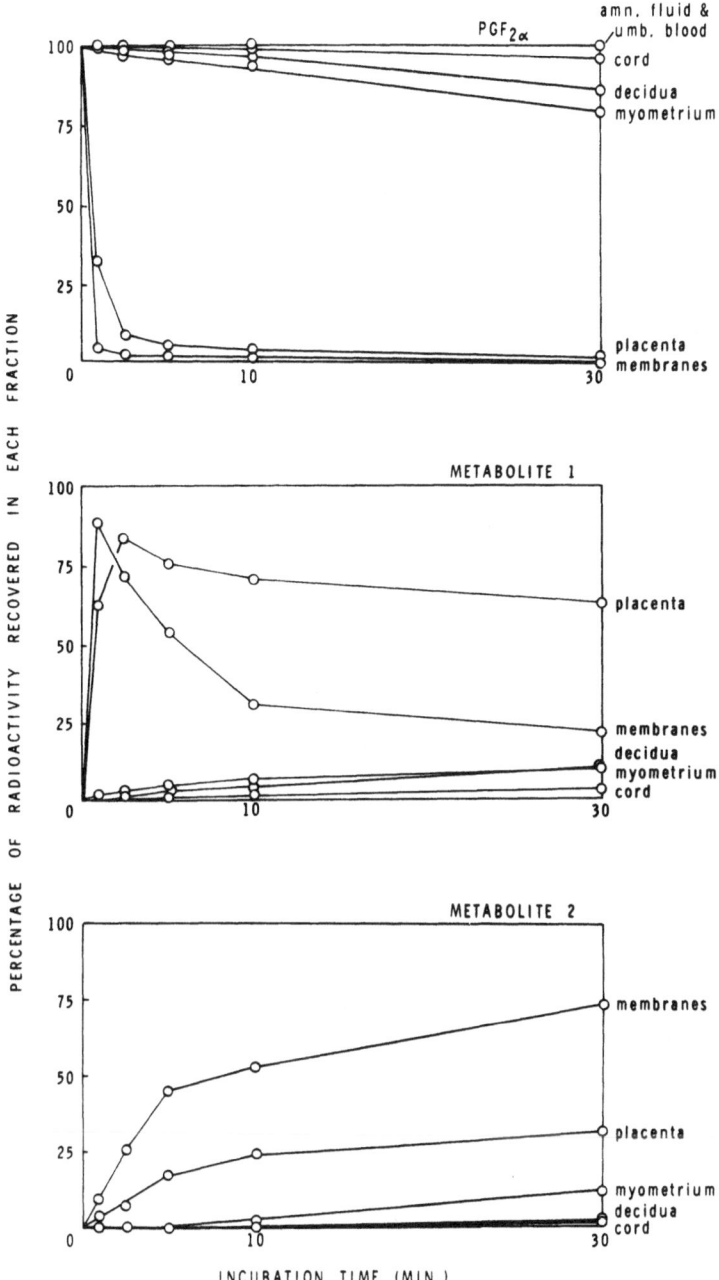

Figure 2.18 Metabolism of ^3H-$PGF_{2\alpha}$ in amniotic fluid, umbilical venous blood and homogenates of membranes, placenta, myometrium, decidua and umbilical cord, all obtained from a same patient at elective Caesarean section at term. Concentrations of $PGF_{2\alpha}$ used were 20 ng ml^{-1} of blood or amniotic fluid and 900 ng g^{-1} of tissue. Incubations were conducted at 37 °C in the presence of NAD (2 mM). Thin layer chromatography was used for the separation of $PGF_{2\alpha}$ from its metabolites. Metabolite 1 was further identified as 15-keto-$PGF_{2\alpha}$ and metabolite 2 as 15-keto-13,14-dihydro-$PGF_{2\alpha}$. (From M. Keirse, unpublished data)

cal cord, placenta and the fetus are involved in the physiology of labour either via their ability to synthesise or metabolise prostaglandins and by effects on other hormones.

The source of prostaglandin in amniotic fluid has been suggested to be of decidual origin because this tissue is rich in prostaglandins (Karim and Devlin, 1967). Endometrial tissue is also able to synthesise prostaglandins from the natural precursor—arachidonic acid. Gustavii (1972) and Gustavii and Green (1972) have suggested that the onset of uterine contractility results from decidual cell stress resulting in the events outlined in Figure 2.17. The key steps of labilisation of lysomes by hypoxia and ischaemia have been demonstrated (Gustavii, 1972); furthermore $PGF_{2\alpha}$ itself can labilise lysomes (Weiner and Kaley, 1972). The chain of events represents an attractive hypothesis for explaining prostaglandin-induced contractility but a number of questions arise:

1. Can decidua synthesise and metabolise prostaglandins ?
2. Can formed prostaglandins pass to their site of action?
3. Can other tissues in the uterine milieu synthesise and metabolise prostaglandins and represent an alternative to a decidual source?

Partial answers to these questions are available. Keirse *et al.* (1974b) have measured the ability of placental villous tissue, membranes, umbilical cord, fetal skin, myometrium and decidua at 16 weeks gestation and myometrium and villous tissue at seven weeks gestation to metabolise exogenous $PGF_{2\alpha}$. ^3H-$PGF_{2\alpha}$ was added to homogenates of tissue at 37 °C for various lengths of time. Thin layer radiochromatography identified various metabolites. With membrane and placental homogenates, added $PGF_{2\alpha}$ concentrations dropped to less than half their original values within three minutes while the

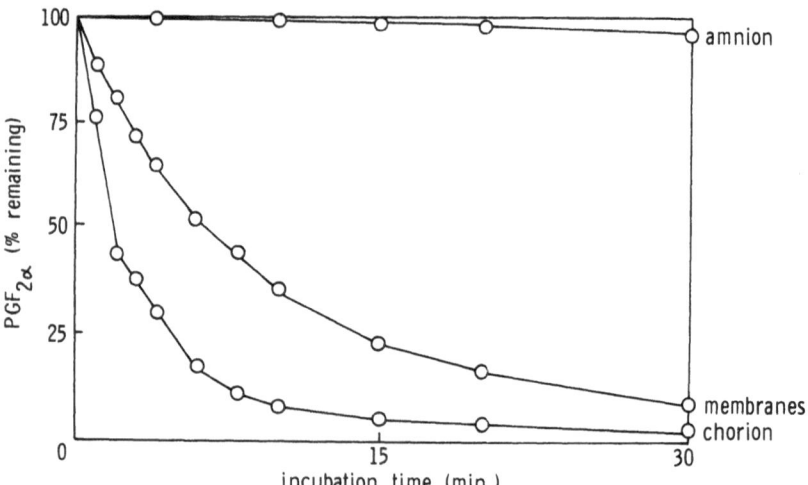

Figure 2.19 Proportional rates of metabolism of ^3H-$PGF_{2\alpha}$ in homogenates of combined fetal membranes and its two components, amnion and chorion. The tissues were incubated at 37 °C in 0.1 M potassium phosphate (pH 7.4) containing 2 mM NAD. Amnion was incubated with a five times lower $PGF_{2\alpha}$ concentration (3 μg g^{-1} tissue) than chorion and membranes (15 μg g^{-1}). (From M. Keirse, unpublished data)

concentrations of two metabolites tentatively identified as 15-keto-PGF$_{2\alpha}$ (metabolite 1) and 15-keto-13,14-dihydro-PGF$_{2\alpha}$ (metabolite 2) increased in the incubation fluid. Myometrial and decidual homogenates metabolised 15 and 5% PGF$_{2\alpha}$ respectively in 30 min. The fetal skin and umbilical cord did not metabolise PGF$_{2\alpha}$ during 60 min incubation. Tissues obtained at term gave similar results. Figure 2.18 shows the metabolising ability of intrauterine tissues at term. Figure 2.19 shows that term chorion has a much greater ability to metabolise PGF$_{2\alpha}$ than the amnion. The low metabolising ability of umbilical cord vessels may explain the findings of Hillier (1970) that the umbilical cord blood vessel prostaglandin is high in specimens from elective Caesarean sections when amniotic fluid prostaglandins are low. Jarabak (1972) and Schlegel et al. (1974) using term placental tissue have also shown high prostaglandin dehydrogenase concentrations.

The observations that membranes obtained from term pregnancies have the same metabolising capacity as early pregnancy tissue do not suggest

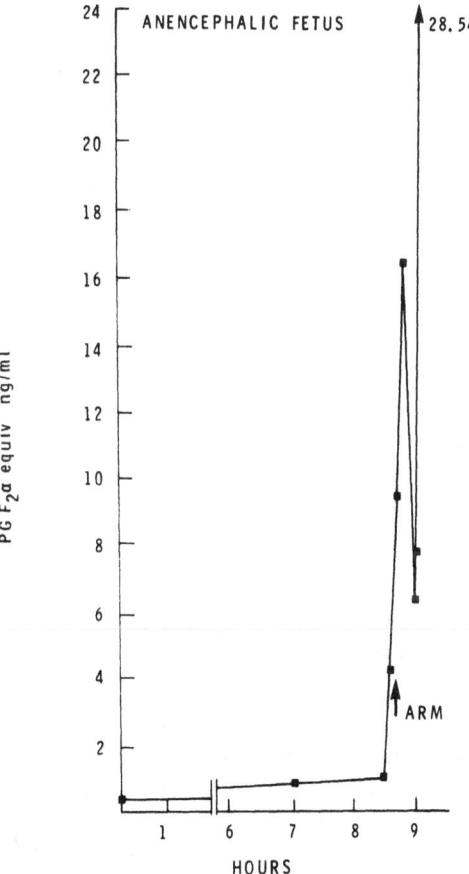

Figure 2.20 Induced labour in a patient with an anencephalic fetus at term. Note the extreme rise in prostaglandin concentrations only occurring at and following ARM. Delivery occurred immediately following the last sample. (From Hillier, 1975, unpublished data)

that a lowering of this capacity and consequent increased prostaglandin levels are important in the onset of labour. The high metabolising ability of fetal tissues suggests they may play a role in the maintenance of pregnancy. It has been shown that the arachidonic acid content of amniotic fluid increases dramatically during labour and appears consistent with elevated prostaglandin in this fluid (Schultz *et al.*, 1974).

The possibility of a fetal source of prostaglandins has been investigated by studying amniotic fluid from patients with anencephalic fetuses or with intra-uterine death of the fetus. Figure 2.20 shows that elevated levels do occur in induced labour complicated by anencephaly but generally not until the membranes have been ruptured after many hours of uterine stimulation. In two patients with intrauterine death of the fetus an increase in liquor levels was noted before rupture of the membranes (Figure 2.21). The results with anencephalic fetuses suggest strongly that membrane stimulation or rupture, or the

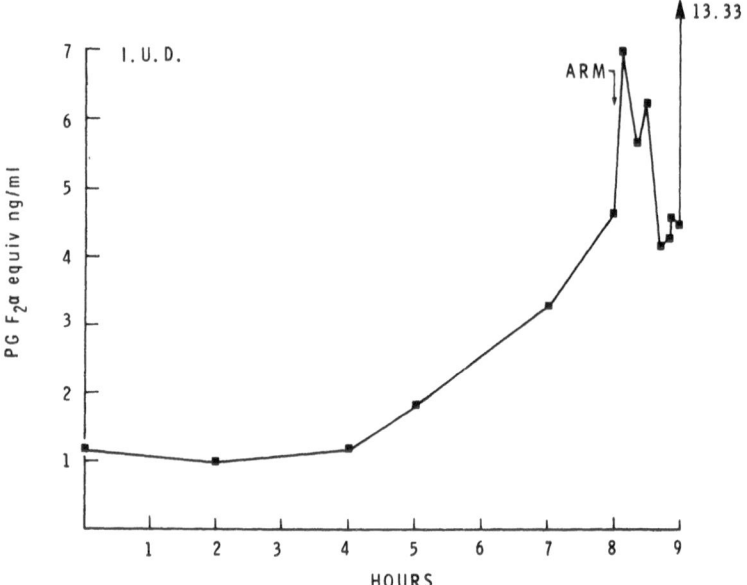

Figure 2.21   Induced labour in a case of intrauterine death of the fetus. Note rise in PGF concentrations before rupture of membranes. Last sample taken at time of delivery (Hillier, 1975, unpublished data)

stimulation of associated tissues and organs may cause increased prostaglandin synthesis or decreased metabolism. The integrity of the membranes in patients with intrauterine death of the fetus would be expected to have diminished, possibly altering their metabolising and synthesising capacity (Hillier *et al.*, 1975). It is possible that within the locale of the uterus prostaglandins may cause a number of vital events. At present some evidence is available to show that it can stimulate oestrogen production by aromatisation of testosterone in the isolated human placenta (Alsat and Cedard, 1973). This and other observations that local prostaglandin concentrations increase before the onset of labour make them strong contenders as one of the mediators in the on-set of labour.

(c) Effect of prostaglandins on pregnant human uterus

Indirect evidence implicating prostaglandins in the process of labour and spontaneous abortion comes from the observation that PGE_2 and $F_{2\alpha}$ have a stimulant action on the pregnant human uterus and can be used for the termin-ation of early and late pregnancies. The subject is discussed in detail in Chapters 3 and 4.

(d) Inhibition of prostaglandins action or synthesis on uterine contractions

Intravenous infusion of 10% ethyl alcohol has been shown to be effective in suppressing uterine activity in premature labour. Karim and Sharma (1970) have shown that ethyl alcohol is also able to abolish prostaglandin induced uterine stimulation without affecting oxytocin induced contractions—the im-plication being that spontaneous uterine contractility is mediated through prostaglandin release. Mantell and Liggins (1970), however, by using a differ-ent experimental approach were able to partially inhibit oxytocin induced uterine activity. Some analgesic drugs may inhibit the oxytocic effect of pros-taglandins. Smith and Temple (1973) noted that the mean time to abortion fol-lowing intra-amniotic $PGF_{2\alpha}$ was significantly prolonged (35 hours v. 14 hours) when a combination of acetaminophen and dextropropoxy-phene was given instead of pethidine. The failure rate was also considerably increased (20% v. 3%). *In vitro* experiments performed by the authors showed that dextropropoxyphene inhibited $PGF_{2\alpha}$ contractions on the rabbit uterus while acetoaminophen and pethidine had no such effect.

Non-steroidal anti-inflammatory drugs (e.g. aspirin and indomethacin) pre-vent biosynthesis of prostaglandins by an inhibitory effect on the prosta-glandin synthetase enzyme system (Vane, 1971). On the rat uterus *in vitro* it has been shown that spontaneous activity is due to a generation of prosta-glandins from the tissue. Both prostaglandin production and spontaneous activity are abolished by aspirin or indomethacin. These drugs also have been shown to prolong parturition in rats presumably by inhibiting the synthesis of prostaglandins (Aiken, 1972; Vane and Williams, 1973; Williams, 1973). Novy *et al.* (1974a) have reported that in pregnant rhesus monkey indo-methacin prolongs gestation and prevents normal initiation of parturition.

Lewis and Schulman (1973) carried out a retrospective study of 103 pa-tients taking high doses of acetylsalicylic acid for at least six months of preg-nancy. Aspirin administration was associated with a highly significant in-crease in the 'average length of gestation, in the frequency of postmaturity and in the mean duration of spontaneous labour' (Table 2.8). Horan (1974) has suggested that the effect of aspirin on gestation and parturition may be the result of delayed rate of deciduoma growth in early weeks of pregnancy.

Direct observation on the effect of prostaglandin synthetase inhibitors on premature and term labour is limited to two reports. Gyory *et al.* (1974)

Table 2.8   Influence of acetylsalicylic acid on the duration of human gestation and labour—Comparisons in three study groups (From Lewis and Schulman, 1973)

Variable	Group I 103 women	Group II 52 women	Group III 50 women
Age (yr)	26.0 ± 5.68	26.7 ± 5.05	26.3 ± 5.18
Gravidity	2.55 ± 1.69	2.69 ± 1.34	2.52 ± 1.60
Parity	1.37 ± 1.52	1.50 ± 1.43	1.62 ± 1.40
Length of gestation days	$286.1* \pm 13.3$	275.2 ± 10.6	278.6 ± 6.91
Length of labour (hours)	$12.1* \pm 10.6$	7.30 ± 4.11	6.96 ± 4.96
Birth weight (g)	3077 ± 597	2972 ± 538	$3379* \pm 460$
Blood loss estimated (ml)	$340* \pm 155$	244 ± 114	235 ± 97

* Mean different ($p < 0.05$) from other two groups. Otherwise difference between groups was not significant at this level.

Group I: Patients taking 50 grains (3250 mg) aspirin daily for at least last six months of gestation for rheumatoid arthritis, non-specific collagen disease or degenerative musculoskeletal disease during gestation

Group II: (First control group) Consists of patients with rheumatoid arthritis, non-specific collagen disease or degenerative musculoskeletal disease during gestation who were not taking aspirin or other compounds known to affect prostaglandin synthesis

Group III: (Second control group) Pregnant patients without known disease who were not taking aspirin or related drugs

studied the effect of salicylate on 50 cases of premature labour and 10 cases of term labour. With intact membranes and cervical dilatation of less than 4 cm in premature cases 1–2.5 mg sodium salicylate diminished uterine activity for five to six hours. Repeated administration abolished uterine contraction. In hormone deficient patients concomitantly administered progesterone therapy became effective after 24–48 hours and contractility could be controlled until this time. At term 2–2.5 mg sodium salicylate suspended uterine activity for 5–6 hours. The overall success rate in preventing premature labour was not stated. Mosler *et al.* (1974) have also implied that aspirin may be of use in delaying premature labour. Larger controlled studies are required to confirm the above findings.

The evidence that the abortifacient action of hypertonic saline is at least partly mediated through prostaglandin release has already been discussed. Waltman and Tricomi (1973) and Waltman *et al.* (1973) have shown that pretreatment (of second trimester patients undergoing therapeutic abortion with hypertonic saline) with prostaglandin synthetase inhibitors (aspirin, indomethacin, or mefenamic acid) significantly prolongs saline instillation to abortion time possibly by inhibiting the synthesis of prostaglandins.

2.3.9 Prostaglandins and lactation

Both inhibitory and stimulant effects of prostaglandins on milk ejection in laboratory animals have been reported. In the rabbit PGE_1 diminished the increase in mammary pressure induced by oxytocin (Turker and Kiran, 1969) while in the rat $PGF_{2\alpha}$ increased the tone of mammary gland strips *in vitro* (Cobo *et al.*, 1974). McNeilly and Fox (1971) have shown that in the guinea-pig PGE_1, E_2, $F_{1\alpha}$ and $F_{2\alpha}$ increase mammary gland pressure.

In the human only one direct study has thus far been reported although some indirect observations have been made. In an investigation on lactating women Cobo *et al.* (1974) showed that $PGF_{2\alpha}$ given intravenously increased mammary pressure. The response varied from patient to patient (Figure 2.22) but overall a clear increasing dose–response relationship existed within the range used (40–200 μg $PGF_{2\alpha}$). A latency of 30–90 s was noted before the patient responded to the injection; the duration of this delay was inversely related to dosage and was two to four times longer than that seen on injection of equiactive amounts of oxytocin. Aspirin ingested in unspecified dosage two to four hours before administration of $PGF_{2\alpha}$ failed to modify the response of the mammary gland.

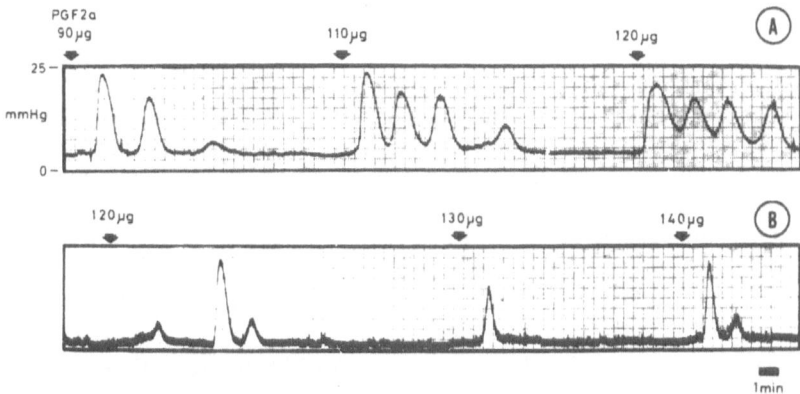

Figure 2.22   Intra mammary pressure in human *in vivo*. Response to $PGF_{2\alpha}$. In the upper recording (A) a dose effect relationship was observed whereas in patient B no clear dose effect response was demonstrated. (From Cobo *et al.*, 1974, by courtesy of *Amer. J. Obstet. Gynecol.*)

The exact mechanism of action of prostaglandins in increasing mammary pressure is not known. The latent period between prostaglandin administration and the response suggests an indirect action (possibly through oxytocin release or due to a metabolite of prostaglandins). The former mechanism has been suggested to exist in the human (Gillespie *et al.*, 1972) although sound evidence is lacking (Hillier, 1972). Another mechanism which may be of importance is the sensitisation of tissues to circulating oxytocin by prostaglandin application (Liggins *et al.*, 1972). It is possible that prostaglandins act by lowering the threshold of the mammary cells to oxytocin. Some metabolites of prostaglandin $F_{2\alpha}$ are also smooth muscle stimulants (Bygdeman *et al.*, 1974; Dawson *et al.*, 1974) and are probably less rapidly broken down than the parent prostaglandins. The observations of Cobo *et al.* (1974) provide some support for the suggestion that the effect of $PGF_{2\alpha}$ is mediated through a metabolite. Following 150 μg $PGF_{2\alpha}$ there is a prolonged increase in mammary pressure and phasic contractility. The duration of action is far longer than the circulating life of natural $PGF_{2\alpha}$. Metabolites with a long half-life in circulation may provide extended stimulation of the posterior pituitary to produce oxytocin release either directly or reflexly through stimulation of mammary gland.

The latency of the onset of response to $PGF_{2\alpha}$ is not confined to the mammary gland but is also seen on the uterus following intravenous administration (Karim et al., 1970). The doses injected by Cobo et al. (1974) are likely to stimulate the uterus which could reflexly cause oxytocin release.

Indirect involvement of prostaglandins with lactation has been reported by Shearman et al. (1973) who showed that almost 100% of a small group of second trimester patients terminated with intra-amniotic or extra-amniotic $PGF_{2\alpha}$ experienced lactation 72–96 hours after abortion. The explanation for this is obscure and the investigators showed that surgical termination of pregnancy did not result in increased lactation. Lauersen and Wilson (1974) and Lauersen et al. (1974) confirmed these observations. Out of 30 patients aborted by intra-amniotic $PGF_{2\alpha}$, 27 (90%) complained of engorged breasts and varying degrees of lactation within one week. For comparison, lactation was observed in only three out of ten women following intra-amniotic instillation of hypertonic saline and intravenous oxytocin combination.

MacKenzie and Hillier (unpublished data) have found an approximately 50% incidence of lactation on questioning patients 6–8 weeks following PGE_2-induced abortion. The postabortal menstrual pattern of women induced with prostaglandins appeared to be normal and was probably not influenced by the induced lactation. The physiology and pharmacological involvement of prostaglandins in lactation require elucidation.

2.3.10 Intrauterine contraceptive device and prostaglandins

The mechanism of action of the IUCD has been attributed to increased concentrations of prostaglandins within the uterine cavity. The hypothesis originally advanced by Chaudhuri (1971, 1973) has been supported by experiments carried out in laboratory animals and is discussed in detail in Chapters 6 and 7.

In the human there is little direct evidence for a prostaglandin involvement in the mechanism of action of the IUCD. Superficially its introduction is often associated with increased uterine contractility and pain; intrauterine administration of prostaglandins also produces these effects.

An inflammatory response to a foreign body could explain the increase. Polymorphonuclear lymphocytes are commonly found in the human uterus and rhesus monkey uterus containing an IUCD (Kelly et al., 1969). These bodies synthesise prostaglandin (Higgs and Youlten, 1972).

The significance of these changes is open to conjecture but indirect observations suggest that the presence of an IUCD can cause changes in steroidal hormonal balance which may be hypothesised as resulting from raised prostaglandin levels (Faucher et al., 1969). Although hysterectomy does not affect menstrual hormone function in the primate this does not preclude the possibility in the intact animal of pharmacological access of endometrial prostaglandins into the uterine vein affecting ovarian function. Faucher et al. (1969) showed that the luteal phase is shorter and urinary pregnanediol output slightly reduced in women with an IUCD when compared to their own preinsertion parameters. However, Eckstein (1970) showed that the length of cycles in monkeys with plastic devices was slightly but insignificantly shorter than in controls without IUCDs.

It has also been suggested that the IUCD causes increased uterine and tubal motility (see Eckstein 1970 for references and critical comments). Eckstein suggests that among the actions involved in the mechanism of action of the IUCD may be expulsion of the ovum prematurely, impairment or destruction of the ovum and interference with implantation. The possibility should be investigated whether these effects are mediated in total or in part by increased concentrations of prostaglandins.

2.3.11 Umbilical cord, placenta and fetal haemodynamics

Prostaglandins have been implicated in the regulation of the fetal and placental circulation and in the dynamic vascular changes occurring in the fetus at birth (Karim, 1967; Hillier, 1970). The evidence, as yet fragmentary, is based on the presence of prostaglandins in the umbilical cord and placenta and on their pharmacological actions. The role of prostaglandins in toxaemia of pregnancy is not clear. Speroff (1973) has suggested that altered utero–placental blood flow may in part be mediated by prostaglandin–angiotensin interactions and that imbalance may result in increased vascular resistance within the system. Ryan et al. (1969) have shown that the toxaemic placenta is deficient in PGE-like substance. Prostaglandins deficiency may also affect the renal system thus exacerbating the problem. Zusman et al. (1973) have reported that circulating A prostaglandins (but not E and F) decrease with high sodium intake and increase with low sodium intake.

(a) Distribution

The blood vessels of the full term umbilical cord and the large surface vessels of the placenta contain prostaglandins E_1, E_2, $F_{1\alpha}$ and $F_{2\alpha}$ (Karim, 1967). The distribution of these prostaglandins in umbilical cord vessels at different stages of gestation has been studied by Hillier (1970) and is shown in Table 2.9.

Table 2.9 Concentrations of prostaglandins E and F in umbilical blood vessels at different stages of gestation measured by biological assay—ng g^{-1} tissue mean± SEM. (From Hillier, 1970, by courtesy of K. Hillier)

	Weeks	N	PGE	PGF
Spontaneous abortion	19–29	8	45 ± 7.6	19.7 ± 7.0
Hysterotomy and termination hysterectomy	13–26	18	4.0 ± 1.0	ND
Spontaneous vaginal delivery	36–44	16	56 ± 6.6	10.8 ± 1.2
Emergency Caesarean section	39–41	3	58.3 ± 11.6	12.5 ± 1.1
Elective Caesarean section	39–41	8	38.4 ± 12.6	10.0 ± 1.6

Key: Not detectable

This work indicates that the prostaglandins are present in the blood vessels immediately prior to the onset of labour at term but not in early pregnancy blood vessels obtained at hysterotomy. They do, however, appear during spontaneous abortion. The stage of gestation at which the prostaglandin concentration increases is not known. Whether prostaglandins are synthesised in the blood vessels *in vivo* is not clear although homogenates of umbilical blood vessels obtained at term can biosynthesise PGE and PGF compounds from arachidonic acid. After incubation of term vessel homogenates with 500 μg g^{-1} arachidonic acid the amount of extractable PGE compounds increased 30–40 fold and PGF 6–12 fold although the actual percentage of arachidonic acid converted to E and F prostaglandins was less than 1%. Homogenates of umbilical blood vessels are not able to metabolise prostaglandins significantly (Keirse *et al.*, 1974b).

The release of prostaglandins from perfused strips of term human umbilical vessels *in vitro* has also been reported. Strips placed in Kreb's solution released 7.5 ng g^{-1} h^{-1} wet weight as measured by radioimmunoassay. The amount released was reduced to 0.5 ng g^{-1} h^{-1} in presence of indomethacin. Strips of umbilical vessels suspended in an organ bath and stretched under tension exhibits spontaneous activity which is probably due to prostaglandin production as it is abolished by indomethacin (Tuvemo and Wide, 1973).

(b) Pharmacological actions

The constrictor action of seminal fluid extracts on perfused human placenta was reported by von Euler (1934). The constrictor action of prostaglandins E_2, $F_{1\alpha}$ and $F_{2\alpha}$ on isolated circular and longitudinal strips of full term human umbilical cord and placental vessels was first reported by Karim (1967) and has since been confirmed by several investigators. Prostaglandin E_1 was shown to have a relaxant effect on the umbilical blood vessels (Karim, 1967) although both relaxation and constriction have since been reported (Hillier, 1970). The dual effect is likely to be a dose dependent phenomenon, i.e. relaxation with small doses and constriction with large doses of PGE_1. The effect of other naturally occurring prostaglandins on umbilical blood vessels has recently been reported. PGA_2 and B_2 are several times more potent than PGE_2 in constricting these vessels (Adaikan and Karim, 1974) (Figure 2.23, Table 2.2).

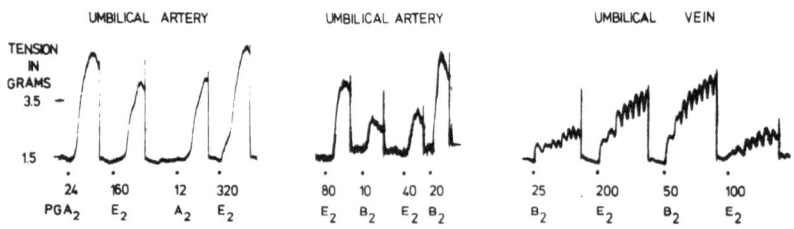

Figure 2.23 Isometric recording of longitudinal strip of human umbilical artery and vein. Krebs solution, 34 °C bubbled with 95% oxygen, 5% CO_2. Doses in ng ml^{-1}. Effect of prostaglandin A_2 (A_2), prostaglandin E_2 (E_2) and prostaglandin B_2 (B_2). (From Adaikan and Karim, 1974, by courtesy of *Prostaglandins*)

Park and Dyer (1973) reported a weak and non-selective antagonism of the action of PGE_2 on umbilical blood vessels with polyphloretin phosphate. Adaikan and Karim (1975) however have shown that PPP 10–40 μg ml^{-1} completely abolished responses to E_2, $F_{2\alpha}$, $F_{1\alpha}$, B_1, A_1, A_2 without affecting responses to 5-HT. The effect of PGB_2 was only partially antagonised. 7-oxa-13-prostynoic acid selectively blocks the constricting effect of PGE_2 after initial stimulation (Park and Dyer, 1973).

Coceani and Olley (1973) investigated the effects of various prostaglandins on strips of lamb ductus arteriosus *in vitro* under anaerobic and aerobic conditions. PGE_1 and E_2 relaxed the anoxic ductus whereas these compounds were without effect on the tissues after exposure to oxygen. The authors have suggested that PGE compounds may have a role in the regulation of the vessel tone during fetal life. This effect is the reverse of prostaglandin-induced contractility of umbilical blood vessels which occurs in aerobic but not anaerobic conditions (Hillier, 1970). PGF compounds contract the ductus arteriosus of the fetal calf *in vitro* (Elliot and Starling, 1972) and PGE compounds dilate the pulmonary vascular bed (Hauge *et al.*, 1967).

As originally postulated by Karim (1967) and Hillier and Karim (1970), these results suggest that the prostaglandins play a role in the circulatory adaptation of the fetus at birth and in haemodynamic control in the fetus.

Novy *et al.* (1974b) have investigated the haemodynamic effect of injecting $PGF_{2\alpha}$, PGE_2 and noradrenaline into fetal lambs. Both $PGF_{2\alpha}$ and noradrenaline increased fetal arterial pressure and umbilical blood flow while umbilical vascular resistance increased slightly with $F_{2\alpha}$ or not at all with noradrenaline. PGE_2 on the other hand increased fetal arterial pressure but decreased umbilical blood flow and exerted a profound vasoconstrictor effect on the fetal placental bed. They suggested that PGE_2 in high concentrations may have a deleterious haemodynamic effect upon the fetus *in utero*.

Beazley *et al.* (1972) have shown that prostaglandins can cross the placenta although it has not been established whether they do so in an active form or as metabolites. Local administration of prostaglandins to induce labour (Calder *et al.*, 1974) may also affect fetal haemodynamics in a different manner to systemic application although some protection is afforded as the placenta and other tissues can rapidly metabolise prostaglandins (Keirse *et al.*, 1974b) or contain a metabolising enzyme (Schlegel *et al.*, 1974). The actions of the prostaglandins upon the fetal circulation may directly affect oxygenation and feto–placental endocrine function. The extent of this may depend upon the prostaglandin used and the route of administration.

Biochemically and clinically there is so far little evidence to suggest that the human fetus *in vivo* is compromised under normal circumstances during prostaglandin administration to the mother. Brosens *et al.* (1974) suggested that a potential hazard may be caused where pre-existing problems such as pre-eclampsia are present. However, Calder *et al.* (1974) have found no evidence for this in intensively monitored patients with pre-eclampsia and hypertension. Thiery and Willighagen (1973) found no effect of prostaglandin $F_{2\alpha}$ administered intravenously or PGE_2 administered orally to induce labour at term upon the morphologic or histochemical profile of the human placenta.

2.3.12 Metabolites of prostaglandins in human reproduction

The first formed metabolites of prostaglandin E_2 and $F_{2\alpha}$ are the 15-keto, 15-keto-13,14-dihydro and 13,14-dihydro compounds respectively. Because the metabolism of PGE_2 and $PGF_{2\alpha}$ to the above compounds is very rapid, it has been suggested that measurements of these metabolites rather than the parent prostaglandins would be preferable in understanding their physiological roles in reproduction. The metabolites are more stable and some are present in higher concentrations in circulation than the parent compounds.

The larger number of urinary excreted metabolites are outlined by Samuelsson (1973) and have been measured in both male and female subjects. Only results which may be relevant to the physiology of reproduction will be discussed in this section. Only 1.5 min after PGE_2 injection, 3% remained unchanged in plasma whereas 40% was recovered as the 15-keto-13,14-dihydro metabolite (Samuelsson, 1973).

During the continuous infusion of 75 μg min^{-1} $PGF_{2\alpha}$ the concentration of the 15-keto-dihydro derivative was 105 ± 29 ng ml^{-1}, while $PGF_{2\alpha}$ was 4.4 ± 2.6 pg ml^{-1}. On the basis of this and other experiments Samuelsson (1973) stated that 2 pg ml^{-1} $PGF_{2\alpha}$ and 50 pg ml^{-1} 15-keto-dihydro-$PGF_{2\alpha}$ would be the calculated basal level in plasma. The major plasma metabolite of $PGF_{2\alpha}$, 15-keto-13,14-dihydro-$PGF_{2\alpha}$ is formed in tissue but not in blood.

Measurement in pooled citrated blood using GLC-mass spectrometry realised concentrations of 0.02 ng ml^{-1} $PGF_{2\alpha}$, undetectable 13,14-dihydro-$PGF_{2\alpha}$ and 0.03 ± 0.05 ng ml^{-1} PGE_2. Of particular relevance is the observation that the 15-keto-13,14-dihydro-$PGF_{2\alpha}$ level was about 25 pg ml^{-1} in male, 18–23 pg ml^{-1} in female and 70 pg ml^{-1} at two months gestation (Green and Granström, 1973).

The above findings take on additional significance following the work of Bygdeman *et al.* (1974) who found that 13,14-dihydro-$PGF_{2\alpha}$ stimulated human uterine contractility during mid-pregnancy following intravenous and intra-amniotic administration. The activity approached that of the parent compound. Another major metabolite, 15-keto-13,14-dihydro-$PGF_{2\alpha}$ was less active than the dihydro derivatives and they suggest that the activity of the former may be due to conversion to the latter. These results may explain the relatively long duration of action of the prostaglandins. It is not clear at this time whether some of the major actions of the prostaglandins may be mediated through their metabolites.

Cornette *et al.* (1974) have established a radioimmunoassay for 15-keto-$PGF_{2\alpha}$ and 13,14-dihydro-15-keto-$PGF_{2\alpha}$. They suggest that 15-keto-$PGF_{2\alpha}$ levels in human are 300 ± 100 pg ml^{-1} and for 13,14-dihydro-15-keto-$F_{2\alpha}$ are 1400 ± 100 pg ml^{-1}. Following intra-amniotic $PGF_{2\alpha}$ (40 mg) in the mid-trimester, within $\frac{1}{2}$-1 hour the level of $F_{2\alpha}$ rose from 1000 pg ml^{-1} to 3000 pg ml^{-1} in peripheral plasma and the 15-keto-dihydro-$PGF_{2\alpha}$ from 3000 pg ml^{-1} to 20 000 pg ml^{-1}. In the amniotic fluid during the same time interval $F_{2\alpha}$ rose to 10^5 ng ml^{-1} and the 15-keto-$F_{2\alpha}$ to 3×10^2 ng ml^{-1}. After eight hours the $PGF_{2\alpha}$ levels started to decline whereas the 15-keto-dihydro-$F_{2\alpha}$ had reached 2×10^3 ng ml^{-1} and was still increasing. The resting concentrations in plasma of the mid-trimester patient are higher than results of a collaborative trial published by Samuelsson (1973). The latter suggested that during the mid-trimester 15-keto-dihydro-PGF$_{2\alpha}$ was less than 500 pg ml^{-1} using GLC-mass spectrometry. They also reported 13,14-dihydro-PGF$_{2\alpha}$ levels of 200 pg ml^{-1} using radioimmunoassay. The level of PGF$_{2\alpha}$ in the midtrimester measured by Cornette *et al.* (1974) was approximately 1000 pg ml^{-1} which is far in excess of mid-trimester levels estimated at 3–11 pg ml^{-1} PGF$_{2\alpha}$ and 37–58 pg ml^{-1} PGE$_2$. The relationship and importance of 15-keto-13,14-dihydro prostaglandin F$_{2\alpha}$ (main PGF$_{2\alpha}$ metabolite in plasma) to endogenous prostaglandin F$_{2\alpha}$ concentrations during pregnancy and labour have been assessed by Green *et al.* (1974) using gas–liquid chromatography-mass spectrometry methods. The implications of their conclusions in pregnancy and labour are of importance. These authors suggest that because of the formation PGF$_{2\alpha}$ from platelets during blood collection its measurement gives an unreliable assessment of endogenous production. 15-keto-13,14-dihydro-PGF$_{2\alpha}$ is not formed during blood collection.

The plasma concentrations of the prostaglandin metabolite although slightly raised during the last month of pregnancy were below 70 pg ml^{-1} and increased significantly during the five hours preceding the onset of labour. During active labour there was a 10–30 fold increase (peak concentration 267–942 pg ml^{-1}) in the prostaglandin metabolite. The increases during labour were related to the degree of cervical dilatation. One hour after delivery the plasma concentration of 15-keto-13,14-dihydro-PGF$_{2\alpha}$ had decreased to 20–75% of the values found prior to parturition (Figure 2.24).

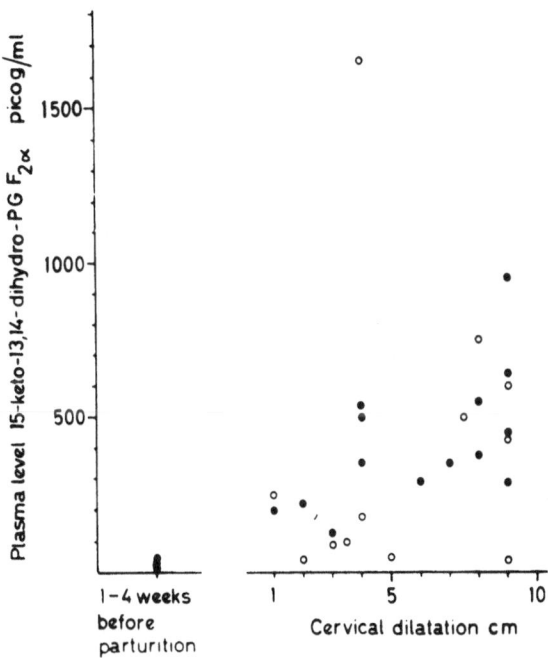

Figure 2.24   Plasma levels of 15-keto-13,14-dihydro-PGF$_{2\alpha}$ plotted *v.* cervical dilatation in patients undergoing normal (•) and oxytocin induced (○) labour. (From Gréen *et al.*, 1974, by courtesy of *Amer. J. Obstet. Gynecol.*)

There was no correlation between the concentration of $PGF_{2\alpha}$ and the stage of labour in two patients studied.

In oxytocin induced labour $PGF_{2\alpha}$ values showed a correlation to those of 15-keto-13,14-dihydro $PGF_{2\alpha}$ except in only one case out of five.

References

Adaikan, G. P. and Karim, S. M. M. (1974). Effects of prostaglandins A_1, A_2, B_1, B_2, E_2 and $F_{2\alpha}$ on human umbilical cord vessels. *Prostaglandins*, **8**, 411–416

Aiken, J. W. (1972). Aspirin and indomethacin prolong parturition in rats: Evidence that prostaglandins contribute to expulsion of foetus. *Nature (London)*, **240**, 21–25

Alsat, E. and Cedard, L. (1973). The stimulatory action of the prostaglandin on the production of oestrogens by the human placenta perfused *in vitro*. *Prostaglandins*, **3**, 145–153

Archer, D. F. and Petrelli, E. S. (1973). Alterations in biosynthesis of progesterone in human corpora lutea of pregnancy by prostaglandins. *Adv. Biosciences*, **9**, 669–672

Beazley, J. M., Brummer, H. C. and Kurjak, A. (1972). Distribution of 9-H^3-prostaglandin $F_{2\alpha}$ in pregnant and non-pregnant subjects. *J. Obstet. Gynaecol. Brit. Cwlth.*, **79**, 800–803

Bitensky, L. and Cohen, S. (1965). The variation of endometrial acid phosphate activity with the menstrual cycle. *J. Obstet. Gynaecol. Brit. Cwlth.*, **72**, 769–774

Bolognese, R. J. and Corson, S. L. (1973). The effect of vaginally administered prostaglandin $F_{2\alpha}$ on corpus luteum function. *Amer. J. Obstet. Gynecol.*, **117**, 240–245

Brosens, I., Dixon, H. G. and Robertson, W. B. (1974). Prostaglandins and Induction of labour. *Lancet*, **1**, 808

Brummer, H. C. (1972). Serum $PGF_{2\alpha}$ levels during late pregnancy, labour and puerperium. *Prostaglandins*, **2**, 185–194

Brummer, H. C. (1973a). Vasectomy and seminal prostaglandins. *Fertility and Sterility*, **24**, 131–133

Brummer, H. C. (1973b). Serum $PGF_{2\alpha}$ levels during human pregnancy. *Prostaglandins*, **3**, 3–5

Bygdeman, M., Fredericsson, B., Svanborg, K. and Samuelsson, B. (1970). The relation between fertility and prostaglandin content of seminal fluid in man. *Fertility and Sterility*, **21**, 622–629

Bygdeman, M., Green, M., Toppozada, M., Wiqvist, N. and Bergström, S. (1974). The influence of prostaglandin metabolites on the uterine response to $PGF_{2\alpha}$. A clinical and pharmacokinetic study. *Life Sci.*, **14**, 521–531

Bygdeman, M., Hamberg, M. and Samuelsson, B. (1966). The content of different prostaglandins in human seminal fluid and their threshold doses on the human myometrium. *Mem. Soc. Endocrinol*, **14**, 49–64

Bygdeman, M. and Samuelsson, B. (1966). Analyses of prostaglandins in human semen. *Clinica chim. Acta*, **13**, 465–474

Bygdeman, M. and Samuelsson, B. (1967). Prostaglandins in human seminal plasma and their effects on human myometrium. *Int. J. Fert.*, **12**, 17–20

Calder, A. A., Bonnar, J., Sheppard, B., Embrey, M. P. and Turnbull, A. C. (1974). Prostaglandins and pre-eclampsia. *Lancet*, **2**, 49

Caldwell, B. V., Burnstein, S., Brock, W. A. and Speroff, L. (1971). Radioimmunoassay of the F prostaglandins. *J. Clin. Endocrinol. Metab.*, **33**, 171–175

Challis, J. R. G., Osathanondh, R., Ryan, K. J. and Tulchinsky, D. (1974). Maternal and fetal plasma prostaglandin levels at vaginal delivery and caesarean section. *Prostaglandins*, **6**, 281–288

Challis, J. R. G. and Tulchinsky, D. (1974). A comparison between the concentration of prostaglandin F in human plasma and serum. *Prostaglandins*, **5**, 27–31

Chaudhuri, G. (1971). Intrauterine device: Possible role of prostaglandins. *Lancet*, **1**, 480

Chaudhuri, G. (1973). Release of prostaglandins by the I.U.C.D. *Prostaglandins*, **3**, 773–785

Clithero, H. J. (1961). The separation of three plain-muscle stimulants present in the human endometrium. *J. Physiol. (London)*, **155**, 62–63

Clithero, H. J. and Pickles, V. R. (1961). The separation of the smooth muscle stimulants in menstrual fluid. *J. Physiol. (London)*, **156**, 255–337

Cobo, E., Rodriguez, A. and deVillamizar, M. (1974). Milk-ejecting activity induced by prostaglandin $F_{2\alpha}$. *Amer. J. Obstet. Gynecol.*, 118, 831–836

Coceani, F. and Olley, P. M. (1973). The response of the ductus arteriosus to prostaglandins. *Cand. J. Physiol. and Pharmacol.*, 51, 220–225

Collier, J. G. and Flower, R. J. (1971). Effect of aspirin on human seminal prostaglandins. *Lancet*, 11, 852–853

Cornette, J. C., Harrison, K. L. and Kirton, K. T. (1974). Measurement of prostaglandin $F_{2\alpha}$ metabolites by radioimmunoassay. *Prostaglandins*, 5, 155–164

Coudert, S. P., Winter, J. S. D. and Faiman, C. (1974). Transient decline in serum progesterone levels during prostaglandin $F_{2\alpha}$ infusion in the mid luteal phase of the normal menstrual cycle. *Amer. J. Obstet. Gynecol.*, 119, 755–761

Coutinho, E. M. (1971). Tubal and uterine motility. *Nobel Symp. 15, Control of Human Fertility*, 97–115 (E. Diczfalusy and U. Borell, editors) (Stockholm: Almqvist and Wiksell)

Coutinho, E. M. (1974). Ovarian contractility and ovulation. In: *Research in Reproduction*, 6, 3–4 (R. G. Edwards, editor) (London: I.P.P.F.)

Coutinho, E. M. and Maia, H. S. (1971). The contractile response of the human uterus, fallopian tubes, and ovary to prostaglandins *in vivo. Fertility and Sterility*, 22, 539–543

Craft, I. L., Fergussan, I. L. C., Smith, B. and Youssefnejadian, E. (1973a). Sex steroid hormone levels in plasma following intra-amniotic injection of urea and prostaglandin E_2. *J. Obstet. Gynaecol. Brit. Cwlth.*, 80, 1095–1099

Craft, I. L., Scrivener, R. and Dewhurst, C. J. (1973b). Prostaglandin $F_{2\alpha}$ levels in the maternal and fetal circulations in late pregnancy. *J. Obstet. Gynaecol. Brit. Cwlth.*, 80, 616–618

Csapo, A. I. (1973). The prospects of prostaglandins in post-conceptional therapy. *Prostaglandins*, 3, 245–289

Csapo, A. I. (1974). Prostaglandin impact for menstrual induction. *Population Report on Prostaglandins Series G No. 4* (Washington, D.C.: George Washington Univ. Medical Centre)

Csapo, A. I., Knobil, E., van de Molen, H. J. and Wiest, W. G. (1971). Peripheral plasma progesterone levels during human pregnancy and labour. *Amer. J. Obstet. Gynecol.*, 110, 630–632

Csapo, A. I., Pulkkinen, M. O. and Kaihola, H. L. (1974). The relationship between the timing of luteectomy and the incidence of complete abortions. *Amer. J. Obstet. Gynecol.*, 118, 985–989

Csapo, A. I., Pulkkinen, M. O., Ruttner, B., Sauvage, J. P. and Wiest, W. G. (1972). The significance of the human corpus luteum in pregnancy maintenance. *Amer. J. Obstet. Gynecol.*, 112, 1061–1067

Currie, W. B., Wong, M. S. F., Cox, R. I. and Thorburn, G. D. (1973). Spontaneous or Dexamethasone induced parturition in the sheep and goat. Changes in plasma concentrations of maternal prostaglandin F and foetal oestrogen sulphate. *Mem. Soc. Endocrinol.*, 20, 95–118

Dawson, W., Lewis, R. L., McMahon, R. E. and Sweatman, W. J. F. (1974). Potent bronchoconstrictor activity of 15-keto prostaglandin $F_{2\alpha}$. *Nature (London)*, 250, 331–332

Dhont, M., Vanderheyden, K., Vandekerckhove, D., Vermeulen, A. and Thiery, M. (1974). Prostaglandin E_2: Effect on cortisol, growth hormone, prolactin, LH, FSH and TSH levels before and after suppression with dexamethasone. *I.R.C.S.*, 2, 1301

Downie, J., Poyser, N. L. and Wunderlich, M. (1974). Levels of prostaglandins in human endometrium during the normal menstrual cycle. *J. Physiol.*, 236, 465–472

Dray, F. and Charbonnel, B. (1973). Dosage radioimmunologique des prostaglandins F_a et E_1 dans le plasma peripherique de l'homme normal. In: *Prostaglandines 1973*. Seminaire les prostaglandins, 133–158 (Paris: Inserm)

Dray, F. and Charbonnel, B. (1974). Radioimmunoassay of PGE and $PGF_{2\alpha}$ in human plasma. *Prostaglandins*, 5, 173–174

Eckstein, P. (1970). Mechanisms of action of intra-uterine contraceptive devices in women and other mammals. *Brit. Med. Bull.*, 26, 52–59

Eglinton, G., Raphael, R. A., Smith, G. N., Hall, W. J.. and Pickles, V. R. (1963). The isolation and identification of two smooth muscles stimulants from menstrual fluid. *Nature (London)*, 200, 960, 993–995

Eliasson, R. (1959). Studies on prostaglandin. Occurrence, formation and biological actions. *Acta Physiol. Scand.*, 46, Suppl. 158, 1–73

Eliasson, R. and Posse, N. (1965). Rubin's test before and after intravaginal application of prostaglandin. *Int. J. Fert.*, **10**, 373–377

Elliot, R. B. and Starling, M. B. (1972). The effect of prostaglandin $F_{2\alpha}$ in the closure of the ductus arteriosus. *Prostaglandins*, **2**, 399–403

Ellis, L. C., Johnson, J. M. and Hargrove, J. L. (1972). Cellular aspects of prostaglandin synthesis and testicular function. In: *Prostaglandins in Cellular Biology*, 385–396 (P. W. Ramwell and B. B. Phariss, editors) (N.Y., London: Plenum Press)

Eskin, B. A. and Azarbal, S. (1973). Effect of $PGF_{2\alpha}$ upon periovular cervical mucus. *Adv. Biosciences*, **9**, 731–735

Eskin, B. A., Azarbal, S., Sepic, R. and Slate, W. G. (1973). *In vitro* response of the spermatozoa–cervical mucus system treated with prostaglandin ($F_{2\alpha}$). *Obstet. Gynecol. (N.Y.)*, **41**, 436–439

Euler, U. S. von (1934). Zur Kenntnis der pharmakologischen Wirkungen von Natirsekreten und Extrackten männlicher accessorischer Geschlechtsdrüsen, Naunyn-Schmiedebergs. *Arch. Path. Pharmak.*, **175**, 78–84

Euler, U. S. von (1936). On the specific vasodilating and plain muscle stimulating substances from accessory genital glands in man and certain animals (Prostaglandin and Vesiglandin). *J. Physiol. (London)*, **88**, 213–234

Faucher, G. L., Ellegood, J. O., Mahesh, V. B. and Greenblatt, R. B. (1969). Urinary estrogens and pregnanediol before and after insertion of an intrauterine contraceptive device. *Amer. J. Obstet. Gynecol.*, **104**, 502–507

Gillespie, A., Brummer, H. C. and Chard, T. (1972). Oxytocin release by infused prostaglandin. *Brit. Med. J.*, **1**, 543–544

Goldblatt, M. W. (1933). A depressor substance in seminal fluid. *J. Soc. Chem. Ind. London*, **52**, 1056–1057

Goldblatt, M. W. (1935). Properties of human seminal plasma. *J. Physiol. (London)*, **84**, 208–218

Gréen, K., Bygdeman, M., Toppozada, M. and Wiqvist, N. (1974). The role of prostaglandin $F_{2\alpha}$ in human parturition. *Amer. J. Obstet. Gynecol.*, **120**, 25–31

Gréen, K. and Granström, E. (1973). Literature data on endogenous levels of prostaglandins in humans measured by bioassay, radioimmunoassay and gas chromatography-mass spectrometry. In: *Prostaglandins and Fertility Control*, 3 (S. Bergström, editor) (Karolinska Institutet, Stockholm: WHO Research and Training Centre)

Gustavii, B. (1972). Labour: A delayed menstruation? *Lancet*, 1149–1150

Gustavii, B. and Gréen, K. (1972). Release of prostaglandin $F_{2\alpha}$ following injection of hypertonic saline for therapeutic abortion. A preliminary study. *Amer. J. Obstet. Gynecol.*, **114**, 1099–1100

Gutierrez-Cernosek, R. M., Zukerman, J. and Levine, L. (1972). Prostaglandin $F_{2\alpha}$ levels in sera during human pregnancy. *Prostaglandins*, **1**, 331–337

Gyory, G., Kiss, Cs., Benyo, T., Bagdány, S., Szalay, J., Kurez, M. and Virág, S. (1974). Inhibition of labour by prostaglandin antagonists in impending abortion and preterm and term labour. *Lancet*, **2**, 293

Hamberg, M. and Samuelsson, B. (1966). Prostaglandins in human seminal plasma. *J. Biol. Chem.*, **241**, 257–263

Hargrove, J. L., Johnson, J. M. and Ellis, L. C. (1971). Prostaglandin E_1 induced inhibition of rabbit testicular contractions *in vitro*. *Proc. Soc. Exp. Biol. Med.*, **136**, 958–961

Hauge, A., Lünde, P. K. M. and Waaler, B. A. (1967). Effects of prostaglandin E_1 and adrenaline on the pulmonary vascular resistance (PVR) in isolated rabbit lungs. *Life Sci.*, **6**, 673–680

Hennam, J. F., Johnson, D. A., Newton, J. R. and Collins, W. P. (1974). Radioimmunoassay of prostaglandin $F_{2\alpha}$ in peripheral venous plasma from men and women. *Prostaglandins*, **5**, 531–542

Henzl, M. R., Ortega, E., Cortés-Gallegos, V., Tomlinson, R. V. and Segre, E. J. (1973). Prostaglandin E_2 and the luteal phase of the menstrual cycle: Effects on blood progesterone, estradiol, cortisol and growth hormone levels. *J. Clin. Endocrinol. Metab.*, **36**, 784–787

Henzl, M. R., Smith, R. E., Boost, G. and Tyler, E. T. (1972). Lysosomal concept of menstrual bleeding in humans. *J. Clin. Endocrinol.*, **34**, 860–875

Hertelendy, F., Woods, R. and Jaffe, B. M. (1973). Prostaglandin E levels in peripheral blood during labour. *Prostaglandins*, **3**, 223–227

Hibbard, B. M., Sharma, S. C., Fitzpatrick, R. J. and Hamlett, J. D. (1974). Prostaglandin $F_{2\alpha}$ concentrations in amniotic fluid in late pregnancy. *J. Obstet. Gynaecol. Brit. Cwlth.*, **81**, 35–38

Higgs, G. A. and Youlten, L. J. F. (1972). Prostaglandin production by rabbit peritoneal polymorphonuclear leukrocytes *in vitro. Brit. J. Pharmacol.*, **44**, 330 P

Hillier, K. (1970). *Occurrence and Actions of some Prostaglandins in Human Umbilical and Placental Blood Vessels.* (University of London: Ph.D Thesis)

Hillier, K. (1972). Oxytocin release by infused prostaglandin. *Brit. Med. J.*, **2**, 46

Hillier, K. (1975). (Unpublished data)

Hillier, K., Calder, A. A. and Embrey, M. P. (1974). Concentrations of prostaglandin $F_{2\alpha}$ in amniotic fluid and plasma in spontaneous and induced labours. *J. Obstet. Gynaecol. Brit. Cwlth.*, **81**, 257–263

Hillier, K. and Dilley, S. R. (1974). Separation and radioimmunoassay of F_α prostaglandins using silica gel micro columns. *Prostaglandins*, **5**, 137–150

Hillier, K., Dutton, A. and Corker, C. S. (1973). The effect of prostaglandin $F_{2\alpha}$ administration on plasma steroid and LH levels in the luteal phase of the menstrual cycle. *Adv. Biosciences*, **9**, 673–678

Hillier, K., Dutton, A., Corker, C. S., Singer, A. and Embrey, M. P. (1972). Plasma steroid and luteinizing hormone levels during prostaglandin $F_{2\alpha}$ administration in luteal phase of menstrual cycle. *Brit. Med. J.*, **4**, 333–336

Hillier, K., Dutton, A., MacKenzie, I. Z. and Embrey, M. P. (1975). (Submitted for publication)

Hillier, K. and Karim, S. M. M. (1968). Effects of prostaglandins E_1, E_2, $F_{1\alpha}$ and $F_{2\alpha}$ on isolated human umbilical and placental blood vessels. *J. Obstet. Gynaecol. Brit. Cwlth.*, **75**, 667–673

Hillier, K. and Karim, S. M. M. (1970). The human isolated cervix: a study of its spontaneous motility and responsiveness to drugs. *Brit. J. Pharmacol.*, **40**, 576–577

Horan, A. H. (1974). Aspirin, Prostaglandin and gestation. *Lancet*, **1**, 31

Horton, E. W., Jones, R. L. and Marr, C. G. (1973). Effects of aspirin on prostaglandin and fructose levels in human semen. *J. Reprod. Fertil.*, **33**, 385–392

Jarabak, J. (1972). Human placental 15-hydroxy-prostaglandin dehydrogenase. *Proc. Nat. Acad. Sci. U.S.A.*, **69**, 533–534

Jewelewicz, R., Cantor, B., Dyrenfurth, I., Warren, M. P. and Vande Wiele, R. L. (1972). Intravenous infusion of prostaglandin $F_{2\alpha}$ in the mid-luteal phase of the normal human menstrual cycle. *Prostaglandins*, **1**, 443–451

Jubiz, W. and Frailey, J. (1974). Prostaglandin E generation during storage of plasma samples. *Prostaglandins*, **7**, 339–344

Jubiz, W., Frailey, J., Child, C. and Bartholomew, K. (1972). Physiologic role of prostaglandins of the E(PGE), F(PGF) and AB(PGAB) groups. Estimation by radioimmunoassay in unextracted human plasma. *Prostaglandins*, **2**, 471–483

Jurgmannova, C., Havranek, F. and Hodr, J. (1972). The effect of prostaglandin $F_{2\alpha}$ on placental vessels *in vitro. J. Reprod. Med.*, **9**, 79–80

Karim, S. M. M. (1966). Identification of prostaglandins in human amniotic fluid. *J. Obstet. Gynaecol. Brit. Cwlth.*, **73**, 903–908

Karim, S. S. M. (1967). The identification of prostaglandins in human umbilical cord. *Brit. J. Pharmacol. Chemother.*, **29**, 230–237

Karim, S. M. M. (1968). Appearance of prostaglandin $F_{2\alpha}$ in human blood during labour. *Brit.. Med. J.*, **4**, 618–621

Karim, S. M. M. (editor) (1972a). *The Prostaglandins: Progress in Research* (Lancaster: M.T.P.)

Karim, S. M. M. (1972b). Prostaglandins and human reproduction. Physiological roles and clinical uses of prostaglandins in relation to human reproduction. In: *Prostaglandins: Progress in Research*, 71–164 (Lancaster: M.T.P.)

Karim, S. M. M. (1973). Intrauterine prostaglandins for outpatient termination of very early pregnancy. *Lancet*, **2**, 794

Karim, S. M. M. and Adaikan, P. G. (1975). Effects of prostaglandins on human penis *in vitro* (In press)

Karim, S. M. M. and Devlin, J. (1967). Prostaglandin content of amniotic fluid during pregnancy and labour. *J. Obstet. Gynaecol. Brit. Cwlth.*, **74**, 230–234

Karim, S. M. M. and Hillier, K. (1970). Prostaglandins and spontaneous abortion. *J. Obstet. Gynaecol. Brit. Cwlth.*, 77, 837–839

Karim, S. M. M. and Sharma, S. D. (1971). The effect of ethyl alcohol on prostaglandins E_2 and $F_{2\alpha}$ induced uterine activity in pregnant women. *J. Obstet. Gynaecol. Brit. Cwlth.*, 78, 251–254

Karim, S. M. M., Trussell, R. R., Hillier, K. and Patel, R. C. (1969). Induction of labour with prostaglandin $F_{2\alpha}$. *J. Obstet. Gynaecol. Brit. Cwlth.*, 76, 769–782

Keirse, M. J. N. C., Flint, A. P. C. and Turnbull, A. C. (1974a). F prostaglandins in amniotic fluid during pregnancy and labour. *J. Obstet. Gynaecol. Brit. Cwlth.*, 81, 131–136

Keirse, M. J. N. C. and Turnbull, A. C. (1973). E prostaglandins in amniotic fluid during late pregnancy and labour. *J. Obstet. Gynaecol. Brit. Cwlth.*, 80, 970–974

Keirse, M. J. N. C., Williamson, J. G. and Turnbull, A. C. (1974b). Metabolism of prostaglandin $F_{2\alpha}$ within the human uterus in early pregnancy. *J. Obstet. Gynaecol. Brit. Cwlth.* (In press)

Kelly, W. A., Marston, J. H., and Eckstein, P. (1969). Effect of an intrauterine device on endometrial morphology and the deciduomal reaction in the rhesus monkey. *J. Reprod. Fert.*, 19, 331–340

Kitorn, K. T. (1973). Prostaglandins and steroidogenesis. *Adv. Biosciences*, 9, 645–650

Kirton, K. T., Cornette, J. C. and Barr, K. L. (1972). Characterisation of antibody to prostaglandin $F_{2\alpha}$. *Biochem. Biophys. Res. Comm.*, 47, 903–909

Labhsetwar, A. P. (1973). Do prostaglandins stimulate LH release and thereby cause luteolysis? *Prostaglandins*, 3, 729–733

Lauerson, N. H. and Wilson, K. (1974). Mid trimester abortion induced with a single intra-amniotic instillation of prostaglandin $F_{2\alpha}$. *Amer. J. Obstet. Gynecol.*, 118, 210–217

Lauerson, N. H., Wilson, K. H., Beling, C. G. and Fuchs, F. (1974). Comparison of prostaglandin $F_{2\alpha}$ and hypertonic saline for induction of midtrimester abortion. (In press)

Lehmann, F., Peters, F., Breckwoldt, M. and Bettendorf, G. (1972). Plasma progesterone levels during infusion of prostaglandin $F_{2\alpha}$ in the human. *Prostaglandins*, 1, 269–277

Lemaire, W. J. and Shapiro, A. G.. (1972). $PGF_{2\alpha}$: its effect on the corpus luteum of the menstrual cycle. *Prostaglandins*, 1, 259–267

Lemaire, W. J., Spellacy, W. N., Shevach, A. B. and Gall, S. A. (1972). Changes in plasma estriol and progesterone during labour induced with prostaglandin $F_{2\alpha}$ or oxytocin. *Prostaglandins*, 2, 93–101

Levine, L. and Gutierrez-Cernosek, R. M. (1973). Levels of 13,14 dihydro-15 keto-$PGF_{2\alpha}$ in biological fluids as measured by radioimmunoassay. *Prostaglandins*, 3, 785–804

Lewis, R. B. and Shulman, J. D. (1973). Influence of acetylsalicylic acid, an inhibitor of prostaglandin synthesis on duration of human gestation and labour. *Lancet*, 2, 1159–1160

Liggins, G. C. (1973). Hormonal interactions in the mechanism of parturition. *Mem. Soc. Endocrinol.*, 20, 119–139

Liggins, G. C., Grieves, S. A., Kendall, J. Z. and Knox, B. S. (1972). The physiological roles of progesterone, oestradiol-17$_\beta$ and prostaglandin $F_{2\alpha}$ in the control of ovine parturition. *J. Reprod. Fertil.*, Suppl. 16, 85–103

Mackenzie, I. Z. (1974). Trancervical fetoscopy. *Lancet*, 2, 346

Mantell, C. D. and Liggins, G. C. (1970). The effect of ethanol of the myometrial response to oxytocin in women at term. *J. Obstet. Brit. Cwlth.*, 77, 976–981

Marsh, J. M. and Lemaire, W. J. (1974). Cyclic AMP accumulation and steroidogenesis in the human corpus luteum. Effect of gonadotrophins and prostaglandins. *J. Clin. Endocrinol. Metab.*, 38, 99–106

McCracken, J. A., Glew, M. E. and Scaramuzzi, R. J. (1970). Corpus luteum regression induced by prostaglandin $F_{2\alpha}$. *J. Clin. Endocrinol. Metab.*, 30, 544–546

McNeilly, A. S. and Fox, C. A. (1971). The effects of prostaglandins on the guinea-pig mammary gland. *J. Endocrinol.*, 51, 603–604

Mocsary, P. and Csapo, A. I. (1973). Delayed menstruation induced by prostaglandin in pregnant patients. *Lancet*, 2, 683

Mosler, K. H., Dornhöfer, W. and Linka, F. (1974). Hemmungvorzeiter wehen. *Med. Klin.*, 69, 97–101

Novy, M. J., Cook, M. J. and Manaugh, L. (1974a). Indomethacin block of normal onset of parturition in primates. *Amer. J. Obstet. Gynecol.*, 118, 412–416

Novy, M. J., Piasecki, G. and Jackson, B. T. (1974b). Effect of prostaglandins E_2 and $F_{2\alpha}$ on umbilical blood flow and fetal haemodynamics. *Prostaglandins*, 5, 543–556

Ogra, S. S., Kirton, K. T., Tomasi, T. B. and Lippes, J. (1974). Prostaglandins in the human fallopian tube. *Fertil. and Steril.*, 25, 250–255

Okamura, H., Aso, T., Yoshida, Y. and Nishimura, T. (1974). Effects of prostaglandin $F_{2\alpha}$ on human corpora lutea. *Obstet. Gynecol. N.Y.*, 44, 127–134

Olley, P. M., Coceani, F. and Kent, G. (1974). Inactivation of prostaglandin E_1 by lungs of the fetal lamb. *Experientia*, 30, 58

Van Orden, D. E. and Farley, D. B. (1973). Prostaglandin $F_{2\alpha}$ radioimmunoassay utilizing polyethylene glycol separation technique. *Prostaglandins*, 4, 215–233

Pace-Asciak, C., Wolfe, L. S., Gillett, P. G. and Kinch, R. A. (1972). Disappearance of $PGF_{2\alpha}$ from human amniotic fluid after intra-amniotic injection. *Prostaglandins*, 1, 469–477

Park, M. K. and Dyer, D. C. (1973). Effect of polyphloretin phosphate and 7-oxa-13 prostynoic acid on the vasoactive actions of prostaglandin E_2 and 5-hydroxytryptamine on isolated human umbilical arteries. *Prostaglandins*, 3, 913–920

Patrona, C., Grossi-Belloni, D., Ciabattoni, G., Serra, G. B. and Dell Acqua (1974). Peripheral plasma concentrations of prostaglandins (PG) $F_{1\alpha}$ and $F_{2\alpha}$ in relation to estradiol (E_2) and progesterone (P) during normal menstrual cycles. *J. Steroid. Biochem.*, 5, 375

Patrona, C. and Serra, G. B. (1974). Do pituitary prostaglandins play an essential role in the action of LH RH in man. *Prostaglandins*, 6, 345–346

Patwardhan, V. V. and Lanthier, A. (1974). Effect of prostaglandins on the *in vitro* steroidogenesis in human ovarian tissues. *Prostaglandins*, 6, 385–388

Pickles, V. R. (1957). A plain muscle stimulant in the menstrual fluid. *Nature (London)*, 1198–1199

Pickles, V. R.. (1967). The prostaglandins. *Biol. Rev.*, 42, 614–652

Pickles, V. R. and Hall, W. J. (1963). Some physiological properties of the menstrual stimulant substances A_1 and A_2. *J. Reprod. Fertil.*, 6, 315–317

Pickles, V. R. and Ward, P. V. F. (1965). Menstrual stimulants component B and possible prostaglandin precursors in the endometrium. *J. Physiol. (London)*, 178, 38–39

Powell, W. S., Hammarström, S. and Samuelsson, B. (1974). Prostaglandin $F_{2\alpha}$ receptor in human corpora lutea. *Lancet*, 1, 1120

Puri, C. P., Hingorani, V. and Laumas, K. R. (1973). Effect of prostaglandin $F_{2\alpha}$ on progestin synthesis in the human and rabbit ovary. *Adv. Biosciences*, 9, 657–663

Rao, B. and Karim, S. M. M. (1975). (Unpublished results)

Ryan, W. L., Coronel, D. M. and Johnson, R. J. (1969). A vasodepressor substance of the human placenta. *Amer. J. Obstet. Gynecol.*, 105, 1201–1206

Salmon, J. A. and Amy, J.-J. (1973). Levels of prostaglandin $F_{2\alpha}$ in amniotic fluid during pregnancy and labour. *Prostaglandins*, 4, 523–533

Samuelsson, B. (1963). Isolation and identification of prostaglandins from human seminal fluid. *J. Biol. Chem.*, 238, 3229–3234

Samuelsson, B. (1973). Methods for determination of prostaglandin formation in man. In: *3rd Conference on Prostaglandins in Fertility Control*, 37–42 (S. Bergström, editor) (Karolinska Institutet Stockholm: WHO Research and Training Centre on human reproduction)

Sandberg, F., Ingelman-Sundberg, A. and Ryden, G. (1963). The effect of prostaglandin E_1 on the human uterus and the fallopian tubes *in vitro*. *Acta Obstet. Gynecol. Scand.*, 42, 269–278

Sandberg, F., Ingelman-Sundberg, A. and Ryden, G. (1964). The effect of prostaglandin E_2 and E_3 on the human uterus and fallopian tubes *in vitro*. *Acta Obstet. Gynecol. Scand.*, 43, 95–102

Sandberg, F., Ingelman-Sundberg, A. and Ryden, G. (1965). The effect of prostaglandin $F_{1\alpha}$, $F_{1\beta}$, $F_{2\alpha}$ and $F_{2\beta}$ on the human uterus and the fallopian tubes *in vitro*. *Acta Obstet. Gynecol. Scand.*, 44, 585–594

Satoh, K. and Ryan, K. J. (1972). Prostaglandins and their effects on human placental adenyl cyclase. *J. Clin. Invest.*, 51, 456–458

Schlegel, W., Demers, L. M., Hildebrant-Stark, H. E., Behrman, H. R. and Greep, R. O. (1974). Partial purification of human placental 15-hydroxy prostaglandin dehydrogenase: Kinetic properties. *Prostaglandins*, 5, 417–433

Schultz, F. M., Macdonald, P. C. and Johnston, J. M. (1974). Arachidonic acid in human amniotic fluid and its relationship to labour. *Gynaecologic. Invest.*, 5, 62

Shaikh, A. A. (1972). Regulation of menstrual cycle and termination of pregnancy in the monkey by estradiol and $PGF_{2\alpha}$. *Prostaglandins*, 2, 227–233

Sharma, S. C., Hibbard, B. M., Hamlett, J. D. and Fitzpatrick, R. J. (1973). Prostaglandin $F_{2\alpha}$ concentrations in peripheral blood during the first stage of normal labour. *Brit. Med. J.*, 1, 709–711

Shearman, R., Smith, I. and Korda, A. (1972). Second trimester termination by intra-uterine prostaglandin $F_{2\alpha}$. Clinical and hormonal results with observations on induced lactation and chronoperiodicity. *J. Reprod. Med.*, 9, 448–452

Sico-Blanco, Y., Rozada, H., Remedio, M. R., Hendricks, C. H. and Alvarez, H. (1970). Human tubal motility *in vivo. J. Obstet. Gynaecol.*, 106, 79–86

Smith, I. D. and Temple, D. M. (1973). The influence of analgesic drugs on the actions of prostaglandin $F_{2\alpha}$ on the human uterus *in vivo* and rabbit myometrial strips *in vitro. Prostaglandins*, 4, 469–477

Speroff, L. (1973). An essay: Prostaglandins and toxaemia of pregnancy. *Prostaglandins*, 3, 721–728

Speroff, L., Caldwell, B. V., Brock, W. A., Anderson, G. G. and Hobbins, J. C. (1972). Hormone levels during $PGF_{2\alpha}$ infusions for therapeutic abortion. *J. Clin. Endocrinol.*, 34, 531–536

Symonds, E. M., Fahmy, D., Morgan, C., Roberts, G., Gomersall, C. R. and Turnbull, A. C. (1972). Maternal plasma oestrogens and progesterone levels during therapeutic abortion induced by intra-amniotic injection of prostaglandin $F_{2\alpha}$. *J. Obstet. Gynaecol. Brit. Cwlth.*, 79, 976–980

Taylor, P. L. and Kelly, R. W. (1974). 19-hydroxylated E prostaglandins as the major prostaglandins of human semen. *Nature (London)*, 250, 665–667

Thiery, M. and Willighagen, R. G. J. (1973). Prostaglandins-effect on the enzyme content of the human placenta. *I.R.C.S.*, (73–9), 10–26–2

Tom, W. K. C., Sribyatta, B., Thorneycroft, I. H. and Mishell, D. R. (1972). Fertility regulation with cyclic luteal phase vaginal administration of prostaglandin $F_{2\alpha}$. *Contraception*, 6, 479–488

Tulchinsky, D. and Hobel, C. J. (1973). Plasma human chorionic gonadotrophin estrone, estradiol, estriol, progesterone and 17α hydroxy progesterone in human pregnancy. *Amer. J. Obstet. Gynecol.*, 117, 884–893

Turker, R. K. and Kiran, B. K. (1969). Interaction of prostaglandin E_1 with oxytocin on mammary gland of the lactating rabbit. *Eur. J. Pharmacol.*, 8, 377–379

Turnbull, A. C. and Anderson, A. B. M. (1968). Uterine contractility and oxytocin sensitivity during human pregnancy in relation to the onset of labour. *J. Obstet. Gynaecol. Brit. Cwlth.*, 75, 278–288

Turnbull, A. C., Flint, A. P. F., Jeremy, J. Y., Patten, P. T., Keirse, M. J. N. C., and Anderson, A. B. M. (1974). Significant fall in progesterone and rise in oestradiol levels in human peripheral plasma before onset of labour. *Lancet*, 1, 101–104

Tuvemo, T. and Wide, L. (1973). Prostaglandin release from the human umbilical artery in vitro. *Prostaglandins*, 4, 689–694

Tyack, A. J., Lambadarios, C., Parsons, R. J., Stewart, C. R. and Cooke, I. D. (1974). Plasma progesterone and oestradiol-17β changes during abortion induced by prostaglandin $F_{2\alpha}$. *J. Obstet. Gynaecol. Brit. Cwlth.*, 81, 52–56

Tyack, A. J., Parsons, R. J., Millar, D. R., Pennington, G. and Hall, R. (1973). Plasma progesterone changes in abortion induced by hypertonic saline in the second trimester of pregnancy. *J. Obstet. Gynaecol. Brit. Cwlth.*, 80, 548–552

Vane, J. R. (1971). Inhibition of prostaglandin synthesis as a mechanism of action for aspirin like drugs. *Nature New Biol.*, 231, 232–235

Vane, J. R. and Williams, K. I. (1973). The contribution of prostaglandin production to contractions of the isolated uterus of the rat. *Brit. J. Pharmacol.*, 48, 629–639

Vanderheyden, K., Dhont, M., VandeKerckhove, D., Vermeulen, A., and Thiery, M. (1974). Prostaglandin $F_{2\alpha}$: effect on cortisol, growth hormone, follicle-stimulating hormone, prolactin and thyroid stimulating hormone. *I.R.C.S.*, 2, 1164

Waltman, R. and Tricomi, V. (1974). Pentazocine, mefenamic acid and hypertonic saline abortion. *Lancet*, 2, 468

Waltman, R., Tricomi, V. and Palav, A. (1973). Aspirin and indomethacin: Effect of prostaglandins on instillation/abortion time of midtrimester hypertonic saline induced abortion. *Prostaglandins*, 3, 47–58

Weiner, R. and Kaley, G. (1972). Lysosomal fragility induced by prostaglandin $F_{2\alpha}$. *Nature New Biol.*, **236**, 46–47

Wentz, A. C. and Jones, G. S. (1973). Transient luteolytic effect of prostaglandin $F_{2\alpha}$ in the human. *Obstet. Gynecol. (N.Y.)*, **42**, 172–181

Williams, K. I. (1973). Prostaglandins synthesis by the pregnant rat uterus at term and its possible relevance in parturition. *Brit. J. Pharmacol.*, **47**, 628–629

Wilks, J. W., Wentz, A. C. and Jones, G. S. (1973). Prostaglandin $F_{2\alpha}$ concentrations in the blood of women during normal menstrual cycles and dysmennorrhoea. *J. Clin. Endocrinol. Metab.*, **37**, 469–471

Wiqvist, N., Bygdeman, M. and Kirton, K. T. (1971). Non-steroidal antifertility agents in the female. In: *Nobel-Symp.*, **15**, 137–155 (E. Diczfalusy and V. Borell, editors) (N.Y.: John Wiley)

Wolfe, L. S. and Pace-Asciak (1972). Measurement of prostaglandin $F_{2\alpha}$ concentration in plasma during clinical evaluation in therapeutic abortion. In: *Prostaglandins in Fertility Control*, **2**, 201–207 (Karolinska Institutet, Stockholm: WHO Research and Training Centre on human reproduction)

Ylikorkala, O., Jouppila, P., Ylöstalo, P. and Järvinen, P. A. (1974). Intrauterine injection of prostaglandin $F_{2\alpha}$ for termination of early pregnancy in outpatient. *Prostaglandins*, **7**, 57–70

Zetler, G. and Wiechell, H. (1969). Pharmakologisch aktive Lipide in Extrakten aus Tube und Ovar des Menschen, Naunyn-Schmeidebergs. *Arch. Pharmak.*, **265**, 101–111

Zusman, R. M., Spector, D., Caldwell, B. V., Speroff, L., Schneider, G. and Mulrow, P. J. (1973). The effect of chronic sodium loading and sodium restriction on plasma prostaglandins A, E and F concentrations in normal humans. *J. Clin. Invest.*, **52**, 1093–1098

3
Interruption of Pregnancy with Prostaglandins

S. M. M. KARIM and J.-J. AMY

Abbreviations

EEG: electroencephalogram
FSH: follicle stimulating hormone
HCG: human chorionic gonadotrophin
HCS: human chorionic somatomammotrophin
        (= human placental lactogen)
i.v.: intravenous, intravenously
LH: luteinising hormone
SGOT: serum glutamic oxalacetic transaminase
SGPT: serum glutamic pyruvic transaminase
WBC: white blood cells

3.1 INTRODUCTION

Few areas in medical research have received such prompt and widespread
clinical acceptance as the use of prostaglandins for termination of early pregnancy. The changing social attitudes in many countries and liberalisation of
abortion laws have contributed to this progress.

The oxytocic activity of some of the naturally occurring prostaglandins on
human pregnant myometrium was first demonstrated *in vitro* by Bygdeman
(1964) and *in vivo* by Bygdeman *et al.* (1968). Karim and collaborators
found elevated levels of prostaglandins in amniotic fluid and in peripheral
plasma during spontaneous labour and abortion (Karim 1966, 1968; Karim
and Devlin, 1967; Karim and Hillier, 1970). Shortly thereafter the successful
use of natural prostaglandins was reported for induction of labour at term
(Karim *et al.*, 1968) and for termination of early pregnancy (Karim and Filshie, 1970a; Roth-Brandel *et al.*, 1970b).

Lately, research in prostaglandin-induced abortions has aimed at defining
the most effective routes of administration and at identifying compounds
with selective oxytocic effect. Some analogues of the naturally occurring prostaglandins have already proved superior in terms of safety, greater uterotonic
potency and duration of action, and lesser side-effects.

Prostaglandins have also been used for 'menstrual induction' during the two weeks following the first missed menstruation, for termination of pregnancies complicated by hydatidiform mole or missed abortion and as a pharmacological means of dilating the cervix prior to suction curettage.

A review of the literature pertaining to these various topics constitutes the essence of this chapter.

3.2 THE USE OF NATURALLY OCCURRING PROSTAGLANDINS FOR INTERRUPTION OF PREGNANCY

Prostaglandins E_1, E_2 and $F_{2\alpha}$ stimulate the human uterus to contract and when given in adequate doses, are capable of effecting expulsion of the products of conception at any stage of gestation. Various routes of administration have proved effective.

Bygdeman et al. (1968) first reported the oxytocic effect of intravenous infusion of 0.6–9.0 μg min^{-1} of PGE_1 and PGE_2 in eight patients at 16–22 weeks' gestation. The two compounds were equipotent, the threshold dose at mid-pregnancy being in the range of 2–4 μg min^{-1}. At these dose levels, the prostaglandins caused an increment in tone and, to some extent, irregular uterine activity. The authors therefore concluded that PGE_1 and PGE_2 would not be suitable agents for the interruption of pregnancy. Soon thereafter, however, the successful use of a prostaglandin for precisely this purpose was reported by Karim and Filshie (1970a) and by Roth-Brandel et al., (1970b).

3.2.1 Intravenous route

Karim and Filshie (1970a) first demonstrated the efficacy of $PGF_{2\alpha}$ for termination of pregnancy, using the continuous infusion regime. $PGF_{2\alpha}$, when given intravenously at the rate of 50 μg min^{-1}, resulted in abortion in 14 out of 15 women at 9–22 weeks' gestation. The mean induction–abortion interval amounted to 12 hours 30 min. Roth-Brandel et al. (1970b), however, failed in terminating pregnancies in two women with 10–15 μg min^{-1} infusion of $PGF_{2\alpha}$ given for six hours. With intravenous infusion of 1–10 μg min^{-1} PGE_1 given for up to six hours on two occasions, these authors terminated pregnancies in two out of five patients.

Karim and Filshie (1970 a, b) and Embrey (1970) reported on the successful use of intravenous infusion of PGE_2 (2–5 μg min^{-1}) for induction of abortion.

These initial reports and those that have followed on the intravenous administration of naturally occurring prostaglandins E_1, E_2 and $F_{2\alpha}$ for interruption of pregnancy have been summarised in Tables 3.1 and 3.2. Analysis of the data has been made difficult because of the use of different dose levels, varying periods of infusion and different criteria for success. Nevertheless, some general conclusions can be drawn. The intravenous infusion of PGE_1, PGE_2 or $PGF_{2\alpha}$, in adequate dosage, accomplishes abortion (i.e. expulsion of the fetus with or without the placenta) in about 80% of cases. In about 40% of

Table 3.1 Termination of pregnancy with $PGF_{2\alpha}$ infusion

Reference	No. of cases	Gestation range (weeks)	Dose schedule	Success* rate (%)	Mean induction–abortion interval
Karim and Filshie, 1970a	4	9–12	50 μg min^{-1} Max. 48 hours	100	10 hours 6 min
Karim and Filshie, 1970a	11	14–22	50 μg min^{-1} Max. 48 hours	91	13 hours 27 min
Roth-Brandel et al., 1970b	2	13–18	10–50 μg min^{-1} for 6 hours	0	—
Bygdeman and Wiqvist, 1971	22	$\leqslant$8	25–100 μg min^{-1} for 7 hours	91	?
Bygdeman and Wiqvist, 1971	19	9–12	25–100 μg min^{-1} Max. 13 hours	32	?
Bygdeman and Wiqvist, 1971	23	13–16	25–100 μg min^{-1} Max. 13 hours	17	?
Karim, 1971	16	8–12	50 μg min^{-1} Max. 48 hours	81 ⎫	
Karim, 1971	34	13–24	50 μg min^{-1} Max. 48 hours	91 ⎭	19 hours
Wiqvist et al., 1971	30	9–20	50 μg min^{-1} Max. 26 hours	27	15 hours
Wiqvist et al., 1971	61	9–20	100 μg min^{-1} Max. 26 hours	75	14 hours 18 min
Wiqvist et al., 1971	44	9–20	75 μg min^{-1} Max. 15 hours	16	?
Wiqvist et al., 1971	31	7–8	75 μg min^{-1} Max. 8 hours	58	?
Kaufman et al., 1971	6	13–16	25–200 μg min^{-1} Max. 2 × 12 hours	83	16 hours 42 min
Hendricks et al., 1971	5	7–20	25–200 μg min^{-1} Max. 2 × 12 hours	80	17 hours 18 min
Csapo et al., 1971	10	12–16	25–200 μg min^{-1} Max. 2 × 12 hours	60	?
Kinoshita et al., 1971	7	6–14	41–55 μg min^{-1} (variable duration)	43	?
Brenner, 1972	5	7–20	25–200 μg min^{-1} Max. 12 hours	40†	10 hours
Brenner, 1972	5	7–20	50 μg min^{-1} Max. 18 hours	100†	9 hours
Gillet et al., 1972a	10	10–15	25–200 μg min^{-1} Max. 2 × 12 hours	100	24 hours 41 min
Hillier and Embrey, 1972	10	12–16	25–200 μg min^{-1} Max. 24 hours	40‡	11 hours 30 min

[continued

Table 3.1 [*continued*]

Reference	No. of cases	Gestation range (weeks)	Dose schedule	Success* rate (%)	Mean induction– abortion interval
Lehmann *et al.*, 1972a	20	10–26	50–100 μg min^{-1} Max. 18 hours	95†	9 hours 18 min
Dreher and Lippert, 1972	12	12–18	25–100 μg min^{-1} Max. 2 × 10 hours	17	19 hours 25 min
Anderson *et al.*, 1972c	10	7–16	25–200 μg min^{-1} Max. 12 hours	60	?
Anderson *et al.*, 1972c	7	10–16	25–100 μg min^{-1} Max. 6 hours	43	?
Anderson *et al.*, 1972c	25	11–21	25–50 μg min^{-1}	44	?

* abortion within 48 hours, unless specified otherwise
† abortion within 18 hours
‡ abortion within 24 hours

Table 3.2 Termination of pregnancy with PGE$_2$ infusion

Reference	No. of cases	Gestation range (weeks)	Dose schedule	Success* rate (%)	Mean induction– abortion interval
Karim and Filshie, 1970a	12	8–20	5 μg min^{-1} Max. 48 hours	100	12 hours 30 min
Karim and Filshie, 1970b	15	9–13	5 μg min^{-1} Max. 48 hours	87	13 hours 30 min
Karim and Filshie, 1970b	37	14–22	5 μg min^{-1} Max. 48 hours	100	16 hours 44 min
Roth-Brandel *et al.*, 1970b	5	13–18	1–10 μg PGE$_1$ min^{-1} Max. 2 × 6 hours	40	?
Embrey, 1971b	30	9–28	2–6 μg PGE$_1$ or PGE$_2$ min^{-1} Max. 29 hours	93	21 hours
Hendricks *et al.*, 1971	5	7–20	2.5–20 μg min^{-1} Max. 2.5 mg PGE$_2$	100	12 hours 12 min
Kaufman *et al.*, 1971	4	13–16	5–20 μg min^{-1} Max. 2 × 12 hours	75	11 hours 40 min
Karim and Filshie, 1972	139	5–24	5–10 μg min^{-1} Max. 48 hours	94†	18 hours
Hillier and Embrey, 1972	10	12–16	2.5–20 μg min^{-1} Max. 24·hours	60	11 hours 30 min

* abortion within 48 hours

successful cases, abortion is incomplete and may require completion by instrumental means. Success depends mainly on three factors: dose level, duration of infusion and parity of the patient. According to Brenner (1972), the useful pharmacological dose range for intravenous $PGF_{2\alpha}$ extends from 25 μg min^{-1} (producing a threshold effect) to 50 μg min^{-1} which produces a ceiling effect. Beyond this dose, an increased incidence of complications is observed without increased efficacy. Csapo et al. (1971), Hendricks et al. (1971), Kaufman et al. (1971), Gillett et al. (1972a) and Hillier and Embrey (1972) indeed observed a lower efficacy and/or a higher rate of side-effects following intravenous infusion of 10–20 μg min^{-1} of PGE_2 or 100–200 μg min^{-1} of $PGE_{2\alpha}$. The constant infusion of about 5 μg min^{-1} of PGE_2 or 50 μg min^{-1} of $PGF_{2\alpha}$ appears most effective and is associated with the least complications (Karim and Filshie, 1970 a, b, 1972; Embrey, 1971b; Brenner, 1972). The possible mechanism by which abortifacient efficacy is decreased with increasing dosage is discussed by Karim (1971d).

The duration of infusion is the second parameter of importance. The best clinical results in large groups of patients have been reported after continuous administration of the compound until abortion or for a maximum of 48 hours (Embrey, 1971b; Karim and Filshie, 1972).

Thirdly, the clinical outcome may be influenced by the parity of the patient: higher success rates (Anderson et al., 1972c) and shorter abortion times (Wiqvist et al., 1971; Karim and Filshie, 1972) were recorded in parous women than in primigravidas. Finally, Karim and Filshie (1972) also reported a racial variance. They noted shorter induction–abortion intervals in Asian patients than in Caucasians. African women had intermediate times.

In their early studies, Bygdeman and Wiqvist (1971) and Wiqvist et al. 71971) obtained higher success rates in early pregnancy (7–8 weeks) than at more advanced stages of gestation. However, it appears now that the stage of gestation does not influence the clinical outcome (Anderson et al., 1972c, Karim and Filshie, 1972): first and second trimester pregnancies are equally successfully terminated.

At effective dose level (5 μg min^{-1} PGE_2 or 50 μg min^{-1} $PGF_{2\alpha}$), infusion of the prostaglandin causes a rapid rise in uterine tone to 20–50 mmHg. Hypertonus gradually decreases to 10–20 mmHg above the original level. Simultaneously there appear rhythmic contractions of increasing amplitude (frequency: initially 10–14/minute, then 4–10/minute). The increased uterine activity in turn may eventually produce effacement and dilatation of the cervix and expulsion of the products of conception. It is clear that cervical resistance plays a major role in determining the clinical outcome of the attempted abortion. Brenner (1972), Hillier and Embrey (1972), Kirshen et al. (1972) and Haspels and Neth (1973) have encountered failures of attempted abortion in cases where 'satisfactory' contraction patterns were monitored, in no way different from these observed in successful cases. Many of these recordings were obtained at higher dose levels (e.g. 10–20 μg PGE_2 min^{-1} or 100–250 μg $PGF_{2\alpha}$ min^{-1}). It is possible that higher doses could reduce the abortifacient efficacy of prostaglandin infusion by causing a loss of the selective action of PGs at the level of the uterine corpus, with production of contractions and increased resistance at the level of the cervix (Karim, 1972, page 121).

(a) Side-effects

Naturally occurring prostaglandins of the E and F series when given intravenously, are rapidly metabolised and have a very short half life. $PGF_{2\alpha}$, for instance, is degraded into three main metabolites: 15-keto-$PGF_{2\alpha}$; 15-keto-13,14-dihydro-$PGF_{2\alpha}$; and 13,14-dihydro-$PGF_{2\alpha}$. The last of these products has an oxytocic activity which approaches that of its parent compound and it probably contributes to the uterine stimulation observed during intravenous infusion of $PGF_{2\alpha}$ (Bygdeman et al., 1974). Be that as it may, the rapid degradation of both PGE_2 and $PGF_{2\alpha}$ necessitates high infusion rates for the successful induction of abortion. This inevitably results in a high incidence of systemic side-effects, which although dose-related, in fact depend more closely on the blood level of prostaglandin in the individual patient (Roth-Brandel, 1971; Gréen et al., 1972; Wiqvist et al., 1972d; Wolfe and Pace-Asciak, 1972).

1. Gastrointestinal side-effects: nausea, vomiting and diarrhoea. They occur frequently and constitute the main limiting factor to the intravenous administration of prostaglandins for therapeutic abortion. They are more common with $PGF_{2\alpha}$ than with PGE_2 (Hendricks et al., 1971). In common with other side-effects, they are dose-related (Hendricks et al., 1971; Anderson et al., 1972c; Gillett et al., 1972a; Hillier and Embrey, 1972) (Table 3.3).

Table 3.3 Gastrointestinal side-effects following intravenous infusion of $PGF_{2\alpha}$ for induction of abortion. (*From Wiqvist et al., 1971, by courtesy of Acta Obstet. Gynecol. Scand.*)

Dose level of $PGF_{2\alpha}$	No. of cases	Mean no. of episodes/hour	
		Vomiting	Diarrhoea
50 μg min^{-1}	30	0.04	0.14
75 μg min^{-1}	75	0.13	0.11
100 μg min^{-1}	61	0.23	0.24

Nausea and vomiting can to a certain point be prevented or controlled by the administration of prochlorperazine (Hendricks et al., 1971) or perphenazine (Karim and Filshie, 1972) but probanthine has proved ineffective (Karim and Filshie, 1972). Opiates (e.g. kaolin and morphine, tincture of opium) were effective against diarrhoea (Karim and Filshie, 1972; Lehmann et al., 1972a).

2. Hyperthermia, of central origin, was more frequently encountered with $PGF_{2\alpha}$ than with PGE_2 (Hendricks et al., 1971).
3. Shivering.
4. Venous erythema, at the site of infusion, more frequently seen and more severe with PGE_2 than with $PGF_{2\alpha}$ (Hendricks et al., 1971; Hillier and Embrey, 1972).
5. Cramping pain of uterine origin, related to the degree of uterine activity

elicited by the prostaglandin. Pethidine, given intramuscularly or intravenously, is effective.

6. Bronchoconstriction, particularly in association with administration of $PGF_{2\alpha}$ (Fishburne et al., 1972; Smith, 1972). It can become symptomatic and troublesome in patients with a history of bronchial asthma (Brenner, 1972; Brenner et al., 1972e; Cantor et al., 1972). Smith (1973), investigating the effect on lung resistance of prostaglandins intravenously infused for interruption of pregnancy, found that both $PGF_{2\alpha}$ (5–200 μg min^{-1}) and PGE_2 (2.5–20 μg min^{-1}) caused a small but significant increase in lung resistance. In view of the fact that E prostaglandins relax human bronchial muscle in vitro and when given by aerosol spray, Smith hypothesised that the bronchoconstriction observed during systemic administration of PGE_2 could result from metabolites of the prostaglandin formed during its passage through the lung. Although none of his patients became symptomatic, Smith warned that it might be preferable to consider alternative means of terminating pregnancy in women with bronchial asthma or chronic bronchitis. Fraser and Brash (1974) have since reported the occurrence of symptomatic bronchospasm in 2/104 (2%) patients aborted with extra-amniotic PGE_2 and in 1/17 (6%) patients given this drug intra-amniotically.

7. Other side-effects are rare. They include:

—vaso-vagal symptoms,
—headache, epigastric or chest pain,
—blurring of the vision,
—facial flush.

Except for a mild tachycardia, related to the elevation of temperature, no alteration of the cardiovascular function was reported but for Gillett et al. (1972a), who described non-specific electrocardiographic changes following infusion of $PGF_{2\alpha}$. Intraocular pressure remained unchanged in patients given $PGF_{2\alpha}$ for induction of abortion (Hendricks et al., 1971; Brenner, 1972; Hillier and Embrey, 1972). Urine output and osmolality are unaffected (Karim and Filshie, 1972). Bullard et al. (1973) found the decidua and the chorionic tissue obtained after abortion at 6–10 weeks by i.v. $PGF_{2\alpha}$, to be no different from those recovered following spontaneous abortion.

(b) Laboratory studies

Extensive laboratory investigations have been carried out (Table 3.4). The only consistent change described was leucocytosis with neutrophilia and lymphocytopenia. It should be particularly emphasised that prostaglandins, when given intravenously, do not cause water retention (unlike oxytocin in high dose) nor affect the blood coagulation mechanisms (unlike intra-amniotically administered hypertonic saline solution).

There is disagreement among the investigators regarding the moment of onset of uterine contractions and the significance of the decrease in plasma steroid levels observed. Csapo et al. (1971) hypothesised that prostaglandins were able to cause a rhythmic uterine activity only after the initial sustained

Table 3.4 Laboratory investigations performed during intravenous infusion of PGE$_2$ or PGF$_{2\alpha}$ for induction of abortion

Investigation	Result	References
Peripheral blood count	No change except for raised WBC counts with neutrophilia and lymphocytopenia	Hendricks et al., 1971 Hillier and Embrey, 1972 Kirshen et al., 1972 Ruppen et al., 1972
Prothrombin time Partial thromboplastin time Plasma fibrinogen Plasma levels of fibrin degradation products Platelet adhesiveness Factors V, VII–X, VIII, X	No change suggestive of consumption coagulopathy	Karim and Filshie, 1972 Badraoui et al., 1973b
Electrolytes Blood urea nitrogen Creatinine SGOT, SGPT Alkaline phosphatase Plasma bilirubin Blood glucose	No consistent change	Hendricks et al., 1971 Dreher and Lippert, 1972 Karim and Filshie, 1972 Kirshen et al., 1972 Ruppen et al., 1972 Cantor et al., 1972
Plasma cortisol	—Tendency to rise at maximum dose level —Drop during the course of abortion	Kirshen et al., 1972 Newton and Collins, 1973
Serum HCG	—Drop during the course of abortion —Drop only after placental separation	Cantor et al., 1972 Newton and Collins, 1973 Karim and Filshie, 1972 Speroff et al., 1972
Serum HCS	Drop during the course of abortion	Speroff et al., 1972
Serum FSH	No change	Cantor et al., 1972
Serum progesterone	–Drop during the course of abortion —Drop only after placental separation	Csapo et al., 1971 Cantor et al., 1972 Lehman et al., 1972 b, c Wentz et al., 1972b Newton and Collins, 1973 Gillett et al., 1972a Karim and Filshie, 1972 Kirshen et al., 1972 Hillier and Embrey, 1972 Speroff et al., 1972
Serum 17-β oestradiol	—Drop during the course of abortion (successful cases) —Drop only after placental separation	Cantor et al., 1972 Speroff et al., 1972 Wentz et al., 1972b Newton and Collins, 1973 Karim and Filshie, 1972
Serum oestriol	Drop during the course of abortion	Speroff et al., 1972 Wentz et al., 1972b Newton and Collins, 1973

contracture they elicited had altered the functional capacity of the placenta, with an ensuing decrease in circulating pregesterone. However, other investigators believe that prostaglandins have a direct oxytocic activity, not mediated by a decrease in progesterone production, and that this is the key to their abortifacient action. Gillett *et al.* (1972a), Hillier and Embrey (1972), Karim and Filshie (1972), Kirshen *et al.* (1972), and Speroff *et al.* (1972) found no drop in serum progesterone and HCG, following infusion with PGE_2 or $PGF_{2\alpha}$, until after placental separation had occurred. The latter authors observed a decline in serum oestriol preceding any alteration of the levels of other hormones and suggested that this reflected a hypoxic effect on the feto–placental unit (Speroff *et al.*, 1972). Wentz *et al.* (1972b) noted decreasing serum levels of oestradiol, oestriol and progesterone in patients infused with $PGF_{2\alpha}$ who eventually aborted. However, patients in whom the attempted termination ultimately failed, demonstrated similar decreases in oestriol and progesterone, these values returning to normal during continued infusion. Wentz and associates concluded that the prostaglandin acted directly upon the myometrium and that the decrease in steroid production observed was a consequence of placental anoxia secondary to uterine contractions. This decrease in steroid production, however, could subsequently enhance myometrial contractility. Lehmann *et al.* (1972 b, c, 1973) and Newton and Collins (1973) made very similar observations and came to the same conclusion.

Cantor *et al.* (1972) studied serum hormone levels during and after a 12 hours intravenous infusion of $PGF_{2\alpha}$ (maximum: 200 μg min^{-1}) in 10 patients at 12–16 weeks' gestation. Abortion was successfully induced in nine subjects; in the tenth, the infusion had to be discontinued because of bronchospasm. Serum HCG began to drop within four hours of drug administration and in all cases a considerable fall had occurred before expulsion or removal of the placenta. After removal of the placenta, levels fell rapidly until the blood was almost cleared of HCG. Serum progesterone and oestrogens showed similar decreases during the course of infusion, but these changes occurred somewhat later than for HCG. FSH levels were unaltered. Cantor *et al.* (1972) concluded—and this probably correctly summarises the present state of knowledge—that although a definite decrease in the functional capacity of the placenta occurred during PG-induced termination of pregnancy, it could not be determined whether this effect was mediated by means of a direct vasoconstrictor action of the drug upon the uteroplacental vessels or through the hypoxia accompanying the strong uterine contractions. The mechanism of abortifacient action of prostaglandin is further discussed in Chapter 2.

(c) Comments

In conclusion, the relatively low efficacy (80%) and the high incidence of side-effects associated with intravenous administration of PGE_2 or $PGF_{2\alpha}$ preclude its use as a generally applicable method for termination of early pregnancy. For first trimester cases, suction curettage is preferred; for second trimester cases, the extra-amniotic and intra-amniotic routes of prostaglandin administration show more promise. However, the method can be used with advantage for terminating pregnancies complicated by missed abortion or hydatidiform mole (see Sections 3.5.1 and 3.5.2).

3.2.2 Intramuscular and subcutaneous routes

Wiqvist et al. (1968) administered 75–100 μg PGE_1 intramuscularly to three mid-trimester patients and observed stimulation of the uterus. The response was considerably delayed (latent period: 10 min) and prolonged (60 min) as compared with the intravenous administration of similar doses of PGE_1. However, the elevation of the baseline was not so marked.

Roth-Brandel et al. (1970b) gave three-hourly subcutaneous injections of 5 mg $PGF_{2\alpha}$ over two days and were able to terminate pregnancy in one out of four women. Karim et al. (1971) administered subcutaneously and intramuscularly 10 mg $PGF_{2\alpha}$ or 2 mg PGE_2 to four women at 14–18 weeks' gestation. Stimulation of uterine activity was seen in all four, similar to that observed with continuous intravenous infusion of PGE_2 or $PGF_{2\alpha}$. The duration of increased activity following each dose was 2–3 hours. With repeated three-hourly subcutaneous injections of PGE_2, it was possible in two patients to maintain the high frequency and amplitude of the contractions and to terminate pregnancy.

The intramuscular and subcutaneous administration of natural prostaglandins causes severe pain at the site of injection, sometimes lasting for days (Wiqvist et al., 1968, Karim et al., 1971). These routes are therefore not suitable for termination of early pregnancy with naturally occurring prostaglandins.

3.2.3 Oral route

Karim (1971a) administered 5.0 mg PGE_2 or 50 mg $PGF_{2\alpha}$ to patients in early pregnancy. The uterine activity elicited was not strong enough to cause abortion. In addition, at this dose, both prostaglandins produced acute watery diarrhoea and vomiting.

3.2.4 Intravaginal route

Systemic administration of naturally occurring prostaglandins for termination of pregnancy is accompanied by an unacceptable rate of side-effects. Three alternative routes of administration have been explored, whereby the drug is delivered into the genital tract, in closer contact with the target organ, the uterus. The vaginal route, which possesses over the extra- and intraamniotic methods the considerable advantage of ease of administration, has been shown to depend on systemic absorption (Sandberg et al., 1968) and causes side-effects of the magnitude seen with intravenous infusion of prostaglandins. Wiqvist et al. (1968) studied the effect of intravaginal administration of 0.2–1.0 mg PGE_1 in second trimester patients. At these doses, no uterine stimulation was observed.

Karim and Sharma (1971a) first successfully terminated pregnancy by vaginal administration of natural prostaglandins. Lactose tablets containing either 20 mg PGE_2 or 50 mg $PGF_{2\alpha}$, were inserted into the posterior fornix at intervals of $2\frac{1}{2}$ hours. Monitoring of uterine activity showed a pattern similar to that obtained during intravenous infusion of prostaglandins. Within 3–7 min, hypertonus appeared upon which high frequency contractions of increasing amplitude were gradually superimposed. Uterine stimulation lasted 2–3 hours following each dose. All of the 45 women treated aborted within 48 hours. The mean abortion time was 12 hours 30 min for the PGE_2 group and 14 hours 50 min for the $PGF_{2\alpha}$ group. Side-effects were limited to vomiting in six patients, diarrhoea in one and pyrexia to 38 °C in two.

Béguin et al. (1972) and Wiqvist et al. (1972c, d) studied the extent and duration of the uterine response of patients at mid-pregnancy to the insertion of a single vaginal suppository (20 mg PGE_2 or 50 mg $PGF_{2\alpha}$ in a lipid base). Intrauterine pressure was monitored during 10 hours. Insertion of a $PGF_{2\alpha}$ suppository was followed after a 45–60 min delay by hypertonus and rhythmic contractile activity. The effect reached a maximum 2–3 hours later, after which a progressive decline in uterine activity took place. After 10 hours, the uterus had become quiescent. Following insertion of a PGE_2 suppository, there was a similar delay before hypertonus, but myometrial stimulation had not abated by the end of the observation period. Abortion occurred within 10 hours in seven of the 10 patients treated with PGE_2, but in only one of the 10 given $PGF_{2\alpha}$. Side-effects were more frequent and more prolonged in the PGE_2 group (up to 1.9 episodes of vomiting or diarrhoea/hour) than in the $PGF_{2\alpha}$ group (up to 1.2 episodes).

Brenner and collaborators (Brenner et al., 1972c, 1972f) investigated the effects of various formulations of $PGF_{2\alpha}$ (THAM salt) for vaginal administration in a total of 36 women at 8–17 weeks' gestation. Five regimens were investigated, wherein use was made of $PGF_{2\alpha}$ in the form of solution (two different strengths), tablets or vaginal suppositories. Independently of the form or concentration of the medication, the incidence of vomiting, diarrhoea, fever and pain was high whenever a dose schedule giving adequate rates of abortion within 24 hours was used. Although the complications were not serious, they were disturbing to the patients.

Other investigators (Naftolin et al., 1972; Pion et al., 1972; Elias, 1973; Sato et al., 1973a; Wentz et al., 1973a) confirmed that successful termination of pregnancy by vaginal administration of $PGF_{2\alpha}$ in various formulations (solution/tablets/suppositories) could be achieved only at the expense of frequent and troublesome side-effects. It was felt that this sharply reduced the clinical usefulness of this route of administration. Wentz et al. (1973a) successfully terminated 19 of 20 pregnancies (9–16 weeks) by hourly insertion of a tablet of 50 mg $PGF_{2\alpha}$ intravaginally. But 18 of their patients had vomiting, 13 had diarrhoea and 11 became febrile with temperatures of 38 °C or more.

Naftolin et al. (1972) described two cases of vulvitis and Pion et al. (1972) encountered severe vaginismus following vaginal administration of $PGF_{2\alpha}$, which rendered subsequent instillation of the drug by means of a tuberculin syringe difficult for several hours.

Bolognese and Corson (1974) administered 2–3 hourly a vaginal suppository of 20 mg PGE_2 to 63 women at 13–17 weeks' gestation. Intravenous oxytocin was started in case of untimely rupture of the membranes. Sixty-two subjects were successfully aborted after a mean total dose of 116 mg PGE$_2$ (range: 40–420 mg) and a mean time of 12 hours 6 min (range: 5–33$\frac{1}{2}$ hours). Fifty-two patients had vomiting and/or diarrhoea, 39 fever (> 37.8° C orally) and 12 headache. The same authors did not succeed in diminishing the incidence of side-effects by lengthening the interval between doses to four hours. Indeed, in a second series of 100 patients at 7–20 weeks' gestation so treated, side-effects remained frequent despite the routine administration of anti-emetic and anti-diarrhoeal drugs. The mean total dose required to effect interruption of pregnancy was reduced to 77 mg PGE$_2$ but 75 patients had vomiting, 66 pyrexia, 17 diarrhoea and 10 experienced transient vaginal spasm. In the latter series 97 of the 100 subjects were aborted after a mean time of 13 hours 24 min (Corson and Bolognese, 1974a, b). The authors felt that the occurrence of side-effects could be related more to the size of the individual dose than to the total dose.

The incomplete abortion rate following vaginal administration of PGE$_2$ or PGF$_{2\alpha}$ has varied between 22 and 63%. Higher rates, in general, were found in series including first trimester cases (Elias, 1973; Sato et al., 1973a; Wentz et al., 1973a; Corson and Bolognese, 1974a, b). Bolognese and Corson (1974) could somewhat improve on their figures (22% incomplete abortions in a series consisting mostly of second trimester cases) by having the patient bear down, in a sitting position, after passage of the fetus. In case of a failure of abortion, the cervix was nearly always found to be dilated, rendering vaginal evacuation of the products of conception feasible (Naftolin et al., 1972; Pion et al., 1972). Prochlorperazine and trimethobenzamide hydrochloride have been ineffective in controlling vomiting, but diphenoxylate hydrochloride was very successful against diarrhoea (Wentz et al., 1973a; Corson and Bolognese, 1974a, b).

(a) Laboratory studies

Systematic laboratory investigations (Brenner et al., 1972c; Wentz et al., 1973a; Bolognese and Corson, 1974) showed no consistent changes in the following values after vaginal administration of PGE$_2$ or PGF$_{2\alpha}$ for therapeutic abortion: haemoglobin, packed-cell volume, platelet count, serum sodium, potassium, chloride, blood sugar, blood-urea nitrogen, serum creatinine, serum bilirubin, SGOT, SGPT and serum alkaline phosphatase. In the majority of cases, however, a marked rise in WBC count was noted, with neutrophilia and lymphocytopenia. The degree of leucocytosis could not be correlated to that of the pyrexia. Intravaginal PGF$_{2\alpha}$ induced no significant changes in prothrombin time, partial thromboplastin time, or levels of fibrin-fibrinogen degradation products, but the activity of factors V, VIII and X was slightly increased (Badraoui et al., 1973b). These changes were not suggestive of disseminated intravascular coagulation. Sato et al. (1973b) observed a decrease in plasma progesterone levels several hours after intravaginal administration of PGF$_{2\alpha}$ to three patients at 6–10 weeks' gestation.

Peripheral blood levels of F prostaglandin, following intravaginal administration of PGF$_{2\alpha}$ for therapeutic abortion, were similar to those found during

Table 3.5 Termination of pregnancy with extra-amniotic PGF$_{2\alpha}$

Reference	No. of cases	Gestational range (weeks)	Dose schedule	Success* rate (%)	Mean induction–abortion interval
Wiqvist and Bygdeman, 1970	9	5–10	0.2–1.0 mg intermittently	100	?
Wiqvist et al., 1972a Bygdeman et al., 1973	20	13	250–750 µg 2-hourly Max. 8 hours	100	?
Wiqvist et al., 1972a Bygdeman et al., 1973	50	14	250–750 µg 2-hourly Max. 30 hours	90	24 hours 12 min
Hingorani and Ganesh, 1972	20	8–22	500–750 µg 2-hourly Max. 30 hours	70†	19 hours
Korda et al., 1972	7	12–16	375–750 µg 2-hourly Max. not stated	100‡	36 hours
Csapo et al., 1972a	12	13	continuous fundal infusion of 2–4 mg/hour until abortion	75	12 hours
Csapo et al., 1972d	10	13	single dose of 10 mg (fundal instillation)	100	11 hours 7 min
WHO collaborative study (in Bergström et al., 1972, p. xv)	129	1st and 2nd trimesters	250–750 µg 2–hourly Max. 30 hours	84†	23 hours
Embrey et al., 1973b	93	1st and 2nd trimesters	250–750 µg 2-hourly Max. 36 hours	85	24 hours 54 min
Järvinen et al., 1973	54	11–20	0.5–2.5 mg 1–2 hourly Max. 6 doses	72§	20 hours 18 min
Lauersen and Wilson, 1973	15	12–16	continuous fundal infusion of 2–4 mg/hour	100	14 hours
Lippert et al., 1973	12	12–16	continuous fundal infusion of 0.75–6.0 mg/hour	100	16 hours 45 min
Lippert and Modly, 1973	6	13–17	initial dose of 5 mg in gel, then 2.5–3.7 mg in gel 2–3 hourly	100	17 hours 38 min
Corson and Bolognese, 1974a	30	12–16	1–4 mg 2–6 hourly Max. 36 hours	70	17 hours 24 min

[continued

Table 3.5 [*continued*]

Reference	No. of cases	Gestational range (weeks)	Dose schedule	Success* rate (%)	Mean induction– abortion interval
Hingorani et al., 1974	81	8–16	250 µg 2-hourly	89	18 hours
Zoltan et al., 1974	30	6–12	initial dose of 10 mg, followed by 5 mg after 8 hours, if necessary	100	14 hours 18 min
Fylling and Refsdal, 1974	100	8–16	single dose of 5 mg	81‖	12 hours 42 min

* abortion within 36 hours, unless specified otherwise
† abortion within 30 hours
‡ abortion within 72 hours
§ abortion within 48 hours
‖ abortion within 24 hours

intravenous infusion of this drug, explaining why comparable incidences of side-effects are encountered with both methods of drug administration. In general, the appearance of side-effects corresponded to the peaks in the blood levels (Caldwell *et al.*, 1972; Gréen *et al.*, 1972).

(b) Comments

To summarise, the abortifacient efficacy of vaginally administered prostaglandins is mediated by systemic absorption. The naturally occurring prostaglandins given by this route cause frequent and sometimes severe general side-effects. The clinical usefulness of the vaginal route could be improved by the use of synthetic prostaglandin analogues, devoid of gastrointestinal stimulant activity.

3.2.5 Extra-amniotic route

The effect of vaginally administered prostaglandin is mediated by systemic absorption and side-effects are similar to those observed during intravenous infusion. Attention therefore has focused upon alternative routes of administration. Prostaglandins possess the unusual property of acting locally, not only after endogenous release, but also—unlike the majority of other drugs—after exogenous administration (Embrey, 1966).

Instillation of PGE_2 or $PGF_{2\alpha}$ into the space between uterine wall and fetal membranes causes direct myometrial stimulation and interruption of pregnancy can be accomplished with a total dose 10–20 times lower than that required by the intravenous route. Side-effects are considerably reduced.

Wiqvist and Bygdeman (1970) initially reported on the extra-amniotic injection of repeated doses of 25–75 µg PGE_2 or 200–1000 µg $PGF_{2\alpha}$ in 12 patients at 5–13 weeks' gestation. Termination of pregnancy was achieved in 11 patients, abortion was inevitable in the twelfth. Embrey and Hillier (1971) independently showed the usefulness of this route in second trimester patients. The efficacy of the extra-amniotic method has since been confirmed by many investigators (Tables 3.5 and 3.6).

Table 3.6   Termination of pregnancy with extra-amniotic PGE$_2$

Reference	No. of cases	Gestational range (weeks)	Dose schedule	Success* rate (%)	Mean induction– abortion interval
Roberts et al., 1971	20	<12	25–600 μg 2–hourly Max. 24 hours	65†	13 hours 23 min
Miller et al., 1972	52	12–20	continuous infusion of 45–270 μg hourly until abortion	90	15 hours 45 min
Embrey et al., 1973b	70	1st and 2nd trimesters	200 μg 2–hourly	93	19 hours 24 min
Midwinter et al., 1973	20	10–20	continuous infusion of 46.5 μg hourly	50	21 hours 54 min
Midwinter et al., 1973	28	10–20	continuous infusion of 66.5 μg hourly	93	13 hours 48 min
Midwinter et al., 1973	24	10–20	continuous infusion of 93 μg hourly	92	15 hours 30 min
Midwinter et al., 1973	16	10–20	continuous infusion of 133.5 μg hourly	63	17 hours 6 min
Lippert and Modly, 1973	14	13–17	1.25 mg in gel 2–3 hourly	100	11 hours 35 min
Fraser and Brash, 1974	104	12–24	100 μg hourly × 3, then 200 μg hourly	89	18 hours 30 min

* abortion within 36 hours, unless specified otherwise
† abortion within 24 hours

Usually after an initial test dose (e.g. 250 μg PGF$_{2\alpha}$), two-hourly doses of 750 μg PGF$_{2\alpha}$ or 200 μg PGE$_2$ are instilled via a transcervically placed extra-amniotic Foley catheter. Embrey et al. (1973b) reported a success rate of 85% within 36 hours in a series of 93 patients given PGF$_{2\alpha}$ and 93% in 70 patients given PGE$_2$. The mean induction–abortion intervals were 24 hours 54 min for PGF$_{2\alpha}$ and 19 hours 24 min for PGE$_2$. Bygdeman et al. (1972c, 1973) terminated 45 (90%) of 50 mid-trimester pregnancies within 36 hours by extra-amniotic administration of PGF$_{2\alpha}$. The mean abortion time was 24 hours 12 min.

Fraser and Brash (1974) attempted to terminate pregnancy in 104 women at 12–14 weeks' gestation by extra-amniotic instillation of PGE_2. After three hourly doses of 100 μg of the drug, the dose was increased to 200 μg administered hourly until expulsion of the conceptus. Ninety-three patients (89%) aborted within 36 hours; the others aborted after i.v. oxytocin was infused for augmentation; (one patient pulled out the Foley catheter, in a bout of mental agitation). The mean induction–abortion interval was $18\frac{1}{2}$ hours; the mean total dose of PGE_2 amounted to 3 mg. Only 19 of the 103 patients successfully aborted had a complete abortion and all others required a curettage. Side-effects included vomiting in 18 cases (17%), diarrhoea in three (3%) and bronchospasm in two (2%). Pyrexia of more than 37.5 °C was noted in 30 subjects (29%).

Wiqvist et al. (1972a) achieved interruption of pregnancy more easily at 7–8 weeks' gestation than at a later stage: a smaller total dose was required and the abortion time was shorter. However, different criteria were used to assess the occurrence of abortion: expulsion of the products of conception, in second trimester cases provided a definite endpoint, while uterine bleeding served as endpoint in the early cases (interruption of pregnancy, in these cases, was later confirmed by a negative immunological pregnancy test). Embrey et al. (1973b) found no significant difference in outcome between first and second trimester cases. The success rate was higher and the mean abortion time shorter in multigravidae than in primigravidae (Embrey et al., 1973b; Järvinen et al., 1973; Lauersen and Wilson, 1973; Lippert et al., 1973; Fraser and Brash, 1974).

Following extraovular injection, two types of responses have been observed which may depend upon the technique of administration. Embrey and Hillier (1971) and MacKenzie et al. (1975) have pointed out that with moderate doses (200 μg PGE_2 or 750 μg $PGF_{2\alpha}$) the usual response is a gradual increase in uterine tone and frequent low amplitude contractions which gradually increase. In certain cases however an immediate rise in uterine tone occurs following injection resulting in strong uterine pain, vomiting and in some cases hypotension. MacKenzie and Hillier (1974), MacKenzie et al., (1975) have attributed the latter effect to a rapid systemic absorption of the drug possibly due to the catheter being close to a uterine sinus or to trauma on inserting the tube resulting in the breakdown of decidual and placental integrity. In cases where blood flows down the tube on insertion, greater side-effects are initially seen. Rapid absorption and dissolution of drug away from its site of action (indicated by initial rapid response) results in delayed abortion whereas conservation at the site of action (characterised by a gradual increase in tone) results in shorter abortion times (MacKenzie et al., 1975).

Fundal (=high intrauterine) administration via a thin polyethylene or a Nelaton catheter (Braaksma et al., 1972; Csapo et al., 1972a) offers no particular advantage over instillation of the drug into the isthmic region via a Foley catheter. Radiological studies with radio-opaque dyes (Wiqvist et al., 1972a; Dillon et al., 1974) have shown that prostaglandin instilled into the isthmic region is forced by local contractions to spread over the major part of the internal surface of the uterus. Besides, high fundal administration is often followed by an immediate uterine contraction of fairly short duration, similar to that seen after a single intravenous injection. This most probably is caused by leakage of the injected material into the systemic circulation (Wiqvist *et al.*, 1972d).

For better results it is advisable to inflate the balloon of the self-retaining catheter to a volume that reduces leakage of prostaglandin via the cervix and expulsion of the catheter before completion of the abortion (Alderman, 1972; Seppälä *et al.*, 1973). The WHO Prostaglandin Task Force following the original study of Embrey *et al.* (1972, 1973b) recommends the use of a Foley catheter (8–16 French) with the balloon filled with 20 ml saline for uteri 12–15 weeks' size and with 30 ml for uteri 16–20 weeks' size (Bergström, 1973, page 29).

(a) Side-effects

For a similar rate of efficacy, the extra-amniotic administration of natural prostaglandins causes about five times less side-effects than the intravenous infusion of these compounds. Following two-hourly injection of 200 μg PGE$_2$ or 750 μg PGF$_{2\alpha}$, occasional vomiting is seen in 25% of the patients, at most (Hingorani and Ganesh, 1972; Wiqvist *et al.*, 1972a; Embrey *et al.*, 1973b; Hingorani *et al.*, 1974). Diarrhoea occurs in 1–2% of cases (same references). No effect on pulse or blood pressure is noted (Wiqvist *et al.*, 1972a). Distressing pain of uterine origin occurs in 20% of patients, but it may be alleviated by injectable analgesics (Midwinter *et al.*, 1972; Wiqvist *et al.*, 1972a). Temperature elevation of 1 °C or more is noted in about 5% of cases (Hingorani and Ganesh, 1972; Midwinter *et al.*, 1972, 1973; Embrey *et al.*, 1973b). Except for Korda *et al.* (1972: three cases diagnosed among seven subjects treated), Naftolin *et al.* (1972: two cases in six subjects) and Lauersen and Wilson (1974b: seven cases among 76 patients), investigators rarely encountered endometritis. With the only exception of Dillon *et al.* (1974: 21% in a series of 34 cases), authors did not encounter haemorrhage (>500 ml blood loss) in a large number of their patients. Fraser and Brash (1974) reported two cases (2%) of bronchospasm in women given hourly extra-amniotic doses of 200 μg PGE$_2$. Increasing the dosage has caused more severe side-effects, without improving the success rate (Roberts *et al.*, 1971; Midwinter *et al.*, 1973; Corson and Bolognese, 1974a).

The incomplete abortion rate is approximately 40% (Wiqvist *et al.*, 1972a; Embrey *et al.*, 1973b). The proportion of incomplete *v.* complete abortions is mainly related to the duration of gestation; to some extent, it is influenced by the skill of the attendant in avoiding placental retention.

The need for repeated instillations and the presence of an indwelling catheter that may cause intrauterine infection somewhat limit the clinical usefulness of the extra-amniotic method. Continuous intrauterine delivery of the prostaglandin can be achieved by making use of an infusion pump (Csapo *et al.*, 1972a; Midwinter *et al.*, 1972, 1973; Miller *et al.*, 1972; Embrey *et al.*, 1973b; Lauersen and Wilson, 1973, 1974b; Lippert *et al.*, 1973). The drawbacks mentioned for the extra-amniotic method could be eliminated altogether by the use of a 'single-shot' technique allowing for removal of the catheter immediately after intrauterine instillation of a large single dose of the compound or alternatively by drug formulation to achieve a slow and sustained local release of prostaglandins. Both these approaches have been tried.

Csapo et al. (1972d) achieved abortion in all of ten first trimester cases by the slow injection of a single dose of 10 mg $PGF_{2\alpha}$ into the extraovular space. The mean induction–abortion interval was 11 hours seven min. However, using the same treatment schedule, Pitkanen and Rauramo (1974) were able to terminate only 44 of a series of 50 pregnancies at 9–14 weeks, despite the administration of oxytocin intravenously to 23 patients who had made slow clinical progress. Similarly, in order to achieve a 100% success rate, Zoltan et al. (1974) had to administer a second dose of 5 mg $PGF_{2\alpha}$, eight hours after the initial 10 mg dose, to 15 of 30 patients at 6–12 weeks' gestation. The mean abortion time in this series was 14 hours 18 min. Enkola (1974), assessing the method in first and second trimester cases, noted accidental rupture of the membranes during instillation of the initial dose in 11 of his 30 patients. The initial dose therefore was increased to as much as 26 mg, and at least part of it was administered into the amniotic fluid. Here too, additional extra-amniotic instillation was often required to achieve abortion. Fylling and Refsdal (1974) injected a single dose of 5 mg $PGF_{2\alpha}$ (in 5 ml solution) into the isthmic region of the uterus. Of 100 women at 8–16 weeks' gestation so treated, 81 aborted within 24 hours. As discussed later, prostaglandin analogues are more suitable and safer for a 'single-shot' technique via the extra-amniotic route.

To prevent the severe side-effects that could follow extra-amniotic instillation of a large dose of natural prostaglandin, as given in the one-shot method advocated by Csapo, patients need to be premedicated. A suitable combination consists of 50 mg pethidine, 10 mg diazepam and 10 mg thiethylperazine maleate, given intramuscularly (Pitkanen and Rauramo, 1974).

Attempts have also been made to overcome the comparative short duration of action of natural prostaglandins by incorporating them into a high viscosity solution. In a preliminary report by MacKenzie et al. (1975) PGE_2 in a dose of 1.5 mg in a 5% viscous solution of hydroxy ethyl methyl cellulose was administered by the extraovular route. Abortion was achieved in 20/24 patients (83%) with a single dose within 24 hours and the remainder aborted within 29 hours on administering oxytocin. The authors claim that the side-effects compared with extra-amniotic administration of 1.5 mg PGE_2 in aqueous solution were considerably reduced and the abortifacient efficacy with a single dose increased.

(b) Laboratory studies

The results of laboratory investigations conducted during extra-amniotic administration of natural prostaglandins have been similar to those obtained during intravenous infusion of these compounds. Seppälä et al. (1973) observed a rise in WBC count and erythrocyte sedimentation rate. Blood cultures were negative in all of 62 patients tested. This confirms that the risk of developing clinical endometritis may be more theoretical than real. Badraoui et al. (1973a, b) and Phillips et al. (1974), studying the blood coagulation system during and after termination of pregnancy by extra-amniotic $PGF_{2\alpha}$, found no changes suggestive of disseminated intravascular coagulation. No significant alterations were noted in prothrombin time, partial thromboplastin time or levels of fibrin–fibrinogen degradation products. An increase in several of the coagulation factors (platelets, fibrinogen, factors V, VIII, X and XI) was interpreted by Phillips and co-workers as a non-specific inflammatory type response to the administration of the prostaglandin.

Csapo and collaborators found significant decreases in plasma progesterone and 17-β oestradiol, which were more marked in patients who eventually aborted completely. They hypothesised that the prostaglandin acted by suppressing the endocrine function of the feto–placental unit and that the ensuing drop in progesterone was necessary to convert the uterus into a reactive organ, susceptible of responding to stimulation (Csapo et al., 1972a; Csapo et al., 1972d; Enkola, 1974; Pitkanen and Rauramo, 1974; Zoltan et al., 1974). Dillon et al. (1974) also observed a progressive decrease in plasma progesterone after extraovular administration of $PGF_{2\alpha}$; cortisol levels were unchanged. Lehmann et al. (1973) felt that the decrease in steroidogenesis was only due to the disturbance of placental function brought about by the uterine contractions. Ylikorkala and Pennanen (1973) observed a significant decrease in serum HCS within two hours following the first extra-amniotic injection of 2 mg $PGF_{2\alpha}$. They concluded that the prostaglandin had a direct effect on the synthesis and/or the secretion of the placental hormone in early pregnancy. Despite the authors' statement to the contrary, the mechanical influence of the uterine contractions upon the placenta should not be overlooked. Pulkkinen et al. (1974) measured the uterine blood flow by the radioactive Indium method in seven patients in the mid-trimester of pregnancy given a single extraovular injection of 10 mg $PGF_{2\alpha}$ and in three untreated subjects. Treatment with the prostaglandin caused a rapid decrease in uteroplacental blood flow. The authors interpreted this as being evidence that interruption of pregnancy was effected by sustained vasoconstriction of the utero–placental vessels, leading to suppression of the endocrine function of the feto–placental unit.

Fraser and Gray (1974a) and Van der Plaetsen et al. (1974) observed no EEG changes after extra-amniotic administration of PGE_2.

(c) Comments

In conclusion, the extra-amniotic instillation of natural prostaglandins appears as a valuable technique of termination of pregnancy, particularly during the late first trimester and early second trimester (12–15 weeks' gestation) when the uterus has become too large for suction curettage, yet is still too small for intra-amniotic injection. The technique is of course contraindicated in case of active infection of the lower genital tract. Results can be further improved by simultaneous infusion of oxytocin, as discussed later (Section 3.4.1). It is likely that with proper drug formulation in case of natural prostaglandins or by using some synthetic analogues of natural prostaglandins a large number of pregnancies can be terminated with a single extra-amniotic dose.

3.2.6 Intra-amniotic route

Wiqvist *et al.* (1968) first attempted to stimulate the uterus by intra-amniotic instillation of 75 μg PGE_1. At this dose, no uterine response was observed. The authors hypothesised that PGE_1 did not cross the fetal membranes to stimulate myometrial contractility. However, using larger single intra-amniotic doses of PGE_2 or $PGF_{2\alpha}$ Karim (1971d) and Karim and Sharma (1971b) were able to induce uterine activity lasting for several hours and terminate pregnancies in second trimester patients. The above findings were independently confirmed by Bygdeman *et al.* (1971) in women and by Kirton and Forbes (1971) in rhesus monkeys.

Following intra-amniotic administration of a single dose of 2.5–5.0 mg PGE_2 or 25 mg $PGF_{2\alpha}$, Karim and Sharma (1971b) could terminate pregnancy within $4\frac{1}{2}$ to 18 hours (mean: 11 hours 24 min) in all of 10 subjects at 13–22 weeks' gestation. Uterine activity, monitored via an epidural catheter transabdominally inserted into the amniotic cavity, showed a gradual increase in tone after a latent period of 15–30 min. Hypertonus was less marked, but the contractions were similar to those induced by prostaglandins given by other routes. The same protocol was used in a later study (Karim *et al.*, 1972b). Pregnancy was interrupted within 48 hours in nine of 10 women given a single intra-amniotic injection of 5 mg PGE_2 and in eight of 10 subjects treated with 25 mg $PGF_{2\alpha}$. The mean times to abortion were 15 hours 12 min and 19 hours 21 min respectively.

Bygdeman *et al.* (1971) and Toppozada *et al.* (1971) successfully interrupted 42 of 46 pregnancies by intra-amniotic instillation of one to 12 doses of 5–25 mg $PGF_{2\alpha}$. The mean abortion time was 24 hours 54 min in their first group of patients (No. = 9), and 28 hours in the second (No. = 33). Side-effects in these initial three series were found to be considerably less frequent than with intravenous infusion of PGE_2 and $PGF_{2\alpha}$ and were acceptable to the patients. Numerous investigators have since confirmed the superiority of the intra-amniotic route over other systems of delivery of prostaglandins for therapeutic abortion in the second trimester of pregnancy (Tables 3.7, 3.8 and 3.9).

Transabdominal puncture of the amniotic sac is a relatively easy procedure after the 14th week of gestation. Single dose schedules allow for immediate withdrawal of the needle (or catheter) used for the injection and bear a lesser risk of infection. However, in order to attain an acceptable rate of efficacy (90% or more abortions within 48 hours; mean abortion time of 20 hours), high doses of natural prostaglandins (e.g. 40–50 mg $PGF_{2\alpha}$) need to be given and side-effects, at these levels, though still minor and acceptable are understandably more frequent (Bergström, 1973, pages 33–35; Brenner *et al.*, 1973a; Wiqvist *et al.*, 1973b). But Laursen and Wilson (1974a) and Corlett and Ballard (1974) had less side-effects with a single instillation of 40 mg $PGF_{2\alpha}$ than with serial injections and Craft (1973g) could inject as much as 75 or 100 mg $PGF_{2\alpha}$ into the amniotic cavity without causing troublesome side-effects. Of 16 patients given 75 mg $PGF_{2\alpha}$, 14 aborted within 24 hours without additional treatment. The two others were given oxytocin supplementation. Five patients had vomiting, none had diarrhoea. Intra-amniotic administration of a single dose of 100 mg $PGF_{2\alpha}$ terminated preg-

Table 3.7 Termination of pregnancy with intra-amniotic $PGF_{2\alpha}$. Multiple dose schedules

Reference	No. of cases	Dose schedule	Success* rate(%)	Mean induction–abortion interval
Brenner et al., 1972b	20	15 mg, repeated after 24 hours	70	28 hours
WHO collaborative study (in Bergström et al., 1972, p. xv)	52	id.	61	35 hours
Ballard and Quilligan, 1973a	10	id.	40	33 hours 18 min
Bygdeman et al., 1973	10	id.	50	?
Brenner et al., 1972b	21	25 mg, repeated after 24 hours	90	22 hours 54 min
Gillett et al., 1972b	20	id.	90	27 hours 30 min
Seppälä et al., 1972	21	id.	86	26 hours 36 min
Ballard and Quilligan, 1973a	20	id.	80	24 hours 24 min
Bygdeman et al., 1973	34	id.	97	28 hours
Bergström, 1973 (pp. 5 & 7)	100	id.	90	?
Wentz et al., 1973b	17	40 mg, repeated after 24 hours	94	22 hours 56 min
Brenner et al., 1973c	24	50 mg, repeated after 24 hours	96	23 hours 48 min
Nyberg, 1973	101	25–35 mg initially; 30–40 mg after 24 hours	100†	33 hours
Korda et al., 1972	7	30 mg initially; 15 mg after 24 hours	100	25 hours
Anderson et al., 1972a	35	40 mg initially; 10–20 mg after 24 hours	100	23 hours 30 min
Anderson et al., 1973	42	id.	100	24 hours 54 min
Brenner et al., 1973f	10	15 mg, repeated after 6 hours	70‡	17 hours 24 min
Bygdeman et al., 1973; Bergström, 1973 (pp. 9 & 10)	89	25 mg, repeated after 6 hours	92	?
Bergström, 1973 (pp. 33 & 34)	123	id.	89	19 hours 30 min
Gillett et al., 1973	20	id.	100	21 hours 20 min

[continued

Table 3.7 [*continued*]

Reference	No. of cases	Dose schedule	Success* rate(%)	Mean induction–abortion interval
Hingorani *et al.*, 1974	43	id.	86	20 hours
Brenner *et al.*, 1973f	22	id.	68‡	13 hours 48 min
Ballard and Quilligan, 1972	20	25 mg initially; 15 mg after 6 hours	85	15 hours 24 min
Brenner *et al.*, 1973f	25	25 mg, repeated after 6 and 12 hours	60‡	15 hours 12 min
Anderson *et al.*, 1973; Behrman and Anderson, 1974	70	40 mg initially; 20 mg after 6 hours; 40 mg after 24 hours	100	19 hours 15 min
Karim *et al.*, 1972b	30	25 mg 10-hourly	93	17 hours
Toppozada *et al.*, 1971	26	5–15 mg repeated at 3–24 hours intervals	85	?
id.	11	25 mg initially; 15–25 mg at 12–24 hours intervals	100	?
Csapo *et al.*, 1972b	14	10 mg initially; then 5 mg 3-hourly	100	15 hours 16 min
Haspels and Neth, 1973	‹ 9	5 mg hourly	100	?
Brenner *et al.*, 1972f	10	15 mg, repeated after 6, 24 and 30 hours	100	22 hours 8 min
Brenner *et al.*, 1973d	22	25 mg, repeated after 6, 24 and 30 hours	95	18 hours 54 min
Brenner *et al.*, 1973e	25	25 mg, repeated after 6, 12, 24, 30 and 36 hours	96	21 hours 30 min
Shutt *et al.*, 1973	10	30 mg, repeated after 24 and 42 hours	100	24 hours
Wentz *et al.*, 1973b	43	30 mg initially; then 25 mg after 6–8 hours and after 24 hours	93	17 hours 12 min

* abortion within 48 hours, unless specified otherwise
† 8 of these cases were given i.v. oxytocin after spontaneous rupture of the membranes had occurred
‡ abortion within 24 hours

Table 3.8 Termination of pregnancy with intra-amniotic PGF$_{2\alpha}$. Single dose schedules

Reference	No. of cases	Dose schedule	Success* rate(%)	Mean induction– abortion interval
Brenner et al., 1973f	20	15 mg single dose	20†	19 hours
id.	31	25 mg single dose	45†	14 hours 30 min
Karim and Sharma, 1971b	3	25 mg single dose	100	13 hours 30 min
Karim et al., 1972b	10	25 mg single dose	80	19 hours 21 min
Roberts et al., 1973	14	25 mg single dose	43	?
Wiqvist et al., 1973b	33	40 mg single dose	76	18 hours 30 min
Bergström, 1973 (pp. 33 & 34)	50	40 mg single dose	92	21 hours 54 min
Corlett and Ballard, 1974	30	40 mg single dose	97	25 hours
Lauersen and Wilson, 1974a	20	40 mg single dose	100‡	16 hours 15 min
Brenner et al., 1973a; Bergström, 1973 (pp. 33 & 35)	46	50 mg single dose	96	19 hours 30 min
Brenner et al., 1973f	24	50 mg single dose	54†	17 hours 36 min
Craft, 1973g	8	100 mg single dose	100	17 hours 23 min

* abortion within 48 hours, unless specified otherwise
† abortion within 24 hours
‡ two patients also given i.v. oxytocin after 24 hours

nancy in all of eight subjects within 24 hours. The mean time to abortion was 17 hours 23 min. One woman vomited, none had diarrhoea.

Repeated intra-amniotic injection of natural prostaglandins requires the maintenance of a catheter for administration of the second and subsequent doses, but it is highly efficacious without causing a disturbing range of side-effects. PGF$_{2\alpha}$, in the dose of 25 mg repeated after 24 hours, if necessary, gives a success rate of 90–95%, with a mean abortion time of 26–28 hours in successful cases (Brenner et al., 1972; Gillett et al., 1972b; Seppälä et al., 1972; Ballard and Quilligan, 1973a; Bergström, 1973, pages 5 and 7; Bygdeman et al., 1972c, 1973). The mean induction–abortion interval can be shortened to about 20 hours, with the same high rate of success being maintained if the second 25 mg dose is given after only six hours (Bergström, 1973, pages 9–10 and 33–34; Bygdeman et al., 1973; Gillett et al., 1973). Karim et al. (1972b) reported a success rate of 93% and a mean abortion time of 17 hours in a group of 30 patients given 10-hourly intra-amniotic injections of 25 mg PGF$_{2\alpha}$ for a maximum of four doses.

Table 3.9 Termination of pregnancy with intra-amniotic PGE$_2$

Reference	No. of cases	Dose schedule	Success rate (%) within 48 hours	Mean induction–abortion interval
Karim and Sharma, 1971b	7	2.5–5.0 mg single dose	100	10 hours 30 min
Karim et al., 1972b	10	5 mg single dose	90	15 hours 12 min
Bergström, 1973 (pp. 9 & 10)	5	10 mg single dose	100	23 hours 48 min
Fraser and Brash, 1974	17	id.	94	14 hours 10 min
Karim et al., 1972b	40	5 mg 10-hourly	95	14 hours
Craft, 1972, 1973g	35	20 mg 24-hourly	100	14 hours 27 min
Craft, 1973c	15	10 mg repeated at intervals	100	26 hours 49 min*
Roberts et al., 1973	13	3 mg repeated at intervals	85	?

* mean induction–abortion interval of all patients, including those who took more than 48 hours to abort

Anderson and collaborators investigated yet another dose schedule. These authors gave 40 mg PGF$_{2\alpha}$ intra-amniotically, followed by a second dose of 20 mg after six hours and, if needed, a third dose of 40 mg 24 hours after the first one. In a series of 70 patients, a success rate of 100% was obtained, with a mean abortion time of 19 hours 15 min. Only 5 ($=7\%$) of patients required reinjection at 24 hours (Anderson et al., 1973; Behrman and Anderson, 1974).

PGE$_2$ has not been as widely used as PGF$_{2\alpha}$ by the intra-amniotic route (initial report: Karim and Sharma, 1971b). Craft (1972, 1973g) successfully terminated within 48 hours all of 35 mid-trimester pregnancies by intra-amniotic instillation of 20 mg PGE$_2$, followed, if needed, by a second identical dose after 24 hours. Epidural analgesia was provided in every case for prevention of the severe pain that would probably have followed administration of these very high doses.

Karim et al. (1972b) could interrupt pregnancy in 38 of 40 women given 10-hourly intra-amniotic injections of 5 mg PGE$_2$, for a maximum of four doses. The mean time to abortion was 14 hours. Fraser and Brash (1974) treated 17 patients at 14–24 weeks with a single intra-amniotic injection of 10 mg PGE$_2$. Abortion took place in 16 (94%), in the mean time of 14 hours 10 min (range: 8–41$\frac{1}{2}$ hours). Troublesome vomiting was noted in three (18%) of the cases, diarrhoea in four (24%) and bronchospasm in one (6%). MacKenzie et al. (1974), using the same regimen, reported successful interruption of pregnancy within 24 hours in nine of 15 patients. Two patients took more than 48 hours to abort. In another 16 women, a second 10 mg dose of PGE$_2$

was given intra-amniotically six hours after the first one. All patients aborted within 24 hours. The mean abortion time amounted to approximately 26 hours in the first group and 13 hours in the second.

Finally, a single series of 10 patients has been described in whom a mixture of 2.5 mg PGE_2 and 12.5 mg $PGF_{2\alpha}$ was administered 10-hourly via the intra-amniotic route. All subjects aborted in a mean time of 14 hours (Karim et al., 1972b).

Studies with intra-amniotic injection of $PGF_{2\alpha}$, containing trace amounts of tritiated $PGF_{2\alpha}$, have shown a slow rate of disappearance of the prostaglandin from the amniotic cavity. The drug partly crosses the fetal membranes to act directly upon the myometrium, and it is partly metabolised by the fetal and placental tissues—probably also by the decidua (see Chapter 2). This results in the production of 15-keto-$PGF_{2\alpha}$; 15-keto-13,14-dihydro-$PGF_{2\alpha}$; and 13, 14-dihydro-$PGF_{2\alpha}$, all of which can be recovered from the amniotic fluid and the maternal plasma. One of these metabolites, 13,14-dihydro-$PGF_{2\alpha}$, has an oxytocic activity of its own (Bygdeman et al., 1974) and it may contribute to the stimulatory effect observed following administration of $PGF_{2\alpha}$. The half-life of $PGF_{2\alpha}$ in the liquor varies widely (6–20 hours) from case to case, and does not correlate with the induction–abortion interval. Low levels of $PGF_{2\alpha}$ are found in maternal plasma (0.2–0.3 ng/ml) explaining why side-effects can be kept to a minimum when use is made of the intra-amniotic route (Caldwell et al., 1972; Gréen et al., 1972; Pace-Asciak et al., 1972; Wolfe and Pace-Asciak, 1972; Anderson et al., 1973; Granström et al., 1973; Gréen et al., 1974).

When uterine activity is being monitored, in a majority of cases, but not in all, hypertonus of about 50 mmHg occurs within 15 min of intra-amniotic injection of the prostaglandin. Rhythmic contractions then appear, which gradually increase in amplitude (to 80–200 mmHg) and decrease in frequency (from 10–14/10 min to 4–10/10 min). Again, the uterine contractile response correlates poorly with the induction–abortion interval: some patients with very marked uterine activity have the longest abortion time or even fail to abort altogether. The length and firmness of the cervix determine the resistance to the expulsion of uterine contents and it has been stated that progressive cervical effacement and dilatation are the most reliable prognostic signs of success (Corson et al., 1973; Wentz et al., 1973b).

Opinions vary as to the effect of parity and of duration of pregnancy on the outcome of abortion. Many authors noted that multiparas aborted faster than nulliparas, but with few exceptions (e.g.: Corlett and Ballard, 1974: $18\frac{1}{2}$ hours $\pm$ 8 hours v. 32 hours $\pm$ 12 hours, after a single intra-amniotic dose of 40 mg $PGF_{2\alpha}$; $p < 0.01$) the difference between the mean induction–abortion intervals for these two groups did not reach statistical significance. Again, individual variations in cervical resistance probably account for these discrepancies.

Smith and collaborators (Smith et al., 1973; Smith, 1974b) studying a group of 240 women in the second trimester of gestation found an association between the time of intra-amniotic injection of $PGF_{2\alpha}$ and the duration of the subsequent interval to abortion. The authors used a standardised procedure in which 30 mg $PGF_{2\alpha}$ was injected transabdominally into the amniotic sac, followed—if necessary—by doses of 15 mg at 24 and 42 hours. The treatment was initiated at various times between 6 a.m. and 2 a.m. The optimal response (in terms of induction–abortion interval, total dose of $PGF_{2\alpha}$ required and duration of hospitalisation) was obtained when the initial dose of prostaglandin was injected at 6 p.m. in nulliparas and at 5 p.m. in the pooled patient group. This difference in timing of about one hour was thought to be associated with differences in activity patterns between nulliparous and parous women. Other factors, such as bed rest or withholding of meals prior to treatment, adversely affected the efficacy of the treatment. Smith and colleagues felt that their observations established the existence of a circadian rhythm in the response to the intra-amniotic injection of $PGF_{2\alpha}$. They suggested that this could possibly be related to circadian variations in plasma steroid levels. If confirmed, these findings should obviously have important consequences. First, many of the data reported in this chapter and elsewhere, might have to be re-evaluated, taking into account the time of administration of prostaglandin, in order to make valid comparisons between different treatment protocols. Second, in the management of the individual patient, administration of the prostaglandin at the optimal time could reduce the total dose of compound required to effect abortion, the duration of hospitalisation and the cost of the procedure.

The rate of incomplete abortions varies considerably between different case materials, even when the same protocol is used, but this may depend on whether the 'third stage of abortion' was managed actively or not. On the whole (Bygdeman and Wiqvist, 1974; Amy, unpublished data), about 40% of successful cases are accounted for by incomplete abortions, as demonstrated by systematic exploration of the uterine cavity following abortion.

(a) Side-effects

Due to the slow transfer of prostaglandins across the fetal membranes and the low levels in maternal plasma, side-effects are less frequent than with other methods of administration. They are dose-related and consist mainly of nausea, vomiting, pyrexia and pain of uterine origin. Diarrhoea is uncommon. Headache, chills and vaso-vagal reactions are rare. Care should be taken to inject the drug slowly, in order to detect in time an adverse reaction. $PGF_{2\alpha}$ particularly may cause bronchospasm (Brenner et al., 1972a; Leslie and Laufe, 1972; Corson et al., 1973). Severe reactions are seen in case of inadvertent intravascular injection (Craft, 1973g; Nyberg, 1973; Wentz et al., 1973; Brown, 1974) or if rapid absorption of the prostaglandin from the uterine cavity takes place (Leslie and Laufe, 1972). This may be seen when use is made of the 'intra-amniotic' method to effect expulsion of a hydatidiform mole (Karim, 1974; Smith, 1974a) or for termination of missed abortion (Anderson et al., 1973). Prochlorperazine or trimethobenzamide hydrochloride are effective against nausea and vomiting (Brenner et al., 1972b; Wentz et al., 1972a; Lauersen and Wilson, 1974a). Pethidine injections or continuous epidural analgesia (Craft, 1972) have been used for relief of pain.

Lyneham et al. (1973) encountered five cases of major convulsions in a series of 320 patients given intra-amniotic $PGF_{2\alpha}$ (30 mg + 15 mg at 24 and 42 hours). Only two of these patients were known epileptics. However, other authors have not encountered this complication and it can be stated that prostaglandins, given by various routes, in the usual doses for induction of labour or for interruption of pregnancy, are not a cause of seizures (Craft, 1973f; MacKenzie et al., 1973; Fraser and Gray, 1974a; Thiery et al. 1974). Shearman et al. (1972) and Smith et al. (1972) noted a high frequency of frank lactation starting a few days after interruption of pregnancy with intra-amniotic $PGF_{2\alpha}$. This was sometimes preceded by copious secretion from the nipple, during prostaglandin administration and before the occurrence of abortion. Lactation occurred significantly more frequently ($p < 0.001$) in patients receiving intra-amniotic $PGF_{2\alpha}$ (75–80%) than in subjects treated by suction curettage (0%) or hysterotomy (4%). The authors concluded that $PGF_{2\alpha}$ could induce lactogenesis following the termination of early pregnancy and that it also possessed milk ejection activity, although the latter effect could have been mediated through the release of endogenous oxytocin (see Chapter 2). Lauersen and Wilson (1974a) and Lauersen et al. (1974) confirmed these observations. Of 30 patients aborted by intra-amniotic $PGF_{2\alpha}$, 27 (90%) complained of engorged breasts and varying degrees of lactation within a few days. For comparison, lactation was observed in only three of 10 women following intra-amniotic instillation of hypertonic salt solution, combined with i.v. oxytocin (see also Chapter 2).

Uterine stimulation in the face of unusual cervical resistance may lead to extreme thinning out of the isthmus and ultimately to transverse rupture of the posterior uterine wall at the level of the cervico–isthmic junction. This was described after intra-amniotic instillation of hypertonic saline (Gordon, 1972; Lowensohn and Ballard, 1974) and urea (Bradley-Watson et al., 1973) but is not specific to those methods. Similar cases have been reported in young primigravidae, after use of intra-amniotic $PGF_{2\alpha}$ and PGE_2 (Shearman et al., 1972; Brenner et al., 1973e; Corson and Bolognese, 1973; Nyberg, 1973; Wentz et al., 1973c; Fraser, 1974; Kajanoja et al., 1974; Lowensohn and Ballard, 1974; Ylöstalo et al., 1974). Even when repaired immediately, this type of cervical rupture may fail to heal and a fistulous tract may develop, interfering with the later reproductive performance of the patient. The complication can be prevented by examination of the cervix at regular intervals during the course of abortion and, in those cases at risk, by gentle instrumental dilatation of the cervical canal or insertion of one or more laminaria tents (Corson et al., 1973; Engel et al., 1973). Extension of this type of injury into the lateral and anterior aspects of the uterus may lead to annular detachment of the cervix, as occurred in the case reported by Bowen-Simpkins (1973), following intra-amniotic injection of 80 g urea and 5 mg PGE_2.

Of less consequence is the longitudinal tear that may involve the lateral aspect of an insufficiently dilated cervix during the expulsion of the conceptus. The handful of cases described occurred after intra-amniotic injection of PGE_2, or $PGF_{2\alpha}$, mostly supplemented by i.v. oxytocin or intra-amniotic urea (Bradley-Watson et al., 1973; Craft, 1974; Craft et al., 1974; Kajanoja et al., 1974). This lesion is easier to repair and—if it does not reach the uterine isthmus—it should not be a cause of cervical incompetence.

To the best of our knowledge, only a single instance of traumatic lesion to the cervix was reported after extra-amniotic administration of prostaglandin $F_{2\alpha}$ (Göretzlehner and Klausch, 1974). It is possible that the Foley catheter (usually resorted to when use is made of this route) has a ripening effect on the cervix which facilitates dilatation.

Some analgesic drugs inhibit the oxytocic effect of prostaglandin and should therefore not be used during attempted termination of pregnancy with these agents. Smith and Temple (1973) noted that the mean time to abortion following intra-amniotic administration of $PGF_{2\alpha}$ was significantly prolonged (35 hours $v.$ 14 hours, $p < 0.001$) when a combination of acetaminophen and dextropropoxyphene (Digesic®) was given instead of pethidine. The failure rate was also considerably increased (20% $v.$ 3%). This difference persisted even when the time of administration was taken into account (Smith et $al.$, 1973). In $vitro$ experiments performed by the authors showed that dextropropoxyphene inhibited $PGF_{2\alpha}$–induced contractions, while acetaminophen and pethidine had no such effect.

(b) Laboratory studies

The results of laboratory investigations have been similar to those obtained after administration of natural prostaglandins by other routes (Table 3.10). Again disagreement is noted among various authors regarding the moment of onset and the significance of the decrease in plasma steroid levels observed. Csapo et $al.$ (1972b) believe that the initial sustained contracture and the ensuing decrease in functional capacity of the placenta are the key to the abortifacient action of the prostaglandin. The drop in progesterone production would allow cyclic intrauterine pressure to increase and clinical progress to evolve. Kochenour et $al.$ (1972), Saldana et $al.$ (1973), Craft and Youssefnejadian (1974) and Tyack et $al.$ (1974) indeed observed significant decrements in plasma levels of progesterone and oestrogens in patients who eventually aborted. Simultaneously, the uterine reactivity to test doses of oxytocin increased. But Shutt et $al.$ (1973) noted wide variations in individual values and Symonds et $al.$ (1972) and Roberts et $al.$ (1973) found no consistent changes in steroid levels until after expulsion of the conceptus. These authors felt that intra-amniotic prostaglandin acted by direct stimulation of the myometrium rather than by interference with placental steroidogenesis. Lauersen et $al.$ (1974) noted a drop in plasma progesterone of only 10% six hours after intra-amniotic instillation of $PGF_{2\alpha}$ in spite of the fact that a high level of uterine activity (about 500 Montevideo Units) had developed within one hour of drug administration. In comparison, a much more pronounced drop in progesterone (27%) was observed six hours after intra-amniotic instillation of hypertonic saline, even though in these patients uterine activity was markedly slower to develop. Lauersen and co-workers therefore felt that it was difficult to maintain that the development of myometrial activity following administration of prostaglandin was dependent on the removal of a 'progesterone block'.

Lyneham et $al.$ (1973) found significant alterations in the electroencephalogram (EEG) after intra-amniotic injection of $PGF_{2\alpha}$ for therapeutic abortion. This could not be confirmed by Fraser and Gray (1974b). Neither were significant changes in the EEG detected after intra-amniotic administration of PGE_2 (Fraser and Gray, 1974a; Van der Plaetsen et $al.$, 1974).

All authors agreed that disseminated intravascular coagulation, as seen

Table 3.10 Laboratory investigations performed after intra-amniotic instillation of PGE$_2$ or PGF$_{2\alpha}$ for induction of abortion

Investigation	Result	References
Peripheral blood count	—No change except for raised WBC counts with neutrophilia and lymphocytopenia	Anderson et al., 1972a Brenner et al., 1972b Brenner et al., 1973c Gillett et al., 1972b, 1973 Wiqvist et al., 1973b Lauersen and Wilson, 1974a Golbus and Erickson, 1974
	—Decreased platelet count	Kochenour et al., 1972
Prothrombin time Partial thromboplastin time Thrombin clotting time Factors V, VIII and X Plasma fibrinogen Fibrinogen survival time Plasma levels of fibrin degradation products	No change indicative of consumption coagulo-pathy	Anderson et al., 1972a, b Brenner et al., 1973c Badraoui et al., 1973b Bell and Wentz, 1973 Phillips et al., 1974 Golbus and Erickson, 1974
Electrolytes Creatinine Blood urea nitrogen Total serum bilirubin Alkaline phosphatase SGOT, SGPT Lactic dehydrogenase	No change	Anderson et al., 1972a Brenner et al., 1972b Kochenour et al., 1972 Gillett et al., 1972b, 1973 Lauersen and Wilson, 1974a Golbus and Erickson, 1974
Plasma cortisol	—No consistent change	Kochenour et al., 1972 Golbus and Erickson, 1974 Lauersen and Wilson, 1974a
	—Rise during the course of abortion	Leslie and Laufe, 1972 Dillon et al., 1974
Plasma progesterone	—Drop during the course of abortion	Kochenour et al., 1972 Saldana et al., 1973 Tyack et al., 1974 Dillon et al., 1974 Craft and Youssefnejadian, 1974 Lauersen et al., 1974
	—Drop only after placental separation	Shearman et al., 1972 Leslie and Laufe, 1972 Symonds et al., 1972 Roberts et al., 1973
Plasma oestrogens	—Drop during the course of abortion	Shearman et al., 1972 Shutt et al., 1973 Craft and Youssefnejadian, 1974
	—Drop only after placental separation	Tyack et al., 1974 Roberts et al. 1973
Serum HCG	Drop, only after abortion	Shearman et al., 1972
Plasma HCS	Drop during the course of abortion	Ylikorkala and Pennanen, 1973 Lauersen et al., 1974
Urine analysis	No change	Gillett et al., 1972b, 1973

[continued

Table 3.10 [*continued*]

Investigation	Result	References
Urine levels of oestrone, oestradiol, oestriol and pregnanediol	Drop during the course of abortion	Lauersen *et al.*, 1974
EEG	$PGF_{2\alpha}$—significant changes	Lyneham *et al.*, 1973
	—no changes	Fraser and Gray, 1974b
	PGE_2 —no changes	Fraser and Gray, 1974a
		Van der Plaetsen *et al.*, 1974

following intrauterine instillation of hypertonic saline, did not take place after intra-amniotic injection of prostaglandin (all studies done with $PGF_{2\alpha}$). Phillips *et al.* (1974) found no soluble fibrin monomer complexes. Several of the coagulation factors were even increased (platelets, fibrinogen, factors V, VIII, X and XI) which these investigators attributed to an inflammatory-type reaction similar to that seen in the postoperative period, in arthritic syndromes, in some malignancies and in infection.

The fetus after abortion with intra-amniotic prostaglandins may occasionally show signs of life (Anderson *et al.*, 1972a; Naftolin *et al.*, 1972; Golbus and Erickson, 1974) but Lauersen and Wilson (1974a), using an ultrasonic Doppler apparatus, showed that—in the majority of cases—the fetal heart was lost $1\frac{1}{2}$ to 2 hours after instillation of $PGF_{2\alpha}$. Golbus and Erickson (1974) studied tissues recovered at abortion induced by intra-amniotic injection of 40 mg $PGF_{2\alpha}$. Twenty-four of the 28 attempts (86%) at tissue culture from fetal skin, lung or thymus were successful and good karyotypes were obtained easily. The four failures were due to bacterial contamination. Assays for fetal intestinal β-galactosidase and β-glucuronidase activities gave results that were comparable to those obtained following hysterotomy. The authors felt that in cases where fetal cell cultures were required for verification of prenatal diagnosis of metabolic or genetic defect, for virus culture or for production of attenuated vaccines, this method of termination of pregnancy was clearly superior to the intra-amniotic instillation of hypertonic saline which makes the establishment of fetal cell cultures virtually impossible.

(c) Comments

To conclude, for termination of second trimester pregnancies with natural prostaglandins, the intra-amniotic route of administration appears as the most satisfactory both in terms of high success rates and low incidence of side-effects.

3.2.7 Other routes

Other routes of administration of natural prostaglandins for interruption of pregnancy have not been systematically evaluated. Wentz and King (1972) established that, when compared to hypertonic saline solutions, $PGF_{2\alpha}$ (5 mg) injected into the myometrium of the pregnant rhesus monkey induced no histologic changes. Possibly, direct intramyometrial injection of small doses of prostaglandins would effect uterine stimulation without causing many systemic side-effects. A transvaginal approach with injection of the drug into the uterine isthmus could be used without undue difficulties. Similarly, the uterine effects of intracervical injections of prostaglandins are worth an investigation. In both cases, however, care should be taken not to inject the drug inadvertently into a maternal vessel.

Intrarectal administration of PGE_2 or $PGF_{2\alpha}$ has been used by Karim and Sharma (1971a) for stimulation of labour at term after spontaneous rupture of the membranes had made the continued use of the vaginal route impractical. To the best of our knowledge, it has not been used for induction of abortion. Most likely it would be effective but would cause side-effects of the same magnitude of those seen following vaginal administration.

Karim et al. (1972b) and Anderson et al. (1973) each reported a case of inadvertent intravesical instillation of $PGF_{2\alpha}$ at attempted amniocentesis. Neither uterine contractions nor side-effects followed, but in one of the cases (Karim et al., 1972b) vesical spasm (50 mmHg) was elicited that lasted for 25–30 min. It is likely that the prostaglandin is being transferred across the transitional epithelium of the bladder in amounts insufficient to stimulate an organ at a distance.

3.3 THE USE OF PROSTAGLANDIN ANALOGUES FOR INTERRUPTION OF PREGNANCY

Naturally occurring prostaglandins are a safer and more effective means of interrupting second trimester pregnancy than methods previously known. Yet in order to avoid an unacceptable rate of side-effects, these compounds need to be administered directly into the target organ, the uterus, making use of the extra- or the intra-amniotic route. Metabolic inactivation of the prostaglandin necessitates administration of a large single dose or smaller multiple doses. To circumvent these drawbacks, synthetic analogues of the natural compounds have been evaluated. The 15-methyl prostaglandins, which are resistant to degradation by the enzyme 15-hydroxydehydrogenase (Yankee and Bundy, 1972), have proved the most effective so far. But as they are not entirely devoid of effects upon other systems, they are best given extra- or intraamniotically. It is hoped that in the near future, other analogues will become available that will be more specifically oxytocic and will permit systemic administration for interruption of pregnancy.

3.3.1 ω-homo-PGE$_1$

Gillespie et al. (1971) first used an 'unnatural' prostaglandin for therapeutic abortion. These authors terminated two of three mid-trimester pregnancies by intravenously infusing 5–6.7 μg min^{-1} of ω-homo-PGE$_1$. In the third case, oxytocin was required for completion of abortion. No side-effects were reported.

3.3.2 15-methyl analogues of PGE_2 and $PGF_{2\alpha}$

(a) 15(S),15-methyl-PGE_2 methyl ester

Karim and collaborators (Karim and Sharma, 1972; Karim et al., 1972a; Karim et al., 1973) first tested 15(S),15-methyl-PGE_2 methyl ester as an abortifacient. Depending upon the route of administration, it proved 80–400 times more oxytocic and—except for the intra-amniotic route—its duration of action was three times longer than that of PGE_2.

Eight-hourly administration of 25–50 μg intramuscularly or of 50 μg intra-vaginally caused abortion in all of 14 patients within 18 hours. Side-effects included nausea, vomiting, occasional diarrhoea, feeling cold and shivering. Three dose schedules of intra-amniotic administration of 15(S),15-methyl-PGE_2 methyl ester were evaluated. Pregnancy was successfully terminated in all of 78 volunteers. The mean abortion time was 14 hours 45 min following 10-hourly instillation of 50 μg; 11 hours 45 min when 100 μg was given 10-hourly, and 14 hours after a single intra-amniotic dose of 200 μg. Side-effects were limited to nausea, vomiting and a rise in temperature in a small number of patients. The main advantage resulting from an increase in dosage was the reduction in need for a further injection. To assess the safety of the drug, 50–75 μg 15(S),15-methyl-PGE_2 methyl ester was injected directly into the placenta or the peritoneal cavity of four women. All were successfully aborted without major complications. Instillation of the prostaglandin into the bladder, in one case, caused a sustained contracture of this organ but had no effect on the uterus. In a later study, Amy et al. (1973) administered 100 μg 15(S),15-methyl-PGE_2 methyl ester at 24-hour intervals to 20 patients at 14–22 weeks' gestation. All were successfully aborted in a mean time of 16 hours 30 min. Only two patients required a second injection of prostaglandin. Three women had a rise in temperature of 1.0–1.5 °C and three had vomiting. Neither diarrhoea nor shivering was observed. The high success rate (90%) and the very low rate of side-effects following a single intra-amniotic injection of 100 μg 15(S),15-methyl-PGE_2 methyl ester puts this technique among the best available for termination of second trimester pregnancy. It is nearly a 'one-shot' method and there is therefore virtually no need for insertion of a catheter into the amniotic cavity. Intra-amniotic administration of 200 μg 15(S),15-methyl-PGE_2 methyl ester (10 patients) offered no advantage and, besides, it was felt that inadvertent intravascular injection of such high dose could cause severe systemic reactions.

Ballard and Quilligan (1974) gave an intramuscular injection of 10 μg 15-methyl-PGE_2 methyl ester to 20 patients every two hours until the fetus was expelled or for a maximum of eight injections. Within 24 hours 95% aborted with a mean injection–abortion time of 9 hours 6 min. Ten women experienced one or more episodes of vomiting (four out of five without chlorpromazine pretreatment and six out of fifteen with chlorpromazine). Seventeen patients had one or more episodes of diarrhoea. All 20 subjects experienced shivering and had a temperature elevation of at least 1.0 °C which returned to normal shortly after abortion.

Salmon et al. (1974) observed a drop in maternal plasma levels of HCG, progesterone and oestrogens following intramuscular administration of

15(S),15-methyl-PGE$_2$ methyl ester to women at 6–11 weeks' gestation who eventually aborted successfully. They attributed this decrease in circulating hormones to a hypoxic insult to the feto–placental unit, secondary to the rise in intrauterine pressure.

A substantial advantage in the use of this analogue resides in the fact that there is a relatively narrow difference between the dosages required for interruption of pregnancy by the intra-amniotic (50–100 μg 10–24 hourly) and the systemic routes (25–37.5 μg eight-hourly). Inadvertent administration or rapid absorption of the compound into the maternal circulation after intra-amniotic injection should, therefore, not have dramatic consequences.

(b) 15(R),15-methyl-PGE$_2$ methyl ester

Karim *et al.* (1973) found this compound to be 10 times less oxytocic than its 15(S) equivalent. With appropriate dosage, these investigators succeeded in terminating pregnancy in all of 10 women given 15(R),15-methyl-PGE$_2$ methyl ester via the intravenous, intramuscular, intravaginal or intra-amniotic route.

(c) 15 (S),15-methyl-PGF$_{2\alpha}$ (free acid)

This compound is 20–100 times more potent as an oxytocic than its parent compound PGF$_{2\alpha}$ and displays a threefold increase in duration of action on the uterus (Karim and Sharma, 1972; Karim *et al.*, 1972a; Wiqvist *et al.*, 1972d). Unlike PGF$_{2\alpha}$, intramuscular injection of this analogue does not cause local irritation.

The Stockholm group of investigators has most extensively reported on the use of 15(S),15-methyl-PGF$_{2\alpha}$ for interruption of pregnancy. They succeeded in terminating mid-trimester pregnancy within 10 hours in eight out of 10 subjects given a continuous infusion of 5 μg min^{-1} of this drug. The incidence of side-effects was comparable to that seen with infusion of an equally efficient dose of PGF$_{2\alpha}$ (i.e. 75 μg min^{-1}) (Toppozada *et al.*, 1972a; Wiqvist *et al.*, 1972d).

Bygdeman and collaborators (Bygdeman *et al.*, 1972c; Bygdeman *et al.*, 1972d) reported on the successful induction of abortion by intrauterine administration of 15(S),15-methyl-PGF$_{2\alpha}$. The experience of the group with intra-amniotic instillation of the analogue was summarised in two later papers (Wiqvist *et al.*, 1973a; Wiqvist *et al.*, 1973b). Hypertonus and rhythmic contractile activity were slower to develop after intra-amniotic injection of the analogue than with PGF$_{2\alpha}$. But uterine activity which—depending on the dose—reached its maximum after 4–9 hours, was subsequently maintained at this level throughout the 24-hour observation period or until abortion. In comparison, intra-amniotic doses of PGF$_{2\alpha}$ caused a rapid uterine response which reached its maximum within 2–3 hours, and then abated progressively. Intra-amniotic instillation of a single dose of 1.0, 2.5 or 5.0 mg 15(S),15-methyl-PGF$_{2\alpha}$ achieved abortion in 46, 98 and 95% of patients in mean times of 20 hours 6 min, 18 hours 48 min and 18 hours 36 min respectively. The authors felt that 2.5 mg of the analogue was the optimal dose for 'single-shot' administration via the intra-amniotic route. It was more effective and caused fewer side-effects (mean of 1.5 episodes of vomiting per patient) than single doses of 40 mg $PGF_{2\alpha}$ (76% success rate in a mean time of 18 hours 30 min; 3.3 episodes of emesis) or doses of 25 mg $PGF_{2\alpha}$ repeated after 24 hours (97% success rate in a mean time of 28 hours; 2.0 episodes of emesis). Intra-amniotic 15(S),15-methyl-$PGF_{2\alpha}$ caused no bronchospasm in asthmatic patients (Toppozada et al., 1972b).

In contrast to the results of the Swedish investigators discussed above, Karim and Sivasamboo (1974) have reported high efficacy with a single intra-amniotic injection of 1 mg 15(S),15-methyl-$PGF_{2\alpha}$. These authors compared the efficacy and side-effects of 1 mg and 2.5 mg of the analogue in 50 second trimester patients (25 in each group). The abortifacient efficacy of 15-methyl-$PGF_{2\alpha}$ was similar in both groups; over 90% of the patients aborted with a single dose. There was a higher incidence of vomiting, diarrhoea and incomplete abortion in the group treated with 2.5 mg of the analogue. Although the mean injection–abortion interval in the 2.5 mg group was slightly shorter, the authors concluded that intra-amniotic administration of 1 mg 15-methyl-$PGF_{2\alpha}$ provides a better regime, giving high efficacy with a single dose, a low incidence of side-effects and a greater safety in case of inadvertent entry of the intra-amniotic dose into the systemic circulation.

Wiqvist et al. (1973a) and Wiqvist et al. (1974) compared the abortifacient efficacy of extra-amniotic $PGF_{2\alpha}$ and 15(S),15-methyl-$PGF_{2\alpha}$ given in three different vehicles:

1. physiological saline,
2. a high molecular weight polysaccharide solution (Hyskon®), and
3. a solid excipient of triglycerides for administration of the prostaglandin in the form of an intrauterine pellet (2×10 mm).

Pellets gave a high rate of failure. The most effective preparation combined 15(S),15-methyl-$PGF_{2\alpha}$ with the viscous Hyskon® solution. This was instilled into the extra-amniotic space via a Nelaton catheter, which was removed immediately afterwards. An initial dose of 200–400 μg of the analogue was usually insufficient to achieve abortion and additional doses were required. However, a single dose of 500–850 μg 15(S),15-methyl-$PGF_{2\alpha}$ in Hyskon® successfully aborted 46 of 55 subjects (84%) within 36 hours. The mean abortion time was 13 hours 36 min. In the majority of failures, some cervical dilatation had been achieved and abortion could be accomplished by supplemental prostaglandin therapy. For comparison, 2–4 hourly administration of 250–750 μg $PGF_{2\alpha}$ (in saline) could terminate 90% of pregnancies in a mean time of 20 hours 54 min. The incidence of side-effects was comparable for both series: each patient had an average of 1.5 episode of vomiting and diarrhoea and required two injections of an analgesic. In both series, 5% of the subjects required a transfusion because of heavy bleeding.

Karim and Sharma (1972) and Karim et al. (1972a) administered 15(S),15-methyl-$PGF_{2\alpha}$ intramuscularly (250–500 μg eight-hourly), intravaginally (500 μg 10-hourly) or intra-amniotically (500 μg 10-hourly) and reported successful abortion in all of their 17 patients. The mean times to abortion were 20 hours, 15 hours 10 min and 16 hours 13 min, respectively. Side-effects were minimal when the intra-amniotic route was used, but when given intravaginally or intramuscularly, the analogue caused more frequent gastrointestinal upset than $PGF_{2\alpha}$ and the authors felt that this would limit its usefulness as a systemic abortifacient.

Lauersen and Wilson (1975) induced mid-trimester abortion in 35 volunteers by two-hourly intramuscular injection of 250–750 μg 15(S),15-methyl-$PGF_{2\alpha}$. All patients aborted within 36 hours, in a mean time of 16 hours. Despite routine treatment with prochlorperazine and diphenoxylate hydrochloride, 32 subjects experienced one or more episodes of vomiting and 25 had diarrhoea. However, the premedication had a sedative effect on the patients who complained of very little discomfort and never required additional analgesic therapy.

Leibman et al. (1974) attempted termination of second trimester pregnancy by intramuscular injection of 15-methyl-$PGF_{2\alpha}$ in 16 patients. Doses of 250 μg were repeated at eight-hourly intervals until a maximum of 750 μg was given. Only nine patients aborted within 48 hours of the first injection. Side-effects were frequent and consisted of nausea (10 patients), vomiting (11 patients), diarrhoea (6 patients) and hot flushes (1 patient). One patient had postpartum haemorrhage requiring blood transfusion.

3.3.3 PGE_2 methyl ester and $PGF_{2\alpha}$ methyl ester

In a preliminary study (Karim et al., 1973), PGE_2 methyl ester, when given by bolus intravenous injection, was found to be five times more potent than PGE_2 (free acid) in stimulating the mid-pregnant human uterus. $PGF_{2\alpha}$ methyl ester and $PGF_{2\alpha}$ (free acid) were equipotent.

Karim and Amy (1974) studied the abortifacient efficacy of PGE_2 methyl ester in 25 volunteers at 12–24 weeks' gestation. Given by the intra-amniotic route, the analogue was five times more potent in its uterine stimulating activity than PGE_2 free acid. When administered vaginally, it was 10 times more active. The latent period between the administration of PGE_2 methyl ester by various routes and the onset of uterine stimulation was considerably shorter, but the duration of uterine response was approximately the same as for PGE_2.

Intra-amniotic administration of 1 mg PGE_2 methyl ester at 12-hourly intervals to eight women caused six to abort in a mean time of 17 hours 24 min. In one patient spontaneous rupture of the membranes occurred after the second intra-amniotic dose and pregnancy was terminated by vaginal instillation of 2.5 mg PGE_2 methyl ester. The eighth patient failed to respond to the prostaglandin as well as to 50% intra-amniotic glucose and intravenous oxytocin. Pregnancy was eventually terminated by hysterotomy.

In a further nine patients, PGE_2 methyl ester was given intra-amniotically in doses of 2 mg 12-hourly. Eight subjects aborted in a mean time of 14 hours 4 min. The ninth one because of untimely rupture of the membranes, was aborted by vaginal administration of 5 mg of the analogue. Three women given a single dose of 2.5 mg PGE_2 methyl ester intra-amniotically aborted in a mean time of 15 hours.

Vaginal administration of a single dose of 2.5 mg PGE_2 methyl ester in three patients interrupted pregnancy in all in a mean time of 12 hours 15 min.

Evaluation of the extra-amniotic route for administration of PGE_2 methyl ester, in two volunteers, was not pursued beyond the first 250 μg dose because of rigors in one and tachycardia in the other.

At effective abortifacient doses of PGE_2 methyl ester, gastrointestinal, central nervous and cardiovascular side-effects considerably more severe than those seen with PGE_2 were observed. Intense shivering and pyrexia were most troublesome. One patient given 2.5 mg PGE_2 methyl ester vaginally developed acute febrile encephalopathy that required immediate treatment. Diarrhoea was more frequently encountered than vomiting. Due to systemmic absorption, side-effects were most severe after vaginal administration. But, whatever the route of delivery used, side-effects appeared within minutes, indicating a rapid passage of the drug into the circulation.

In conclusion, it was felt that PGE_2 methyl ester did not compare favourably with PGE_2 or its 15-methyl analogues.

3.3.4 16,16-dimethyl-PGE₂ methyl ester

Karim and Amy (1973) administered this compound by different routes to 23 patients in the second trimester of pregnancy. The highest rate of abortifacient efficacy was attained by intravenous injection of one or more doses of 25 μg of the analogue and amounted to only 66%. Vomiting, diarrhoea, pyrexia and shivering were frequently associated with the use of the oral, intravenous and intramuscular routes. Intra-amniotic instillation of 16,16-dimethyl-PGE_2 methyl ester was free of side-effects but required as much as 800 μg (i.e. 32 times the effective intravenous dose). Inadvertent injection or rapid absorption of this amount of the drug into the maternal vascular compartment would undoubtedly cause severe systemic reactions. In view of these drawbacks, the authors felt that this analogue was not suitable for induction of abortion.

16,16-dimethyl-PGE_2 (free acid and methyl ester) administered orally have a stimulant effect on the pregnant human uterus (Karim et al., 1974b). Pregnancy was terminated in 12 out of 20 second trimester patients with two-hourly oral doses of 100 μg of these analogues. The authors concluded that the relatively high incidence of gastrointestinal side-effects—nausea, vomiting and diarrhoea—would tend to limit the usefulness of orally administered 16,16-dimethyl PGE_2 and its methyl ester as abortifacients.

3.3.5 20-ethyl-PGF₂ₐ

Sharp and Burslem (1973) intravenously infused 5–125 μg min^{-1} racemic 20-ethyl-$PGF_{2\alpha}$ (ICI 74 205) to six patients at 9–17 weeks' gestation. Five subjects aborted within 49 hours, the sixth required oxytocin augmentation. The mean interval to abortion for the entire group was 25 hours 15 min. No effect was noted on blood pressure, respiratory rate or body temperature, but all patients had venous erythema at the site of infusion and frequent bouts of vomiting and diarrhoea. Diphenoxylate was given without effect to two of the subjects.

Embrey *et al.* (1973a) terminated early first trimester pregnancy (38–64 days amenorrhoea) in six of eight volunteers with 0.5–1.0 mg ICI 74 205 given two-hourly by the intrauterine route for 12 hours. For comparison, all of seven women aborted after administration of 0.5–1.0 mg $PGF_{2\alpha}$ two-hourly via the same route. All patients complained of moderate to severe uterine cramps; four women given $PGF_{2\alpha}$ and two given the analogue vomited. Uterine bleeding lasted for 5–21 days. The authors felt this method offered no advantage over conventional first trimester termination.

Conclusion

Only a limited number of synthetic analogues of prostaglandins have been evaluated for their abortifacient effect. Results so far are encouraging. There is very little doubt that given by the intrauterine routes the 15-methyl analogues of PGE_2 and $PGF_{2\alpha}$ are safer and more efficacious than the natural compounds for the termination of late first trimester and second trimester pregnancies. Results of studies involving non-invasive (non-uterine) routes have not been very encouraging. Given by the oral route only the 16,16-dimethyl analogues show a limited efficacy. The efficacy of the various 15-methyl analogues, given by the intramuscular route, is high but once again side-effects are prohibitive. It is hoped that the newer analogues now being evaluated will provide better compounds.

3.4 COMBINATION OF PROSTAGLANDINS WITH ACCESSORY MEANS FOR TERMINATING PREGNANCY

3.4.1 Intravenous oxytocin

The uterotonic effect of oxytocin is negligible during the first half of pregnancy, but it is markedly enhanced after exposure of the myometrium to prostaglandins (Brummer, 1971; Embrey, 1971a). This observation led Brummer to suggest that infusion of a low dose of prostaglandin, for priming of the uterus, followed by that of oxytocin might be clinically effective in promoting abortion without causing the side-effects usually associated with high systemic doses of prostaglandins. Various regimens combining the two oxytocics have been tested.

Gillespie (1973) succeeded in interrupting 14 out of 20 pregnancies by intravenously infusing 1 μg min^{-1} PGE_2 or 10 μg min^{-1} $PGF_{2\alpha}$ (i.e. one-fifth of the usual dose) in combination with oxytocin (64 mU min^{-1}). The infusion rate was doubled after 24 hours. The mean induction–abortion interval was 32 hours 15 min. No side-effects were noted. The same protocol, but without oxytocin, caused only one out of 17 women to abort. Five additional subjects were treated with an infusion of 2 μg min^{-1} PGE_2 or 20 μg min^{-1} $PGF_{2\alpha}$ concomitantly with 128 mU min^{-1} oxytocin. All aborted in a mean time of 13 hours 45 min. Again, there were no side-effects.

The combination of intra-amniotic prostaglandin with intravenous oxytocin was evaluated by Anderson *et al.* (1972b). These authors were unable to shorten the induction–abortion interval by infusing 66 mU min^{-1} oxytocin after intra-amniotic injection of 40 mg PGF$_{2\alpha}$, but gastrointestinal side-effects were two to three times more frequent. Kochenour *et al.* (1972) could terminate eight of 10 mid-trimester pregnancies by intravenous administration of 250–333 mU min^{-1} oxytocin, after intra-amniotic instillation of a low dose (10 or 15 mg) PGF$_{2\alpha}$. The mean abortion time amounted to 17 hours 52 min. Seppälä *et al.* (1972) observed a marked shortening of the mean induction–abortion interval (from 26 hours 36 min to 17 hours 18 min), an increase in cumulative abortion rates (from 43 to 81% within 24 hours) and a reduction in the mean total dose of prostaglandin (from 36.6 mg to 26.4 mg PGF$_{2\alpha}$) when 133 mU min^{-1} oxytocin was given intravenously in association with the intra-amniotic injection of 25 mg PGF$_{2\alpha}$ (repeated after 24 hours, if necessary). Corson and Bolognese (1974c) compared the efficacy of a regimen combining intra-amniotic PGF$_{2\alpha}$ (40 mg, repeated after 24 hours if necessary) and intravenous oxytocin (83 mU min^{-1}, starting six hours after prostaglandin administration) with that of intra-amniotic PGF$_{2\alpha}$ alone. The mean abortion time (authors' definition: time to placental expulsion) was shortened from 21 hours 30 min to 15 hours 54 min. MacKenzie *et al.* (1975) observed a marked shortening of the abortion time when oxytocin was given together with two intra-amniotic doses of 10 mg PGE$_2$, injected at six-hourly intervals.

Similarly, Embrey *et al.* (1973b) noted a substantial decrease in mean abortion time (primigravidas: from 20 hours 42 min to 14 hours 42 min; multigravidas: from 18 to 12$\frac{1}{2}$ hours) when intravenous oxytocin (80 mU min^{-1}, begun after six hours) was combined with extra-amniotic administration of 200 μg PGE$_2$, two-hourly. Morewood (1973) terminated pregnancy in all of 38 patients by the extra-amniotic administration of 200 μg PGE$_2$, two-hourly, combined with intravenous infusion of 55 mU min^{-1} oxytocin (started 2–3 hours after the initial dose of PGE$_2$). The mean induction–abortion interval was 13 hours 42 min. Alderman and Thelwall-Jones (1973) combining hourly extra-amniotic administration of 200 μg PGE$_2$ with infusion of 100 mU min^{-1} oxytocin succeeded in aborting all of 28 women in a mean time of 10 hours 6 min. Seppälä *et al.* (1973) reduced the mean abortion time following hourly extra-amniotic administration of 500 μg PGF$_{2\alpha}$ from 26 hours 54 min to 22 hours 6 min by the simultaneous infusion of 100–133 mU min^{-1} oxytocin.

Empirically it was found that oxytocin was often effective in accelerating or reactivating the process of abortion, in cases where progress was poor following prostaglandin administration. The above mentioned prospective studies—that of Anderson and collaborators excepted—clearly establish that prostaglandin and oxytocin work synergistically when given in the second trimester of pregnancy.

The combination of both drugs could be particularly valuable when prostaglandins need to be given systemically (e.g. intravenously, for missed abortion, untimely rupture of the membranes, etc.). The dose of prostaglandin could thus be reduced to a level (e.g. 2 μg min^{-1} PGE$_2$) causing little or no side-effects. Combining intravenous oxytocin with extra- or intra-amniotic prostaglandin somewhat complicates the procedure and requires more nursing supervision. Administration of such high doses of oxytocin as used by many investigators (100 mU min⁻¹ and more during several hours) exposes the patient to the risk of developing water retention, hyponatraemia and convulsions. At these dose levels, oxytocin should be given in electrolyte mixtures (e.g. normal or half-normal saline, Ringer's lactate solution) and a careful record of fluid intake and output should be kept.

3.4.2 Intra-amniotic urea

For termination of mid-trimester pregnancy, intra-amniotic urea is safer but less effective than hypertonic saline. When given alone, it has a 20% failure rate for inducing abortion within 72 hours. Infusion of high doses of oxytocin shortens the time to abortion and increases the success rate. Craft and Musa (1971) reported on two groups of 15 patients each treated with intra-amniotic urea in conjunction with either 137.5 or 275 mU min⁻¹ oxytocin intravenously. All patients aborted. The mean induction abortion intervals were 26 hours 25 min in the first group and 18 hours 48 min in the second. Twelve patients had one or more episodes of vomiting.

At these dose levels, oxytocin may cause water intoxication and close supervision is required. In an attempt to develop a safe and effective 'single-shot' technique, Craft combined the intra-amniotic administration of urea with that of PGE_2 (Craft, 1973b, c, d, e; 1974). The procedure involved aspiration of 100–140 ml amniotic fluid, followed by intra-amniotic injection of 80 g urea (in 80 ml Hartman's solution) and 5 or 10 mg PGE_2. Opiates or epidural block were provided for analgesia.

Twenty patients at 15–22 weeks' gestation were given 80 g urea and 10 mg PGE_2 intra-amniotically. Abortion occurred within 24 hours in all, with a mean time of 10 hours 23 min. Fourteen patients had vomiting and four had diarrhoea. In a second group of 23 patients, administration of 80 g urea and 5 mg PGE_2 proved just as effective. Again, all patients aborted within 24 hours, with a mean time of 9 hours 53 min. But side-effects remained frequent: 16 patients had vomiting and two had diarrhoea, one patient suffered a lateral cervical tear requiring repair. Clearly, the combination of intra-amniotic urea and prostaglandin was more effective than administration of prostaglandin alone, but it was accompanied by a higher incidence of side-effects, probably due to an acceleration of the systemic absorption of PGE_2.

Bowen-Simpkins' data (1973) are in complete agreement with those of Craft. By administering 80 g urea and 5 mg PGE_2 intra-amniotically, this author could terminate pregnancy in 29 of 30 patients within 24 hours. The 30th woman aborted in 26 hours, after stimulation with intravenous oxytocin was started at 24 hours. The mean induction–abortion interval was 10 hours 30 min. Nine patients vomited on one or more occasions, one had diarrhoea. In one case, a partial annular detachment of the cervix was noted.

Craft and Youssefnejadian (1974) have now evaluated a regimen combining intra-amniotic injection of 80 g urea and 2.5 mg PGE_2. Of the 25 patients treated, all aborted in a mean time of 8 hours 57 min. Vomiting was noted in 11 subjects and diarrhoea in one. There was no cervical injury in this series.

In another study, Craft et al. (1974) administered 80 g urea and 20 mg $PGF_{2\alpha}$ to 20 patients at 15–22 weeks' gestation. All patients aborted within 24 hours, in a mean time of 12 hours 38 min; 12 had vomiting and two diarrhoea. Two subjects required suturing of cervical lacerations. Radio-immunoassays of plasma progesterone and oestriol showed markedly de-creased levels only one hour after injection of urea and prostaglandin, suggest-ing an early insult to the feto–placental unit (Craft *et al.*, 1973; Craft *et al.*, 1974). The efficacy of the 'single-shot' method developed by Craft compares favourably with other techniques of interruption of mid-trimester preg-nancy. Further reduction in the dose of prostaglandin (and possibly urea), or the use of a more selective analogue, might bring about a more acceptable rate of side-effects.

3.4.3 Laminaria tents

Manabe's paper (1971) caused—particularly in the United States—a resur-gence of interest in the use of laminaria tents as part of abortive procedures. The dried out stem of laminaria digitata is highly hygrophilic, and, when in-serted into the moist cervical canal, exerts a slow, progressive dilating effect. This advantageously replaces acute instrumental dilatation, often the most difficult and traumatising part of a vaginal termination procedure (Eaton *et al.*, 1972; Newton, 1972—see also Section 3.5.3). In the second trimester, the treatment–abortion interval is substantially reduced when intra-amnio-tic instillation of hypertonic saline is combined with the insertion of laminar-ia tents into the cervical canal. At the same time, the risk of posterior isthmic tear caused by cervical dystocia may be avoided (Hale and Pion, 1972; Lischke and Goodlin, 1972). A logical development has consisted in the exploration of a possible facilitating effect of laminaria tents upon prosta-glandin–induced interruption of pregnancy.

Brenner *et al.* (1973d) reported on the intra-amniotic injection of 25 mg $PGF_{2\alpha}$ (repeated, if necessary after 6, 24 and 30 hours). In half of their pa-tients, 1–5 laminaria tents were inserted into the cervix 30 min before amnio-centesis. Subjects pretreated with laminaria had a shorter mean abortion time (14 hours 36 min *v.* 18 hours 54 min), higher cumulative abortion rates (95% aborted within 24 hours *v.* 68%) and a higher ultimate success rate (100% aborted within 48 hours *v.* 96%). The frequency of side-effects was similar in both groups. Despite a sharper increase in leucocytosis and neutrophilia in the 'laminaria group', there was no concomitant increase in clinical infection. Monitoring of uterine activity revealed that laminaria tents had no oxytocic ef-fect but facilitated abortion by dilating the cervix. The latter statement is not in agreement with the observations of Manabe *et al.* (1973) who found that the presence of 2–4 laminaria tents in the cervix (without any other form of stimulation) caused an increase in uterine activity after 12 hours.

Stubblefield *et al.* (1974) inserted 1–3 laminaria tents into the cervix 14–19 hours before intra-amniotic instillation of 40 mg $PGF_{2\alpha}$. In their series of 11 patients, the mean prostaglandin administration–abortion interval was nine hours 36 min. There was no clinical evidence of infection in any of the subjects. Golbus (1974) placed 1–2 laminaria tents into the cervix imme-diately before amniocentesis in 20 out of 40 patients given 40 mg $PGF_{2\alpha}$ intra-amniotically. The mean abortion time was significantly shorter (15 hours *v.* 21 hours 42 min) in the 'laminaria group', in which there was also a decreased demand for narcotic analgesics and a 50% reduction in gastrointestinal side-effects.

Engel *et al.* (1973) combined in an elaborate protocol the use of a laminaria tent (inserted on the evening prior to prostaglandin administration), intravenous oxytocin (105–250 mU min^{-1}, commenced one hour before prostaglandin administration) and intra-amniotic instillation of 15 mg $PGF_{2\alpha}$. All 20 patients aborted within 24 hours of prostaglandin administration, in a mean time of 9 hours 24 min. However, Corson and Bolognese (1974c) found no advantage in inserting a laminaria tent (at the time of amniocentesis) in patients given 40 mg $PGF_{2\alpha}$ intra-amniotically and 83–166 mU min^{-1} oxytocin, starting six hours after amniocentesis. The mean abortion time in the 'laminaria group' was 16 hours 6 min as compared to 15 hours 54 min in the other group.

It has been stated elsewhere (Section 3.2) that cervical resistance accounts for a major part in determining the outcome of the attempted termination procedure. The preceding data—those of Corson and Bolognese excepted—indicate that cervically placed laminaria tents facilitate prostaglandin-induced abortions. They also seem to offer a satisfactory mode of prevention of cervico–vaginal fistulae, a complication that follows uterine stimulation in the presence of a rigid cervical os.

So far laminaria tents have been used solely in conjunction with intra-amniotic prostaglandin and a criticism that can be made is that both the placement of the laminaria tents and the amniocentesis require expertise. A possible improvement would consist in the incorporation of a prostaglandin (preferably an analogue with long duration of action) into the laminaria stem or into synthetic hygrophilic material for slow intrauterine release, making it a one-step procedure.

3.5 SPECIAL APPLICATIONS

3.5.1 Management of hydatidiform mole

Hydatidiform mole predisposes to the development of pre-eclamptic toxaemia, uterine haemorrhage and choriocarcinoma. Evacuation of the uterine contents is advisable once the diagnosis is made. Hysterectomy is still exceptionally resorted to in older multiparas, but, in view of the availability of newer techniques, hysterotomy, once the standard form of treatment, is progressively being abandoned. Oxytocin infusion has met with a certain success, but a high dosage needs to be given, which may result in water retention, hyponatraemia and convulsions. At present suction curettage and administration of prostaglandins appear as the two most promising alternatives for dealing with hydatidiform mole.

The successful use of prostaglandins to effect expulsion of molar tissue was first reported by Karim (1970), who administered an infusion of PGE_2 at the rate of 5 μg min^{-1} to one patient and observed abortion after 10 hours. Additional data from Filshie (1971), Karim and Trussell (1971), Karim (1972), Embrey *et al.* (1974), Roberts (1974) and Thiery and Amy (unpublished) have confirmed the efficacy of prostaglandin therapy for this specific indication. All 15 cases were successfully dealt with, within a maximum of 20 hours 30 min, making use of the intravenous, the intravaginal or the extraovular (intrauterine) route. The same dosages were employed as for termination of second trimester pregnancy; side-effects were limited to vomiting and diarrhoea. One patient developed a deep vein thrombosis eight weeks after intrauterine administration of prostaglandin and following her third curettage (Embrey et al., 1974). It is difficult to determine what part, if any, prostaglandin therapy played in the genesis of this complication.

Naismith and Barr (1974) gave simultaneously $0.5-12$ μg min^{-1} PGE$_2$ and oxytocin (2 mU min^{-1} and up) by intravenous infusion to five patients with hydatidiform mole. Expulsion was complete in one patient; in the remaining four, surgical evacuation was required. In no case did the blood loss amount to more than 400 ml. Despite their success, the authors felt that prostaglandins probably had no great clinical application in subjects with a hydatidiform mole because of the efficacy of suction in evacuating the molar tissue.

Karim et al. (1974a) treated 20 patients with hydatidiform mole by intrauterine injection of 30 μg 15(S),15-methyl-PGE$_2$ methyl ester via a transcervically inserted epidural catheter. Five of the 20 patients required a second 30 μg dose after eight hours. Treatment was successful in all cases in a mean time of 9 hours 4 min (range: $2\frac{3}{4}-16$ hours). Curettage was carried out following expulsion of the molar tissue. Side-effects included vomiting (single episode) in three patients, diarrhoea in one, shivering in three and pyrexia in five. Nine of the subjects experienced no side-effects. Blood loss amounted to less than 100 ml in 17 women. In only two cases was a transfusion required for blood loss of 400–500 ml. One of these patients eventually was submitted to hysterectomy because of protracted bleeding of uterine origin that could not be controlled by repeated curettage. The authors felt that termination of molar pregnancy was greatly simplified by the use of this analogue, which proved effective after intrauterine administration of only one or at most two doses.

Recently, Smith (1974a) described a severe systemic reaction consisting of shock with hypotension, bradycardia and rigors, followed by severe suprapubic pain, vomiting, tachycardia (180/min), pyrexia and generalised flushing after transabdominal injection of 20 mg PGE$_2$ into the substance of a hydatidiform mole. Karim (1974), discussing this report, reiterated that intra-amniotic administration of prostaglandin is safe and practical in pregnancies not complicated by molar disease because the amniotic fluid acts as a depot for the drug. The latter then slowly passes across the fetal membranes to stimulate the myometrium. In molar pregnancy, fetal membranes are absent and intrauterine instillation in this situation amounts to extraovular administration. To further emphasise this point, it may be worth reminding that rapid disappearance of the injected contrast material from the uterine cavity is observed when 'amniography' is employed for radiologic confirmation of hydatidiform mole. Instantaneous migration of the dye through the intervesicular septa is followed by prompt absorption into the systemic circulation. The dose of 20 mg PGE$_2$, in the case mentioned above, is 100 times greater than the usual extra-amniotic dose. It is reassuring that even such a massive dose did not prove fatal (Karim, 1974).

In conclusion, evidence to date indicates that prostaglandins when given by the intravenous, intravaginal, or extraovular routes, can safely and effectively terminate molar pregnancy. Definite confirmation of the value of this method of management still awaits a large-scale clinical trial, which could be forthcoming from South-East Asia, where this complication of pregnancy is most frequently encountered. The 'intra-amniotic' method is not of application for termination of molar pregnancy, because of the likelihood of severe systemic reactions. Every effort should be made to rule out hydatidiform mole when the intra-amniotic technique is to be resorted to for interruption of second trimester pregnancy with prostaglandins and injection should be withheld if no free flow of amniotic fluid is obtained after puncture of the uterine cavity. This risk may be minimised in these centres which have ultrasound facilities to diagnose hydatidiform mole.

3.5.2 Management of missed abortion

Fetal death is usually followed within a relatively short time by spontaneous expulsion of the products of conception, but these may, in a number of cases, be retained *in utero* for prolonged periods of time. This occurrence may eventually lead to a syndrome of disseminated intravascular coagulation, hypofibrinogenaemia (together with a depletion in other factors involved in the coagulation process) and haemorrhage. It is therefore advisable to terminate pregnancy once fetal death is confirmed. Medical methods are preferable to surgical evacuation which is attended by a higher risk of trauma, haemorrhage and infection. The use of concentrated solutions of oxytocin has often been disappointing. Intrauterine instillation of hypertonic saline solutions may cause hypernatraemia and augments the risk of coagulopathy. Prostaglandins, so far, have given consistently satisfactory results.

Karim (1970) and Karim and Trussell (1971) first described the use of an intravenous infusion of 5 μg min^{-1} PGE$_2$ in 12 cases of missed abortion (duration intrauterine death: 4–12 weeks). Pregnancy was successfully terminated in all cases after a mean time of 8 hours 30 min. Side-effects comprised vomiting in three patients, diarrhoea in one and venous erythema in four. Filshie (1971), Kinoshita *et al.* (1971), Pedersen *et al.* (1972), Ruppen *et al.* (1972), Miller (1973), Roberts (1974) and Thiery and Amy (unpublished) confirmed the value of natural prostaglandins given intravenously (0.5–5 μg min^{-1} PGE$_2$, 3–6 μg min^{-1} PGE$_1$ or 11–140 μg min^{-1} PGF$_{2\alpha}$) for termination of missed abortion. Of a total of 56 cases, 55 were aborted within 48 hours. Side-effects consisted mainly of vomiting (diarrhoea was less frequent), pyrexia and venous erythema. In the great majority of cases, abortion was complete and no further instrumentation was required. The intra-amniotic instillation of PGE$_2$ (5 mg 10-hourly) has been equally effective. All of 10 cases of missed abortion reported by Karim *et al.* (1972b) were terminated in a mean time of 10 hours. Nausea and vomiting in two women were the only side-effects noted. Thiery and Amy (unpublished) had equal success in five cases treated with various dosages of intra-amniotic PGE$_2$ or PGF$_{2\alpha}$.

Karim (1972, page 110) administered three-hourly doses of 20 mg PGE$_2$ or 50 mg PGF$_{2\alpha}$ intravaginally in six cases of missed abortion and noted expulsion of uterine contents in all after a mean interval of nine hours. Two patients had nausea and vomiting and one developed pyrexia. Southern (personal communication) collected a series of 72 cases of intrauterine death (second and third trimesters combined) which were treated with PGE$_2$ vaginal suppositories (20 mg at 2–3 hours intervals). Seventy of the 72 cases were successfully aborted. The mean time to abortion was 6 hours 54 min when the fetus had been retained for less than three weeks; it was $14\frac{1}{2}$ hours in patients who retained a dead fetus *in utero* for more than three weeks. Side-effects consisted in vomiting in 44% of the patients, diarrhoea in 33% and temperature elevation of more than 1.1 °C in 30%.

Embrey *et al.* (1974) reported favourably on the extra-amniotic administration of PGE$_2$ (200 μg two-hourly) or PGF$_{2\alpha}$ (600 μg two-hourly). Using this form of therapy in 10 cases of missed abortion (seven patients were also given oxytocin intravenously) they succeeded in terminating pregnancy in nine. The mean induction–abortion interval was 14 hours and 12 min. Vomiting occurred occasionally, but less frequently than with intravenous therapy; pyrexia did not occur.

Finally, Naismith and Barr (1974) gave oxytocin (2 mU min^{-1} and up) and PGE$_2$ (0.5–12 μg min^{-1}) simultaneously by the intravenous route for termination of missed abortion. Abortion was successfully induced in all of 28 patients and was complete in 12. Blood loss never exceeded 100 ml. Some of the patients (number not specified) developed pyrexia in excess of 37.7 °C. There was no evidence of water intoxication. The authors felt that the combined use of i.v. oxytocin and PGE$_2$ increased the efficacy of the procedure and allowed for the reduction in the dose of prostaglandin to a level that does not cause gastrointestinal upset. Abortion was achieved faster, the average induction–abortion interval being less than 10 hours and the longest single infusion lasting 13 hours. The mean infusion rates were 6.7 μg min^{-1} for PGE$_2$ and 884 mU min^{-1} [*sic*] for oxytocin. It can be debated whether in order to avoid trivial side-effects such as pyrexia, vomiting, diarrhoea and venous erythema, the patient should be exposed to the risk of developing a lethal complication such as water intoxication, secondary to the administration of these high doses of oxytocin.

To conclude, the intravenous, vaginal, intra-amniotic and extra-amniotic routes of administration of prostaglandins are all effective in terminating pregnancy after missed abortion. The latter two techniques cause fewer systemic side-effects and should be given the preference in the days following intrauterine demise. Later, with further necrosis of the products of conception, the risk of infection increases and strictly non-invasive routes of administration ought to be considered first. Besides, the intra-amniotic method may become technically difficult due to resorption of part or all of the amniotic fluid. Puncture of the altered fetal membranes may also cause leakage of thromboplastin-rich material into the maternal circulation and precipitate the occurrence of defibrination.

3.5.3 Preoperative dilatation of the cervix

For all practical purposes, at present, interruption of pregnancy before the 13th week remains a surgical procedure. Medical methods of abortion (uterine stimulants, feto-toxic drugs) have failed to provide an effective and safe method. The conventional, difficult and frequently used dilatation and curettage (D & C) is rapidly being replaced by vacuum aspiration using the flexible polyethylene Karman catheter 4–10 mm diameter although wider bore metal curettes are still employed. The operation is both rapid and relatively safe. Immediate complications such as bleeding, trauma and infection are infrequent. However, the cervix needs to be mechanically dilated in some women (particularly in nulliparae and during the late first trimester of pregnancy) and cervical incompetence may occur leading to spontaneous abortion or premature labour during subsequent pregnancy (see Toppozada et al. (1973b) for references). There are, therefore, reasons to believe that if drugs or techniques could be developed to achieve gradual dilatation, trauma to the cervix could be minimised.

In case of failure of prostaglandin-induced therapeutic abortion, it is commonly found that the cervix has dilated sufficiently to allow easy vaginal evacuation of the uterine contents, with little or no instrumental dilatation (Naftolin et al., 1972; Pion et al., 1972; Igel et al., 1973; Wentz et al., 1973b; Pitkanen and Rauramo, 1974). This observation has led Béguin et al. (1972) and Haspels and Neth (1973) to suggest that surgical evacuation of late first trimester pregnancies (11–13 weeks) could be facilitated by the preoperative administration of a prostaglandin via the vaginal or the extra-amniotic route.

(a) Prostaglandins E_2 and $F_{2\alpha}$

Wiqvist et al. (1972a) injected 250–750 μg $PGF_{2\alpha}$ or 25–75 μg PGE_2 at intervals of 1–4 hours into the extraovular space for a maximum of eight hours to 10 patients at 12 weeks' gestation. At suction curettage, the cervix was found to be sufficiently dilated for easy insertion of the curette. The only side-effect reported by these authors was one to three episodes of vomiting in three patients. Haspels and Neth (1973) administered a single extra-amniotic dose of 0.5 mg $PGF_{2\alpha}$ to 11 women (gestation 7–13 weeks, parity 0–5) $4\frac{1}{2}$ to 20 hours prior to vacuum aspiration. Varying degree of cervical dilatation was achieved in most women. Side-effects included nausea (2 cases), vomiting (3 cases) and hypotension (1 case).

Three studies utilising vaginal administration of $PGF_{2\alpha}$ for cervical dilatation have been reported. Craft (1973a) inserted two 100 mg pessaries on two occasions within 24 hours of vaginal termination of pregnancy in 10 subjects. Gestational age ranged from 9 to 12 weeks and parity from 0 to 9. Adequate cervical dilatation for vacuum aspiration was achieved in only two cases. Side-effects included headache (1 case), flushing (5 cases), diarrhoea (5 cases), difficulty in breathing and retrosternal discomfort (1 case). All patients had uterine cramps.

In a controlled study reported by Brenner et al. (1973b) 40 nulliparous women were given 50 mg $PGF_{2\alpha}$ in the form of vaginal pessaries three hours prior to vacuum aspiration. Twenty nulliparae served as controls (no prostaglandin administered). Fifty-five per cent of the treated patients were dilated sufficiently to perform suction curettage compared with 5% in the control group. Those $PGF_{2\alpha}$ subjects needing further dilatation to perform suction curettage required less dilatation than did subjects of similar gestational age in the control group. Side-effects related to $PGF_{2\alpha}$ treatment included vomiting and diarrhoea (43%). Severe uterine cramps requiring analgesia were recorded in 13% of the patients. Minor cervical trauma was observed in one treated patient (3%) and in three (15%) of the control group.

Ostergard (1973) attempted to extend this particular application of prostaglandin therapy to non-pregnant patients. This author measured cervical dilatation before and 12 hours after insertion of a single vaginal suppository of 20 mg PGE_2 in five subjects in the mid-luteal phase of the menstrual cycle. The drug had no effect on the cervix in four patients and caused an increment of only 1 mm in the fifth. All patients suffered severe side-effects including rigor (5), nausea (4), fever of 38 °C or more (4), abdominal cramps (4), vomiting (3), diarrhoea (2) and hypotension (1) and required therapy.

(b) Synthetic analogues

Toppozada et al. (1973b) studied the effect of a single extra-amniotic injection of 200–500 μg 15(S),15-methyl-$PGF_{2\alpha}$ on cervical dilatation in 45 women. The gestation varied from 9 to 13 weeks and 60% of the patients were nulliparous. Operative procedure was carried out $17\frac{1}{2}$ hours (mean time lag) after extra-amniotic injection of the prostaglandin analogue. Twenty-one patients (47%) aborted before the scheduled time of operation. The cervix dilated to 10 mm or more in 38 (84%) of the patients. Side-effects associated with the procedure included vomiting in 15 patients (total 45 episodes) and a single episode of diarrhoea was recorded in two cases. A mean of 1.45 analgesic injections per patient was required to alleviate uterine pain. Operative bleeding was less than 100 ml in 32 patients, 100–500 ml in 11 patients and more than 500 ml in two patients.

A similar study by Choo et al. (1973) utilised the 15-methyl analogue of PGE_2. Dilatation of the cervix by a single extra-amniotic dose of 25 μg of 15(S),15-methyl-PGE_2 methyl ester was attempted in 425 women prior to vacuum aspiration or curettage. The procedure resulted in cervical dilatation of 10 mm or more in 385 patients and a dilatation of 8 mm in a further 21 women. Vacuum aspiration or curettage was possible in these patients without mechanical dilatation of the cervix. Gestational age varied between 7 and 16 weeks and parity 0–4 +. Operative blood loss was less than 30 ml in 420 patients, 100 ml in three, 300 ml in one and 500 ml in one. Although most patients experienced uterine cramps, only 22 women out of 425 requested analgesia. Side-effects included vomiting (17 women), diarrhoea (31 women) and pyrexia of 1 °C (18 women). Pyrexia usually appeared two hours after prostaglandin administration and lasted for 2–3 hours.

Karim and Choo (1974) have evaluated the effect of several prostaglandin analogues for preoperative cervical dilatation in 125 nulliparous women in the first trimester of pregnancy. The patients, divided into five groups of 25 women, were given a single extra-amniotic dose of one of the following compounds 14–10 hours prior to evacuation of the uterus by vacuum aspiration: 15(S),15-methyl-PGE_2 (free acid); 15(S),15-methyl-PGE_2 methyl ester; 15(S),15-methyl-$PGF_{2\alpha}$ (acid); 15(S),15-methyl-$PGF_{2\alpha}$ methyl ester or a mixture of 15(S),15-methyl-PGE$_2$ methyl ester and 15(S),15-methyl-PGF$_{2\alpha}$ methyl ester. Evacuation of the uterus without mechanical dilatation of the cervix was possible in 111 (90%) of the patients. In an additional 10 patients (8%) there was some degree of cervical dilatation and further mechanical dilatation could be performed easily. The group treated with a mixture of PGE$_2$ and PGF$_{2\alpha}$ analogues showed the highest efficacy and lowest incidence of side-effects.

Attempts to use a non-invasive route for prostaglandin analogues administration as a means of preoperative cervical dilatation have so far proved disappointing. Intramuscular administration of 300–800 μg of 15(S),15-methyl-PGF$_{2\alpha}$ every sixth hour in 22 women resulted in cervical dilatation of 10 mm or more in 16 patients but the incidence of gastrointestinal side-effects (vomiting and diarrhoea) was high (Toppozada et al., 1973b). With 25 μg 15(S),15-methyl-PGE$_2$ methyl ester administered intramuscularly, adequate cervical dilatation was achieved in 70% of the patients but again diarrhoea and pyrexia were recorded in over 35% of the patients (Karim and Choo, unpublished results).

The mechanism by which prostaglandins produce cervical dilatation is not known but is most likely the result of myometrial stimulation. Most investigators have reported uterine cramps as side-effects when prostaglandins are used for cervical dilatation. Also in a proportion of patients the prostaglandin induced abortion. A direct relaxant effect of prostaglandins on the cervix cannot be completely ruled out. A relaxant effect of some prostaglandins on the non-pregnant cervix in vitro has been reported (Najak et al., 1970) (see Table 3.11 for detailed results).

Table 3.11 Use of prostaglandins as a means of cervical dilatation prior to vacuum aspiration or curettage

Reference	No. of cases	Gestation (weeks)	Parity	PG/dose/route	Interval between PG administration and evacuation (hours)	Results* —success rate	Side-effects
Wiqvist et al., 1972a	10	12	0–4	PGE$_2$ 175–220 μg in 5–10 E/O doses. PGF$_{2\alpha}$ 1–3.5 mg in 3–5 E/O doses	1½–8	100%	Vomiting (3), Uterine cramps
Haspels and Neth, 1973	11	7–13	0–5	0.5 mg PGF$_{2\alpha}$ E/O S.D.	4½–20	Varying degree of dilatation in most patients	Nausea (2), Vomiting (3), Hypertension (1), Uterine cramps
Craft, 1973a	10	9–12	0–9	2 × 100 mg PGF$_{2\alpha}$ vaginal pessaries during 24 hours	24	20%	Headache (1), Pyrexia (5), Diarrhoea (5), Chest pain (1), Uterine cramps

[continued

Table 3.11 *[continued]*

Reference	No. of cases	Gestation (weeks)	Parity	PG/dose/route	Interval between PG administration and evacuation (hours)	Results* —success rate	Side-effects
Brenner et al., 1973b	40	5–12	0	50 mg $PGF_{2\alpha}$ vaginal solution S.D.	3	55%	Vomiting and diarrhoea (17), Uterine cramps
Ostergard, 1973	5	non-pregnant		20 mg PGE_2 vaginal solution S.D.	12	0	Rigor (5), Nausea (4), Pyrexia (4), Vomiting (3), Diarrhoea (2), Hypertension (1), Uterine cramps
Toppozada et al., 1973c	45	9–13	0–4	200–500 μg 15-methyl-$PGF_{2\alpha}$ S.D.	17½ (mean)	84%	Vomiting (15), Diarrhoea (2), Uterine cramps
Toppozada et al., 1973c	22	9–13	0–4	300–800 μg 15-methyl-$PGF_{2\alpha}$ I/M every 6th hour (3 doses)	17½ (mean)	73%	High incidence of vomiting and diarrhoea. Uterine cramps
Choo et al., 1973	425	7–16	0–4	15(S),15-methyl-PGE_2 methyl ester 25 μg E/O S.D.	12–14	95%	Vomiting (17), Diarrhoea (31), Pyrexia (18), Uterine cramps
Karim and Choo, 1974	25	8–13	0	15(S),15-methyl-PGE_2 25 μg E/O	12–14	92%	Vomiting (7), Diarrhoea (12), Pyrexia (11), Shivering (8)
	25	8–13	0	15(S),15-methyl-PGE_2 methyl ester 25 μg E/O	12–14	88%	
	25	8–13	0	15(S),15-methyl-$PGF_{2\alpha}$ 250 μg E/O	12–14	84%	Vomiting (21), Diarrhoea (5), Pyrexia (2)
	25	8–13	0	15(S),15-methyl-$PGF_{2\alpha}$ methyl ester 250 μg E/O	12–14	84%	
	25	8–13	0	15(S),15-methyl-PGE_2 methyl ester 12.5 μg + 15(S),15-methyl-$PGF_{2\alpha}$ 125 μg E/O	12–14	96%	Vomiting (4), Diarrhoea (4)

S.D.—Single doses; E/O—Extra-ovular; I/M—Intramuscular
* Success rate: Adequate cervical dilatation to enable evacuation of the uterus without mechanical dilatation of the cervix.

(c) Comments

The limiting factors in the use of naturally occurring prostaglandins for preoperative cervical dilatation are low efficacy and high incidence of side-effects. The efficacy of 15-methyl analogues given as a single extra-amniotic dose is high and side-effects are minimal. The procedure, however, requires hospitalisation of the patient.

It is generally agreed that preoperative cervical dilatation is necessary when large metallic curettes are used for the evacuation of the uterus during the first trimester of pregnancy. In this situation prostaglandin analogues given by the extra-amniotic route can be usefully employed to achieve gradual cervical dilatation as a substitute for acute dilatation by mechanical means. There is some disagreement whether dilatation of the cervix is necessary when using the flexible polyethylene Karman catheter of 4–10 mm diameter. Some consider that a great majority of first trimester pregnancies can be terminated with Karman catheters without mechanical dilatation of the cervix (Lewis *et al.*, 1971; Amy, 1974). Others, however, find the need to dilate the cervix (even when using Karman catheters) particularly in nulliparae and during the late first trimester of pregnancy (Choo *et al.*, 1973; Toppozada *et al.*, 1973b; Liu and Hudson, 1974). The controversy can be resolved by carrying out comparative studies, i.e. vacuum aspiration using Karman catheter with and without prior treatment with prostaglandin analogues. Factors such as cervical laceration, total blood loss, completeness of evacuation and cervical incompetence will have to be evaluated. For a wider and more practical application it would be necessary to explore other prostaglandin analogues which would be effective in dilating the cervix when given by a non-uterine route.

3.5.4 Menstrual regulation

'Menstrual regulation' is a new and promising approach to fertility control which may fill the present gap between conventional contraceptives and late abortion. The procedure involves evacuation of the uterus within a few days of delayed menstruation. This can be achieved in one of two ways:
1. Surgically, i.e. by vacuum aspiration of uterine contents (usually referred to as menstrual regulation).
2. By administration of drugs, e.g. prostaglandins (referred to as menstrual induction).

Since the procedure is usually carried out during the first two weeks of missed menstruation, it is not always possible to confirm pregnancy and it is likely to include a proportion of women who are not pregnant. This, however, could be an advantage in countries with restrictive abortion laws. There are two main reasons for exploring the use of prostaglandins for menstrual induction: (1) in several subprimate species prostaglandins have a luteolytic effect; (2) prostaglandins through their uterine muscle stimulant action act as early abortifacients.

The various mechanisms by which prostaglandins can terminate early pregnancy and induce menstrual-like bleeding are discussed in Chapter 2. Only the results of clinical studies are reviewed in this section.

(a) Vaginal route

Karim (1971 b, d) originally showed that prostaglandins E_2 or $F_{2\alpha}$ could terminate very early pregnancy and could be used for menstrual induction. Vaginal administration of two 20 mg doses of PGE_2 or two 50 mg doses of $PGF_{2\alpha}$ four hours apart resulted in menstrual-like bleeding and a state of non-pregnancy in eleven out of twelve women. Side-effects included nausea and uterine cramps. Jones et al. (1974) reported similar efficacy. In 10 women with last menstrual period between 42 and 50 days prior to treatment, vaginal suppositories of 20 mg PGE_2 in a hydrophilic base were administered every two hours until abortion or until a maximum of 120 mg was given. Complete abortion was effected in eight, incomplete abortion in one and there was one failure. Seven of the subjects had temperature elevation greater than 38.0 °C. All patients experienced nausea, eight had vomiting and four diarrhoea. Tredway and Mishell (1973) reported a success rate of 70–80% using $PGF_{2\alpha}$ vaginal suppositories.

Bygdeman et al. (1972a) treated eight women with up to 14 days delay in menstruation with 25–50 mg $PGF_{2\alpha}$ administered vaginally and repeated one to four times at 2–4 hour intervals for up to eight hours. Only three had a negative pregnancy test two weeks after treatment. Some patients experienced two to three episodes of vomiting and/or diarrhoea during the treatment period.

In a group of 22 women with a delay in menstruation of 4–12 days Cheng et al. (1973) administered vaginal pessaries containing 20 mg PGE_2 or 50 mg $PGF_{2\alpha}$ every two hours until the onset of uterine bleeding. Menstrual-like bleeding was induced in thirteen while pregnancy continued and was terminated by vacuum aspiration in eight. Side-effects included diarrhoea and abdominal pain.

Bolognese and Corson (1973b) found that the result of attempted early pregnancy termination by vaginal administration of $PGF_{2\alpha}$ depended upon the concentration of the drug. With 25–50 mg $PGF_{2\alpha}$ (50 mg ml^{-1} solution) every two hours for an 8–12 hour period these investigators failed to terminate pregnancy in all four subjects. Using 50 mg every two to three hours (200 mg ml^{-1} solution) for 10–16 hours, they succeeded in terminating six out of eight pregnancies. Emesis and diarrhoea were common side-effects. 'Minor complaints of vaginal burning or pulsation and generalised flushing were encountered' (see Table 3.12 for detailed results).

(b) Intrauterine route

The results of menstrual induction by this route are more consistent. By administering a large single dose of either PGE_2 or $PGF_{2\alpha}$ into the uterine cavity it is possible to induce menstruation when this is delayed by up to two weeks. The first recorded study utilising the intrauterine route for menstrual induction was reported by Bygdeman et al. (1972a). Four women with a delay in menstruation of up to 14 days were given a single intrauterine dose of 500 μg $PGF_{2\alpha}$. The treatment was successful in two. With the use of higher doses of PGE_2 or $PGF_{2\alpha}$ given as a single intrauterine injection several inves-

Table 3.12   Results of menstrual induction with prostaglandins

Reference	No. of cases	Delay in onset of menstruation	PU/dose/route	Results—success rate*	Side-effects
Karim, 1971b	12	2–7 days delay	PGE$_2$ 20 mg or PGF$_{2\alpha}$ 50 mg 2 vaginal tablets 4 hours apart	90%	Nausea (4), Abdominal cramps
Jones et al., 1974	10	LMP 42–50 days before treatment	PGE$_2$ 20 mg vaginal pessaries 2-hourly (Max. 6 doses)	80%	Vaginal pain (8), Pyrexia (7), Nausea (10), Vomiting (8), Diarrhoea (5)
Bygdeman et al., 1972a	8	14 days delay	25 to 50 mg PGF$_{2\alpha}$ 1–4 doses at 2–4 hours interval vaginally	37%	Vomiting and diarrhoea
Cheng et al., 1973	22	4–12 days delay	20 mg PGE$_2$ or 50 mg PGF$_{2\alpha}$. Vaginal pessaries 2-hourly (Max. 5 doses)	60%	Diarrhoea (22), Abdominal pain (22)
Bolognese and Corson, 1973b	12	7–17 days delay	25–50 mg PGF$_{2\alpha}$ 2–3 hours. Vaginal solution for 8–16 hours	50%	Vomiting, diarrhoea, vaginal burning, flushing
Tredway and Mishell, 1973	10	LMP 36–42 days	50 mg PGF$_{2\alpha}$ vaginal suppositories every 2–4 hours (Max. 24 hours)	70%	Nausea, vomiting, diarrhoea, vaginismus, peripheral cyanosis
Bygdeman et al., 1972a	4	up to 14 days delay	0.5 mg PGF$_{2\alpha}$ intrauterine single dose	50%	—
Csapo et al., 1972c	22	11.9 ± 0.4 days	5 mg PGF$_{2\alpha}$ intrauterine single dose	90%	BP change (3), Headache (2), Uterine pain (3), Hyperventilation (1)
Mocsary and Csapo, 1973	65	10–12 days	5 mg PGF$_{2\alpha}$ or 1 mg PGE$_2$ single intrauterine dose	100%	Vomiting (18), BP (1)
Karim, 1973	16	6–14 days delay	PGF$_{2\alpha}$ 4 mg or PGE$_2$ 1 mg single intrauterine dose	100%	Vomiting (6), Uterine cramps
Csapo and Mocsary, 1974	20	11.6 ± 0.4 days	2.5 mg PGF$_{2\alpha}$ (pellet)	100%	Vomiting (2), Bleeding (1)
Ylikorkala et al., 1974	34		PGF$_{2\alpha}$ 1–4 mg single intra-uterine dose	90%	Vomiting (18), BP (1)
Lichtman et al., 1974	20	38–46 days from LMP	PGF$_{2\alpha}$ 5 mg single intra-uterine dose	65%	BP (20), Vomiting (16)

* Usually negative pregnancy test 7–14 days after treatment

tigators have reported almost 100% efficacy. Csapo *et al.* (1973) administered 5 mg $PGF_{2\alpha}$ into the uterus in 22 patients who had passed their expected menstrual period by 11.9 ± 0.4 days and in all of whom pregnancy test was positive. The 5 mg dose of $PGF_{2\alpha}$ contained in 5 ml of physiological saline was administered over a 10 min period. Pregnancy test was negative in 20 out of the 22 patients 14 days after treatment. Twelve out of the 22 patients were sedated prior to prostaglandin administration. For this purpose a combination of analgesic (100 mg pethidine hydrochloride i.v.), tranquilliser (10 mg diazepam + 4 mg lidocain hydrochloride i.v.) and antiemetic drugs (a suppository containing 6.5 mg thiethylperazine maleate) were used. Of the sedated patients 'none had severe uterine pain, diarrhoea, significant changes in blood pressure or in heart rate'. Only three episodes of nausea and vomiting occurred. In the 10 non-sedated patients side-effects were more pronounced and included transient changes of blood pressure (3 instances), headache (2 instances), uterine pain (3 instances) and hyperventilation (1 instance). Mocsary and Csapo (1973) have extended the above study to an additional 65 patients. All were sedated with diazepam 20 mg, pethidine 100 mg and atropine 0.4 mg intravenously 'to reduce prostaglandin-provoked uterine pain, nausea and vomiting'. Fifty were given 5 mg $PGF_{2\alpha}$ and 15 received 1 mg PGE_2. The drug was dissolved in 2 ml physiological saline. Pregnancy test was negative in all women 10 days after treatment. Side-effects with $PGF_{2\alpha}$ included one episode of vomiting in 13 patients shortly after treatment and a transient increase in blood pressure in one subject. 'There were no complaints of uterine pain (most patients did not remember being treated).' The only side-effect in the PGE_2 treated group was vomiting in five patients. Follow-up was normal in all and subsequent spontaneous menstruation started in all within 32 days of treatment and was heavier than normal in five patients. All above studies were carried out on in-patient basis. Karim (1973) has reported on the use of PGE_2 and $PGF_{2\alpha}$ for menstrual induction carried out on an out-patient basis. Sixteen women with a delay in onset of menstruation of 6–14 days and with a positive pregnancy test were given a single intrauterine dose of $PGF_{2\alpha}$ (4 mg) or PGE_2 (1 mg) in an outpatient clinic. After an observation period of two hours they were discharged and asked to return for first follow-up seven days later. Uterine bleeding was initiated within 2–5 hours of drug administration and continued for 8–12 days. Pregnancy test was negative 5–14 days after drug treatment. In one patient slight uterine bleeding continued for 18 days and curettage was performed. Three patients required pethidine for severe uterine cramps. Vomiting occurred in six women. An additional six patients were given 8.0 mg $PGF_{2\alpha}$ or 2 mg PGE_2. All experienced severe uterine cramps and vomiting. One (with PGE_2) had hypotension and one ($PGF_{2\alpha}$) had bronchoconstriction which was reversed with salbutamol. Treatment was successful in all. Ylikorkala *et al.* (1974) used single doses of 1–4 mg $PGF_{2\alpha}$ in 34 women for menstrual induction on out-patient basis. Four patients treated with 4 mg $PGF_{2\alpha}$ started to bleed from the uterus within $1\frac{1}{2}$–8 hours after prostaglandin administration. Pregnancy test was negative in all seven days later although uterine bleeding lasted for 12–14 days. In the group treated with 2.0 mg $PGF_{2\alpha}$ (18 cases) uterine bleeding started on the average $5\frac{3}{4}$ hours after drug administration (range $1\frac{1}{2}$–14 hours) and lasted for 8 to 21 days (mean 13.1 days). Pregnancy test was negative in all after 1–11 days (mean 5.6 days). In one patient curettage was performed and blood transfusion subsequently given two weeks after prostaglandin treatment because of heavy bleeding and anaemia (Hb 6.8 g%). Spontaneous menstruation started on the average in the above groups within 36.3 days (range 25–61 days) after prostaglandin treatment. Twelve patients were treated with 1 mg dose of $PGF_{2\alpha}$. Uterine bleeding lasted for 8–16 days. Because of heavy bleeding, an emergency curettage was performed in one. Pregnancy test was negative in 10 out of 12 cases after three weeks. Curettage was performed in two further cases, one for continued bleeding and one for treatment failure.

The only pretreatment used in the above study was a 'weak spasmolytic', (Litalgin® 5.0 ml) given i.v. 15 min before prostaglandin administration. All patients experienced uterine pains but only one was treated with analgesics. Vomiting 1–6 episodes was observed in 58% in the 1 mg group, 1–8 episodes in 50% in the 2 mg group. A marked decrease in blood pressure and diarrhoea occurred in one patient induced with 2.0 mg $PGF_{2\alpha}$. One case of possible endometritis was treated uneventfully with antibiotics without hospitalisation.

Lichtman et al. (1974) gave a single intrauterine dose of 5 mg $PGF_{2\alpha}$ to a group of 20 women between 38 and 46 days after the onset of last menses. Thirteen (65%) had a successful termination of pregnancy. Seven patients (including two who aborted) had severe adverse reaction including fever, haemorrhage and hypertension. Three of the five women who did not abort developed septic incomplete abortions. Csapo and Mocsary (1974) successfully induced menstruation in all of 20 women with mean menstrual delay of 12 days and a positive pregnancy test, by intrauterine insertion of a semi-solid pellet (7×2 mm) containing 2.5 mg $PGF_{2\alpha}$. Patients were routinely sedated. There were no complications except heavy bleeding requiring curettage (1 case) and vomiting (2 cases). Detailed results are presented in Table 3.12.

(c) Comments

Studies on menstrual induction with vaginally administered prostaglandins E_2 and $F_{2\alpha}$ have given inconsistent results in terms of efficacy and resulted in an unacceptable incidence of side-effects. The difference in success rate reported by various investigators could be due to different dosage and drug formulation employed. There is very little doubt that vaginally administered prostaglandins produce their effects on the uterus after systemic absorption. Factors such as dose of prostaglandin, formulation (i.e. solution, concentration, base used for making vaginal pessaries and tablets), the pH and moisture content of the vagina would all affect absorption. For the present, therefore, attempts to develop prostaglandins as postconceptional abortifacients which could be self-administered have not proved very successful. Further efforts with different types of drug formulation and the use of synthetic analogues (Toppozada et al., 1973a) may improve the situation.

Studies with the intrauterine route have given high and consistent efficacy. However, this route does not easily lend itself to self-medication. For this reason and because of the associated side-effects, the procedure would have limited application.

3.6 PRACTICAL HINTS ON THE CONDUCT OF TERMINATION OF PREGNANCY WITH PROSTAGLANDINS

In the following section, certain aspects specific to the use of prostaglandins for interruption of pregnancy will be very briefly commented upon. It goes without saying that measures applying to therapeutic abortion in general should also be observed when pregnancy is terminated with prostaglandins (e.g. treatment of genital tract infection and correction of severe anaemia prior to abortion; prevention of Rh iso-immunisation).

3.6.1 Contraindications to the use of prostaglandins for termination of pregnancy

An exhaustive list of disorders which may contraindicate the use of prostaglandins for therapeutic abortion is listed in Bergström (1973, page 67). It includes:

—organic heart disease;
—hypertension (blood pressure higher than 140/90);
—respiratory ailment (asthma, allergic bronchitis, emphysema, fibrocystic disease, pulmonary surgery as pneumonectomy or thoracoplasty, bronchiectasis);
—severe hypersensitivity (previous anaphylactic reaction);
—ulcerative colitis;
—diabetes mellitus;
—disorders of blood coagulation;
—severe kidney disease;
—severe liver disease;
—sickle-cell anaemia;
—any serious systemic disease.

At present, however, it can be stated that only bronchial disease (Smith, 1973), and perhaps sickle-cell trait or anaemia constitute major contraindications to the administration of prostaglandins. In case prostaglandins are to be administered for interruption of pregnancy to a patient with one of these disorders, the intra-amniotic route should be preferred, as it gives only very low levels of circulating prostaglandin.

Relative contraindications to the transabdominal intrauterine (='intra-amniotic') administration of prostaglandins include (Bergström, 1973, page 67):

—previous abdominal surgery;
—previous surgery on the uterus (Caesarean section, myomectomy, hysterotomy, Strassman procedure, uterine suspension, repair of uterine or deep cervical lacerations);
—large uterine myomata or other pelvic tumours;
—major congenital anomalies of the uterus;
—rupture of the membranes;
—failed saline induction.

It should be emphatically reiterated that hydatidiform mole constitutes an absolute contraindication to the use of this particular route (Karim, 1974) unless dosage is drastically reduced.

A last word of caution regarding the possible expulsion of a live fetus: Anderson et al. (1972a), Naftolin et al. (1972) and Golbus and Erickson (1974), among others, have mentioned that the fetus may occasionally show signs of life, at abortion. In case termination of a late second trimester pregnancy is contemplated (e.g. for severe fetal malformation), it may be preferable to use a method of abortion which causes fetal death in utero, e.g. the intra-amniotic injection of prostaglandin combined with hypertonic urea (Craft et al., 1973; Craft et al., 1974).

3.6.2 Prevention and treatment of side-effects and complications

Most commonly, only trivial side-effects are encountered during the course of prostaglandin-induced abortion. Cramping pain of uterine origin can be fairly effectively controlled with pethidine (Demerol®); nausea and vomiting with prochlorperazine (Compazine®). Diarrhoea is best treated with diphenoxylate hydrochloride and atropine sulphate (Lomotil®), and drug-induced fever with aspirin. None of these medications seem to affect adversely the outcome of abortion.

In order to prevent the occurrence of severe reactions, including shock or severe bronchoconstriction, both of which are extremely rare, a small initial test dose of prostaglandin should be administered slowly. Should bronchospasm occur, clinical trials have shown that it responds rapidly to the administration of isoprenaline by inhalation (Isuprel®—Bergström, 1973, page 67).

During the course of abortion, pelvic examination should be performed at regular intervals (e.g. 4–6 hourly) in order to assess progress. Abortion often takes place insidiously and the conceptus may otherwise remain in the vagina for a prolonged period of time (Alderman, 1972). More important still, routine vaginal examination allows the observer to detect in time failure of cervical dilatation that may lead eventually to rupture of the posterior uterine wall at the cervico–isthmic junction. This complication can be prevented by gentle instrumental dilatation or by insertion of laminaria tents into the cervical canal (Engel et al., 1973; Corson et al., 1973). Beta-mimetic adrenergic agents such as orciprenaline (i.v. infusion of $10–20$ μg min^{-1}) or ritodrine ($100–300$ μg min^{-1}) inhibit uterine activity induced in the second trimester of pregnancy by prostaglandins (Lindmark et al., 1973). These compounds could therefore prove useful in the prevention of impending uterine rupture.

In case of failure of abortion, intravenous infusion of oxytocin at a dose-level of $50–200$ mU min^{-1} will generally reactivate adequate myometrial activity. If the pregnancy has not progressed beyond 14–16 weeks, it can also be terminated vaginally with a Karman catheter (diameter 10 mm) or a ring forceps, as in the majority of cases, the cervix will have dilated sufficiently to allow safe passage of these instruments into the uterine cavity.

Following abortion, the uterine cavity should be instrumentally explored (ring forceps or Karman curette) in every case in order to remove any retained products of conception and to rule out the presence of a second conceptus. The cervix, at the same time, is examined to exclude possible traumatic lesions.

3.7 COMPARISON WITH OTHER METHODS OF INTERRUPTION OF PREGNANCY

Suction curettage (in the first trimester) and intra-amniotic instillation of 20% saline (in the second trimester of pregnancy) are presently the most commonly used techniques of abortion in the western world. In the following section, an attempt will be made to compare the efficacy and safety of each of these methods with those of prostaglandin-induced abortions.

3.7.1 Suction curettage

Suction curettage consists in evacuation of the uterine contents by means of a rigid (plastic, glass or metallic) or flexible (polyethylene) suction curette connected to a vacuum pump. Insertion of a rigid curette into the uterus requires dilatation of the cervix beforehand. This usually is effected, immediately before curettage, by forcing metallic dilatators through the cervical canal, a procedure which may cause cervical laceration, uterine perforation or isthmic incompetence (Stallworthy et al., 1971; Wright et al., 1972). Nevertheless, the morbidity and mortality among patients submitted to dilatation and suction curettage compare very favourably with those accompanying other currently used techniques of abortion. Berger et al. (1974) calculated that the mortality associated with suction curettages performed in New York State during the period extending from July 1, 1970 to June 30, 1972 was seven times lower than that following 'salting-out' and 100 times less than that of hysterotomy.

The development by Karman of a flexible polyethylene cannula (diameter 4, 5, 6, 8 or 10 mm), which can be inserted into the uterus without cervical dilatation beforehand, has made suction curettage even safer. First trimester pregnancy (4–12 weeks' menstrual age) can be terminated under paracervical anaesthesia, on an out-patient basis and in a matter of minutes (Goldsmith and Margolis, 1971: Lewis et al., 1971; Karman and Potts, 1972; Landesman et al., 1973; Amy, 1974). The cost of the procedure is extremely low. In the hands of the experienced operator, the frequency of incomplete abortion is less than 1% (Landesman et al., 1973; Amy, 1974); besides, the recovery of trophoblastic tissue virtually eliminates the possibility of an ectopic pregnancy.

The administration by various routes of prostaglandins for interruption of first trimester pregnancy has proved successful in a great number of cases. From a practical point of view, however, it appears that at present prostaglandins cannot compete with suction curettage for menstrual induction or termination of first trimester pregnancy:

1. the cost of these drugs is not negligible;
2. presently available prostaglandins, according to the type of compound

and the route of administration, frequently cause vomiting, diarrhoea, rigor, pyrexia, vaginismus or uterine cramps. Because of the possible occurrence of these side-effects, it is preferable to hospitalise the patient during the course of abortion and this further augments the cost of the procedure;

3. abortion is often incomplete and surgical evacuation of the uterine contents is then required as a second procedure;

4. interruption of pregnancy may fail altogether, even in case uterine bleeding was successfully induced and it is advisable to perform an immunologic pregnancy test 1–2 weeks after induction of first trimester abortion with prostaglandins. If pregnancy continues, it is conceivable that the intense uterine contractions elicited by the prostaglandin and the ensuing tissular hypoxia of the early conceptus could have damaging effects.

3.7.2 Intra-amniotic instillation of hypertonic saline

This technique, applicable from the 14–16th week of gestation on, consists in the removal of 50–500 ml amniotic fluid followed by the intra-amniotic instillation of 150-250 ml 20% saline. The transabdominal puncture of the amniotic sac is preferred to the transvaginal approach which carries a higher risk of infection. The potential complications of this method have now been well-documented. Injection of the hypertonic solution into the myometrium causes local necrosis (Wentz and King, 1972; Rovinsky and Amy, unpublished). Inadvertent intravascular administration on the other hand, has led to convulsions, congestive heart failure, renal shut-down, cerebral dehydration and death (Kerenyi, 1969; Berger et al., 1974). In nearly all patients, significant changes in platelets, fibrinogen, fibrinogen survival time, fibrin degradation products, prothrombin time and factors V and VIII are observed following 'salting out' (Stander et al., 1971; Weiss et al., 1972; Laros et al., 1973). These alterations indicate that a generally mild and self-limited form of disseminated intravascular coagulopathy develops. In some cases, however, this defibrination syndrome may lead to a clinically significant bleeding diathesis (Lemkin and Kattlove, 1973; Cohen and Ballard, 1974). Finally, Edström and Odar-Cederlöf (1974) reported that haemolysis frequently occurs following intrauterine instillation of 20% saline.

'Salting out' is a highly efficacious method of interruption of second trimester pregnancy: in 93–100% of the cases, abortion is effected in a mean time of 35–40 hours (Ballard and Quilligan, 1973b). The addition of i.v. oxytocin shortens the induction–abortion interval to 20–25 hours (Ballard and Quilligan, 1973b; Kerenyi et al., 1973; Lauersen and Schulman, 1973) but it augments the risk of uterine rupture (Goodlin, 1972; Kerenyi et al., 1973; Horwitz, 1974) and of consumption coagulopathy (Cohen and Ballard, 1974), and it may be a cause of water intoxication (Gupta and Cohen, 1972; Mann et al., 1973). Other investigators have resorted to the insertion of laminaria tents into the cervical canal in order to facilitate the process of abortion, but divergent results have been reported (Lischke and Goodlin, 1972; Hanson et al., 1974).

Prostaglandins, especially when administered by the intra- or extra-amniotic routes, have proved far superior to the intra-amniotic instillation of hypertonic saline alone and have had an efficacy comparable to that of hypertonic saline combined with intravenous oxytocin. Further, side-effects and complications have generally been trivial and not a single case of mortality has been reported. The Prostaglandin Task Force of the World Health Organisation has recently finished a multicentre randomised investigation comparing the intra-amniotic administration of 200 ml of 20% saline with that of two doses of 25 mg $PGF_{2\alpha}$ given at a six-hour interval. The preliminary results were reported at the Prostaglandin Task Force Meeting in Moscow (September, 1974). The study comprised 1525 patients. Subjects treated with $PGF_{2\alpha}$ had a significantly higher success rate within 48 hours and a highly significant shorter induction abortion interval. Side-effects such as vomiting and diarrhoea were slightly more frequent among women treated with the prostaglandin than in those given hypertonic saline (Bygdeman, personal communication).

Finally, it seems likely that hypertonic saline acts partly by releasing endogenous prostaglandin. Indeed, Gustavii and Green (1972) found a definite rise in amniotic fluid-$PGF_{2\alpha}$ after intrauterine administration of hypertonic saline. The rise preceded the occurrence of effective uterine contractions. Waltman et al. (1972) observed a prolongation of the mean induction–abortion interval from 36 to 70 hours when indomethacin—an inhibitor of prostaglandin synthesis—was administered orally in the dose of 25 mg six-hourly ($\times 8$) starting from four to six hours after intra-amniotic instillation of hypertonic saline. These data have since been confirmed (Waltman et al., 1973; Waltman and Tricomi, 1974). It therefore seems logical to resort directly to prostaglandin for termination of second trimester pregnancy.

Acknowledgements

The authors are particularly grateful to Drs W. E. Brenner, M. Bygdeman, S. L. Corson, I. Craft, A. I. Csapo, M. P. Embrey, N. H. Lauersen, F. Naftolin, G. Roberts, R. P. Shearman, E. M. Southern and M. Thiery for bibliographic assistance.

The expert secretarial assistance of Mrs J. Sagerman and Miss Lily Koh is gratefully acknowledged.

References

Alderman, B. (1972). Abortion with prostaglandins. *Lancet*, 2, 279

Alderman, B. and Thelwall-Jones, H. (1973). Application of the potentiating effect of prostaglandin E₂ and oxytocin to induced second trimester abortion. *J. Obstet. Gynaecol. Brit. Cwlth.*, **80**, 1021–1024

Amy, J.-J. (1974). On the administration of prostaglandins as a pre-operative means of cervical dilatation. *Prostaglandins*, 5, 302–303

Amy, J.-J., Karim, S. M. M. and Sivasamboo, R. (1973). Intra-amniotic administration of prostaglandin 15(S)15-methyl-E₂ methyl ester for termination of pregnancy. *J. Obstet. Gynaecol. Brit. Cwlth.*, **80**, 1017–1020

Anderson, G. G., Hobbins, J. C., Rajkovic, V., Goldstein, L., Speroff, L. and Caldwell, B. V.

(1973). Midtrimester therapeutic abortion using intraamniotic PGF$_{2\alpha}$. *Adv. Biosciences*, 9, 539–543

Anderson, G. G., Hobbins, J. C., Rajkovic, V., Speroff, L. and Caldwell, B. V. (1972a). Midtrimester abortion, using intraamniotic prostaglandin F$_{2\alpha}$. *Prostaglandins*, 1, 147–155

Anderson, G. G., Hobbins, J. C., Rajkovic, V., Speroff, L. and Caldwell, B. V. (1972b). Midtrimester abortion using intra-amniotic prostaglandin F$_{2\alpha}$ with intravenous Syntocinon. In: *The Prostaglandins—Clinical Applications in Human Reproduction*, 417–422 (E. M. Southern, editor) (Mount Kisco, N.Y.: Futura)

Anderson, G. G., Hobbins, J. C., Speroff, L. and Caldwell, B. V. (1972c). The induction of therapeutic abortion using intravenous prostaglandin F$_{2\alpha}$. *Contraception*, 5, 303–311

Badraoui, M. H. H., Bonnar, J., Hillier, K. and Embrey, M. P. (1973a). Coagulation changes during termination of pregnancy by prostaglandins and by vacuum aspiration. *Brit. Med. J.*, 1, 19–21

Badraoui, M. H. H., Bonnar, J., Hillier, K. and Embrey M. P. (1973b). Blood coagulation changes during mid-trimester abortion induced by prostaglandin F$_{2\alpha}$. *Brit. Med. J.*, 3, 375–378

Ballard, C. A. and Quilligan, E. J. (1972). Therapeutic abortion in midtrimester using intra-amniotic instillation of prostaglandin F$_{2\alpha}$. In: *The Prostaglandins—Clinical Applications in Human Reproduction*, 333–336 (E. M. Southern, editor) (Mount Kisco, N.Y.: Futura)

Ballard, C. A. and Quilligan, E. J. (1973a). Intraamniotic prostaglandin F$_{2\alpha}$ for midtrimester abortion. *Adv. Biosciences*, 9, 551–554

Ballard, C. A. and Quilligan, E. J. (1973b). Midtrimester abortion with intra-amniotic saline and intravenous oxytocin. *Obstet. Gynecol. (N.Y.)*, 41, 447–450

Ballard, C. A. and Quilligan, E. J. (1974). Midtrimester abortion with intramuscular injection of 15-methyl prostaglandin E$_2$. *Contraception*, 9, 523–529

Béguin, F., Bygdeman, M., Toppozada, M. and Wiqvist, N. (1972). The response of the midpregnant human uterus to vaginal administration of prostaglandin suppositories. *Prostaglandins*, 1, 397–405

Behrman, H. R. and Anderson, G. G. (1974). Prostaglandins in reproduction. *Arch. Int. Med.*, 133, 77–84

Bell, W. R. and Wentz, A. C. (1973). Abortion and coagulation by prostaglandin—Intra-amniotic Dinoprost Tromethamine effect on the coagulation and fibrinolytic systems. *J.A.M.A.*, 225, 1082–1084

Berger, G. S., Tietze, C., Pakter, J. and Katz, S. H. (1974). Maternal mortality associated with legal abortion in New York State: July 1, 1970–June 30, 1972. *Obstet. Gynecol. (N.Y.)*, 43, 315–326

Bergström, S. (1973). *Prostaglandins in Fertility Control*, Vol. 3 (Stockholm: WHO Research and Training Centre on Human Reproduction)

Bolognese, R. J. and Corson, S. L. (1973a). The effect of vaginally administered prostaglandin F$_{2\alpha}$ on corpus luteum function. *Amer. J. Obstet. Gynecol.*, 117, 240–245

Bolognese, R. J. and Corson, S. L. (1973b). Abortion of early pregnancy by the intravaginal administration of prostaglandin F$_{2\alpha}$. *Amer. J. Obstet. Gynecol.*, 117, 246–250

Bolognese, R. J. and Corson, S. L. (1974). Prostaglandin E$_2$ vaginal suppository as an early second trimester abortifacient. *Obstet. Gynecol. (N.Y.)*, 43, 104–108

Bowen-Simpkins, P. (1973) The induction of second trimester abortion using an intra-amniotic injection of urea and prostaglandin E$_2$. *J. Obstet. Gynaecol. Brit. Cwlth.*, 80, 824–826

Braaksma, J. T., Brenner, W. E., Fishburne, J. I. Jr and Staurovsky, L. (1972). Intrauterine extra-amniotic administration of prostaglandin F$_{2\alpha}$ for therapeutic abortion. Early myometrial effects. *Amer. J. Obstet. Gynecol.*, 114, 511–515

Bradley-Watson, P. J., Beard, R. J. and Craft, I. L. (1973). Injuries of the cervix after induced midtrimester abortion. *J. Obstet. Gynaecol. Brit. Cwlth.*, 80, 284–285

Brenner, W. E. (1972). Intravenous prostaglandin F$_{2\alpha}$ for therapeutic abortion: The efficacy and tolerance of three dosage schedules. *Amer. J. Obstet. Gynecol.*, 113, 1037–1045

Brenner, W. E., Dingfelder, J. R., Hendricks, C. H. and Staurovsky, L. (1973a). Induction of therapeutic abortion with a single dose of intra-amniotically administered prostaglandin F$_{2\alpha}$. *Prostaglandins*, 4, 485–498

Brenner, W. E., Dingfelder, J. R., Staurovsky, L. G. and Hendricks, C. H. (1973b). Vaginally administered PGF$_{2\alpha}$ for cervical dilatation in nulliparas prior to suction curettage. *Prostaglandins*, 4, 819–836

Brenner, W. E., Fishburne, J. I., McMillan, C. W., Johnson, A. M. and Hendricks, C. H. (1973c). Coagulation changes during abortion induced by prostaglandin $F_{2\alpha}$. *Amer. J. Obstet. Gynecol.*, **117**, 1080–1087

Brenner, W. E., Hendricks, C. H., Braaksma, J. T. and Fishburne, J. I. Jr (1972a). The abortifacient efficacy and tolerance of prostaglandin $F_{2\alpha}$ administered by the intraamniotic and intrauterine–extraamniotic routes. In: *Prostaglandins in Fertility Control*, Vol. 2, 139–153 (S. Bergström, K. Gréen and B. Samuelsson, editors) (Stockholm: WHO Research and Training Centre on Human Reproduction)

Brenner, W. E., Hendricks, C. H., Braaksma, J. T., Fishburne, J. I. Jr, Kroncke, F. G. Jr and Staurovsky, L. (1972b). Intra-amniotic administration of prostaglandin $F_{2\alpha}$ to induce therapeutic abortion. Efficacy and tolerance of two dosage schedules. *Amer. J. Obstet. Gynecol.*, **114**, 781–787

Brenner, W. E., Hendricks, C. H., Braaksma, J. T., Fishburne, J. I. Jr and Staurovsky, L. G. (1972c). Vaginal administration of prostaglandin $F_{2\alpha}$ for inducing therapeutic abortion. *Prostaglandins*, **1**, 455–467

Brenner, W. E., Hendricks, C. H., Braaksma, J. T., Fishburne, J. I. Jr and Staurovsky, L. G. (1972d). Intra-amniotic administration of prostaglandin $F_{2\alpha}$ for induction of therapeutic abortion—A comparison of four dosage schedules. In: *The Prostaglandins—Clinical Applications in Human Reproduction*, 457–470 (E. M. Southern, Editor) (Mount Kisco, N.Y.: Futura)

Brenner, W. E., Hendricks, C. H., Dingfelder, J. and Staurovsky, L. (1973d). Laminaria augmentation of intra-amniotic prostaglandin $F_{2\alpha}$ for the induction of mid-trimester abortion. *Prostaglandins*, **3**, 879–894

Brenner, W. E., Hendricks, C. H., Fishburne, J. I. Jr and Braaksma, J. T. (1972e). Intravenous prostaglandin $F_{2\alpha}$ for therapeutic abortion: Cardiovascular and respiratory effects. In: *Prostaglandins in Fertility Control*, Vol. 2, 156–163 (S. Bergström, K. Gréen and B. Samuelsson, editors) (Stockholm: WHO Research and Training Centre on Human Reproduction)

Brenner, W. E., Hendricks, C. H., Fishburne, J. I. Jr and Braaksma, J. T. (1972f). Prostaglandin $F_{2\alpha}$ administered vaginally for inducing therapeutic abortion. In: *Prostaglandins in Fertility Control*, Vol. 2, 170–174 (S. Bergström, K. Gréen and B. Samuelsson, editors) (Stockholm: WHO Research and Training Centre on Human Reproduction)

Brenner, W. E., Hendricks, C. H., Fishburne, J. I. Jr, Braaksma, J. T., Staurovsky, L. G. and Harrell, L. C. (1973e). Induction of therapeutic abortion with intra-amniotically administered prostaglandin $F_{2\alpha}$. A comparison of three repeated-injection dose schedules. *Amer. J. Obstet. Gynecol.*, **116**, 923–930

Brenner, W. E., Hendricks, C. H., Fishburne, J. I. Jr, Staurovsky, L., Braaksma, J. and Taft, R. (1973f). Intraamniotic prostaglandin $F_{2\alpha}$ dose-twenty-four-hour abortifacient response. *J. Pharm. Sci.*, **62**, 1278–1282

Brown, R. (1974). Adverse reactions to intra-amniotic prostaglandin. *Brit. Med. J.*, **2**, 382

Brummer, H. C. (1971). Interaction of E prostaglandins and Syntocinon on the pregnant human myometrium. *J. Obstet. Gynaecol. Brit. Cwlth.*, **78**, 305–309

Bullard, P. D., Herrick, C. N., Hindle, W. H., Hale, R. W. and Pion, R. J. (1973). Histopathologic changes associated with prostaglandin induced abortion. *Contraception*, **7**, 133–144

Bygdeman, M. (1964). The effect of different prostaglandins on the human myometrium *in vitro*. *Acta Physiol. Scand.*, **63**, Suppl. 242, 1–78

Bygdeman, M., Béguin, F., Toppozada, M., Wide, L. and Wiqvist, N. (1972a). Postconceptional fertility control by prostaglandin $F_{2\alpha}$. In: *Prostaglandins in Fertility Control*, Vol. 2, 175–181 (S. Bergström, K. Gréen and B. Samuelsson, editors) (Stockholm: WHO Research and Training Centre on Human Reproduction)

Bygdeman, M., Béguin, F., Toppozada, M. and Wiqvist, N. (1972b). Intra-amniotic administration of prostaglandin $F_{2\alpha}$ for the induction of second trimester abortion. In: *Prostaglandins in Fertility Control*, Vol. 2, 129–136 (S. Bergström, K. Gréen and B. Samuelsson, editors) (Stockholm: WHO Research and Training Centre on Human Reproduction)

Bygdeman, M., Béguin, F., Toppozada, M. and Wiqvist, N. (1972c). Further experience with intrauterine prostaglandin administration. In: *The Prostaglandins—Clinical Applications in Human Reproduction*, 323–332 (Mount Kisco, N.Y.: Futura)

Bygdeman, M., Béguin, F., Toppozada, M. and Wiqvist, N. (1973). Intrauterine administration of prostaglandin $F_{2\alpha}$ for induction of abortion. *Adv. Biosciences*, **9**, 525–531

Bygdeman, M., Béguin, F., Toppozada, M., Wiqvist, N. and Bergström, S. (1972d). Intrauterine administration of 15(S)-15-methyl-prostaglandin $F_{2\alpha}$ for induction of abortion. *Lancet*, **1**, 1336–1337

Bygdeman, M., Gréen, K., Toppozada, M., Wiqvist, N. and Bergström, S. (1974). The influence of prostaglandin metabolites on the uterine response to $PGF_{2\alpha}$. A clinical and pharmacokinetic study. *Life Sci.*, **14**, 521–531

Bygdeman, M., Kwon, S. U., Mukherjee, T. and Wiqvist, N. (1968). Effect of intravenous infusion of prostaglandin E_1 and E_2 on the pregnant human uterus. *Amer. J. Obstet. Gynecol.*, **102**, 317–325

Bygdeman, M. and Wiqvist, N. (1971). Early abortion in the human. *Ann. N.Y. Acad. Sci.*, **180**, 473–482

Bygdeman, M. and Wiqvist, N. (1974). The use of prostaglandins for the control of human fertility. In: *Avortement et Parturition Provoqués*, 145–162 (J. M. Bosc, R. Palmer and C. Sureau, editors) (Paris: Masson)

Bygdeman, M., Wiqvist, N. and Toppozada, M. (1971). Induction of mid-trimester abortion by intraamniotic administration of prostaglandin $F_{2\alpha}$. *Acta Physiol. Scand.*, **82**, 415–416

Caldwell, B. V., Anderson, G. G., Hobbins, J. C. and Speroff, L. (1972). F prostaglandin levels in women receiving $PGF_{2\alpha}$ for therapeutic abortion. In: *Prostaglandins in Fertility Control*, Vol. 2, 182–188 (S. Bergström, K. Gréen and B. Samuelsson, editors) (Stockholm: WHO Research and Training Centre on Human Reproduction)

Cantor, B., Jewelewicz, R., Warren, M., Dyrenfurth, I., Patner, A. and Vande Wiele, R. L. (1972). Hormonal changes during induction of midtrimester abortion by prostaglandin $F_{2\alpha}$. *Amer. J. Obstet. Gynecol.*, **113**, 607–615

Cheng, M. C. E., Tan, P. M. and Ratnam, S. S. (1973). Prostaglandin vaginal pessary as a fertility regulating agent. *Proc. 8th Singapore-Malaysia Congress of Medicine*, **8**, 111–114

Choo, H. T., Karim, S. M. M. and Cheng, P. (1973). Extra-amniotic administration of single dose of 15 (S) 15 methyl prostaglandin E_2 methyl ester for pre-operative cervical dilatation. *J. Asian Fed. Obstet. Gynaecol.*, **4**, 71–73

Cohen, E. and Ballard, C. A. (1974). Consumptive coagulopathy associated with intra-amniotic saline instillation and the effect of intravenous oxytocin. *Obstet. Gynecol. (N.Y.)*, **43**, 300–303

Corlett, R. C. Jr and Ballard, C. A. (1974). The induction of midtrimester abortion with intraamniotic prostaglandin $F_{2\alpha}$. A single-dose technique. *Amer. J. Obstet. Gynecol.*, **118**, 353–357

Corson, S. L. and Bolognese, R. J. (1973). Cervical rupture following induced abortion. *Amer. J. Obstet. Gynecol.*, **116**, 893

Corson, S. L. and Bolognese, R. J. (1974a). Comparison of two prostaglandin routes of administration to induce midtrimester abortion. *J. Reprod. Med.*, **12**, 169–171

Corson, S. L. and Bolognese, R. J. (1974b). Vaginally administered prostaglandin E_2 as a first and second trimester abortifacient. (In press)

Corson, S. L. and Bolognese, R. J. (1974c). Intra-amniotic prostaglandin $F_{2\alpha}$ as a mid-trimester abortifacient: Effect of oxytocin and laminaria. (In press)

Corson, S. L., Bolognese, R. J. and Merola, J. (1973). Intra-amniotic prostaglandin $F_{2\alpha}$ to induce midtrimester abortion. *Amer. J. Obstet. Gynecol.*, **117**, 27–34

Craft, I. (1972). Abortion: use of prostaglandins and epidural analgesia. *Lancet*, **2**, 41

Craft, I. (1973a). The use of prostaglandin pessaries prior to vaginal termination. *Prostaglandins*, **3**, 377–381

Craft, I. (1973b). Intra-amniotic prostaglandin E_2 and urea for abortion. *Lancet*, **1**, 779

Craft, I. (1973c). Induction of abortion by combined intra-amniotic urea and prostaglandin E_2 or prostaglandin E_2 alone. *Lancet*, **1**, 1344

Craft, I. (1973d). Intra-amniotic prostaglandins and urea for abortion. *Lancet*, **2**, 207

Craft, I. (1973e). Intra-amniotic urea and prostaglandin E_2 for abortion. A clinical study to determine the efficacy of using a variable prostaglandin dosage. *Prostaglandins*, **4**, 755–763

Craft, I. (1973f). Prostaglandins and convulsions. *Lancet*, **2**, 1389

Craft, I. (1973g). Intra-amniotic prostaglandin E_2 and $F_{2\alpha}$ for induction of abortion: a dose-response study. *J. Obstet. Gynaecol. Brit. Cwlth.*, **80**, 46–47

Craft, I. (1974). Induction of midtrimester abortion: intra-amniotic prostaglandins and urea. *Contemporary OB/GYN*, April, 1974

Craft, I., Ferguson, I. L. C., Smith, B. and Youssefnejadian, E. (1973). Sex steroid hormone levels in plasma following intra-amniotic injection of urea and prostaglandin E_2. *J. Obstet. Gynaecol. Brit. Cwlth.*, **80**, 1095–1099

Craft, I. and Musa, B. (1971). Induction of mid-trimester therapeutic abortion by intraamniotic urea and intravenous oxytocin. *Lancet*, **2**, 1058–1060

Craft, I., Walker, E. and Youssefnejadian, E. (1974). Intra-amniotic prostaglandin $F_{2\alpha}$ and urea for abortion. *Prostaglandins*, **5**, 397–407

Craft, I. and Youssefnejadian, E. (1974). Intra-amniotic prostaglandin techniques for induction of mid-trimester abortion and associated changes in plasma steroid hormones. (In press)

Csapo, A. I. (1973). The prospects of PGs in postconceptional therapy. *Prostaglandins*, **3**, 245–289

Csapo, A. I. (1974). 'Prostaglandin impact' for menstrual induction. *Population Report (Prostaglandins)*, **G**, 33–40

Csapo, A. I., Kivikoski, A., Pulkkinen, M. O. and Wiest, W. G. (1972a). First trimester abortions induced by the extraovular infusion of prostaglandin $F_{2\alpha}$. *Prostaglandins*, **1**, 295–303

Csapo, A. I., Kivikoski, A. and Wiest, W. G. (1972b). Midtrimester abortions induced by intraamniotic prostaglandin $F_{2\alpha}$ treatment. *Prostaglandins*, **1**, 305–318

Csapo, A. I., Kivikoski, A. and Wiest, W. G. (1972b). Massive initial prostaglandin impact in postconceptional therapy. *Prostaglandins*, **2**, 125–134

Csapo, A. I. and Mocsary, P. (1974). Termination by prostaglandin pellets in very early pregnancy. *Lancet*, **2**, 789–790

Csapo, A. I., Mocsary, P., Nagy, T. and Kaihola, H. L. (1973). The efficacy and acceptability of the 'prostaglandin impact' in inducing complete abortion during the second week after the missed menstrual period. *Prostaglandins*, **3**, 125–139

Csapo, A. I., Ruttner, B. and Wiest, W. G. (1972d). First trimester abortions induced by a single extraovular injection of prostaglandin $F_{2\alpha}$. *Prostaglandins*, **1**, 365–371

Csapo, A. I., Sauvage, J. P. and Wiest, W. G. (1971). The efficacy and acceptability of intravenously administered prostaglandin $F_{2\alpha}$ as an abortifacient. *Amer. J. Obstet. Gynecol.*, **111**, 1059–1063

Csapo, A. I. and Wiest, W. G. (1972). On the mechanism of the abortifacient action of prostaglandin $F_{2\alpha}$. *Prostaglandins*, **1**, 158–165

Dillon, T. F., Phillips, L. L., Risk, A., Horiguchi, T., Mohajer-Shojai, E. and Mootabar, H. (1974). The efficacy of prostaglandin $F_{2\alpha}$ in second-trimester abortion—Coagulation and hormonal aspects. *Amer. J. Obstet. Gynecol.*, **118**, 688–698

Dreher, E. and Lippert, T. H. (1972). Induction of abortion by intravenous infusions of prostaglandin $F_{2\alpha}$. *Arch. Gynäk.*, **213**, 48–53

Eaton, C. J., Cohn, F. and Bollinger, C. C. (1972). Laminaria tent as a cervical dilator prior to aspiration-type therapeutic abortion. *Obstet. Gynecol. (N.Y.)*, **39**, 533–537

Edström, K. and Odar-Cederlöf, I. (1974). Therapeutic abortion by means of intrauterine instillation of hypertonic saline. The occurrence of hemolysis following intravascular injection. *Int. J. Gynaecol. Obstet.*, **12**, 35–45

Elias, J. (1973). Prostaglandin $F_{2\alpha}$ vaginal pessaries for midtrimester abortion. *Adv. Biosciences*, **9**, 581–584

Embrey, M. P., quoted by Pickles, V. R., Hall, W. J., Clegg, P. C. and Sullivan, T. J. (1966). Some experiments on the mechanism of action of prostaglandins on the guinea-pig and rat myometrium. *Mem. Soc. Endocrinol.*, **14**, 89–103

Embrey, M. P. (1970). Induction of abortion by prostaglandin E_1 and E_2. *Brit. Med. J.*, **2**, 258–260

Embrey, M. P. (1971a). PGE compounds for induction of labour and abortion. *Ann. N.Y. Acad. Sci.*, **180**, 518–523

Embrey, M. P. (1971b). Induction of abortion by prostaglandins E (PGE_1 and PGE_2). *J. Reprod. Med.*, **6**, 256–259

Embrey, M. P. (1972). Extra-amniotic prostaglandins. In: *Prostaglandins in Fertility Control*, Vol. 2, 109–117 (S. Bergström, K. Gréen and B. Samuelsson, editors) (Stockholm: WHO Research and Training Centre on Human Reproduction)

Embrey, M. P., Calder, A. A. and Hillier, K. (1974). Extra-amniotic prostaglandins in the management of intrauterine fetal death, anencephaly and hydatidiform mole. *J. Obstet. Gynaecol. Brit. Cwlth.*, **81**, 47–51

Embrey, M. P. and Hillier, K. (1971). Therapeutic abortion by intrauterine instillation of prostaglandins. *Brit. Med. J.*, **1**, 588–590

Embrey, M. P., Hillier, K. and Calder, A. A. (1973a). Early abortion induced with prostaglandin $F_{2\alpha}$ and a prostaglandin analogue I.C.I. 74, 205. *Lancet*, **2**, 1100

Embrey, M. P., Hillier, K. and Mahendran, P. (1972). Induction of abortion by extra-amniotic administration of prostaglandins E_2 and $F_{2\alpha}$. *Brit. Med. J.*, **3**, 146–149

Embrey, M. P., Hillier, K. and Mahendran, P. (1973b). Termination of pregnancy by extra-amniotic prostaglandins and the synergistic action of oxytocin. *Adv. Biosciences*, **9**, 507–513

Engel, T., Greer, B., Kochenour, N. and Droegemueller, W. (1973). Midtrimester abortion using prostaglandin $F_{2\alpha}$, oxytocin and laminaria. *Fertility and Sterility*, **24**, 565–568

Enkola, K. (1974). The abortifacient action of the extraovular 'prostaglandin impact' during the first half of human pregnancy. *Prostaglandins*, **5**, 115–121

Filshie, G. M. (1971). The use of prostaglandin E_2 in the management of intrauterine death, missed abortion and hydatidiform mole. *J. Obstet. Gynaecol. Brit. Cwlth.*, **78**, 87–90

Fishburne, J. I. Jr, Brenner, W. E., Braaksma, J. T., Staurovsky, L. G., Mueller, R. A., Hoffer, J. L. and Hendricks, C. H. (1972). Cardiovascular and respiratory responses to intravenous infusion of prostaglandin $F_{2\alpha}$ in the pregnant woman. *Amer. J. Obstet. Gynecol.*, **114**, 765–772

Fraser, I. S. (1974). Complications of prostaglandin-induced abortion. *Brit. Med. J.*, **2**, 404

Fraser, I. S. and Brash, J. H. (1974). Comparison of extra- and intra-amniotic prostaglandins for therapeutic abortion. *Obstet. Gynecol. (N.Y.)*, **43**, 97–103

Fraser, I. S. and Gray, C. (1974a). Electroencephalogram changes after prostaglandin. *Lancet*, **1**, 360

Fraser, I. S. and Gray, C. (1974b). Prostaglandin $F_{2\alpha}$ and electroencephalogram changes. *Lancet*, **2**, 49–50

Freid, N. D., Tredway, D. R. and Mishell, D. R. (1973). Termination of early pregnancy with prostaglandin E_2 vaginal suppositories. *Contraception*, **8**, 255–263

Fylling, P. and Refsdal, A. (1974). Therapeutic abortion by a single extra-amniotic instillation of prostaglandin $F_{2\alpha}$. *Arch. Gynäk.*, **217**, 119–125

Gillespie, A. (1973). Interrelationship between oxytocin (endogenous and exogenous) and prostaglandins. *Adv. Biosciences*, **9**, 761–766

Gillespie, A., Beazley, J. M. and Van Dorp, D. A. (1971). The use of an 'unnatural' prostaglandin in the termination of pregnancy. *J. Obstet. Gynaecol. Brit. Cwlth.*, **78**, 301–304

Gillett, P. G., Kinch, R. A. H., Wolfe, L. S. and Pace-Asciak, C. (1972a). Therapeutic abortion with the use of prostaglandin $F_{2\alpha}$. A study of efficacy, tolerance, and plasma levels with intravenous administration. *Amer. J. Obstet. Gynecol.*, **112**, 330–338

Gillett, P. G., Kinch, R. A. H., Wolfe, L. S. and Pace-Asciak, C. (1972b). Therapeutic abortion in the second trimester by intra-amniotic prostaglandin $F_{2\alpha}$. In: *The Prostaglandins—Clinical Applications in Human Reproduction*, 373–380 (E. M. Southern, editor) (Mount Kisco, N.Y.: Futura)

Gillett, P. G., Kinch, R. A. H., Wolfe, L. S. and Pace-Asciak, C. (1973). Induction of abortion by intra-amniotic $PGF_{2\alpha}$: a comparison of dose schedules. *Adv. Biosciences*, **9**, 545–550

Golbus, M. S. (1974). Laminaria and intra-amniotic prostaglandin $F_{2\alpha}$ for induction of mid-trimester abortions. *Amer. J. Obstet. Gynecol.*, **119**, 569–571

Golbus, M. S. and Erickson, R. P. (1974). Mid-trimester abortion induced by intra-amniotic prostaglandin $F_{2\alpha}$: Fetal tissue viability. *Amer. J. Obstet. Gynecol.*, **119**, 268–270

Goldsmith, S. and Margolis, A. (1971). Aspiration abortion without cervical dilatation. *Amer. J. Obstet. Gynecol.*, **110**, 580–582

Goodlin, R. C. (1972). Risks of legal abortion. *Lancet*, **1**, 97

Gordon, R. T. (1972). Cervicovaginal fistula as a result of saline abortion. *Amer. J. Obstet. Gynecol.*, **112**, 578–579

Göretzlehner, G. and Klausch, B. (1974). Transverse cervical rupture following extra-amniotic prostaglandin $F_{2\alpha}$-induced abortion. *Amer. J. Obstet. Gynecol.*, **119**, 865

Granström, E. (1973). Metabolism and analysis of $PGF_{2\alpha}$ given by the intraamniotic route. In: *Prostaglandins in Fertility Control*, Vol. 3, 62–64 (S. Bergström, editor) (Stockholm: WHO Research and Training Centre on Human Reproduction)

Granström, E., Gréen, K., Bygdeman, M., Toppozada, M. and Wiqvist, N. (1973). Metabolic and quantitative studies in connection with intraamniotic administration of prostaglandin $F_{2\alpha}$ for induction of therapeutic abortion. *Life Sci.*, **12**, 219–229

Gréen, K., Béguin, F., Bygdeman, M., Toppozada, M. and Wiqvist, N. (1972). Analysis of prostaglandin $F_{2\alpha}$ and metabolites following intravenous, intra-amniotic and vaginal administration of prostaglandin $F_{2\alpha}$. In: *Prostaglandins in Fertility Control*, Vol. 2, 189–200 (S. Bergström, K. Gréen and B. Samuelsson, editors) (Stockholm: WHO Research and Training Centre on Human Reproduction)

Gréen, K., Bygdeman, M. and Wiqvist, N. (1974). Kinetic and metabolic studies of prostaglandin $F_{2\alpha}$ administered intra-amniotically for induction of abortion. *Life Sci.*, **14**, 2285–2297

Gupta, D. R. and Cohen, N. H. (1972). Oxytocin, 'salting out', and water intoxication. *J.A.M.A.*, **220**, 681–683

Gustavii, B. and Gréen, K. (1972). Release of prostaglandin $F_{2\alpha}$ following injection of hypertonic saline for therapeutic abortion: A preliminary study. *Amer. J. Obstet. Gynecol.*, **114**, 1099–1100

Hale, R. W. and Pion, R. J. (1972). Laminaria: an underutilized clinical adjunct. *Clin. Obstet. Gynaecol.*, **15**, 829–850

Hanson, F. W., Haslett, E. O. and Sacks, D. A. (1974). Laminaria digitata in saline abortions. *Obstet. Gynecol. (N.Y.)*, **43**, 761–764

Haspels, A. A. and Neth, F. (1973). Induction of abortion. 1. by intravenous and 2. by intrauterine administration of $PGF_{2\alpha}$ (extra- and intraamniotic). *Adv. Biosciences*, **9**, 515–524

Hendricks, C. H., Brenner, W. E., Ekbladh, L., Brotanek, V. and Fishburne, J. I. Jr (1971). Efficacy and tolerance of intravenous prostaglandins $F_{2\alpha}$ and E_2. *Amer. J. Obstet. Gynecol.*, **111**, 564–578

Hillier, K. and Embrey, M. P. (1972). High-dose intravenous administration of prostaglandin E_2 and $F_{2\alpha}$ for the termination of mid-trimester pregnancies. *J. Obstet. Gynaecol. Brit. Cwlth.*, **79**, 14–22

Hingorani, V., Dua, A. and Bhuyan, U. N. (1974). Induction of abortion by intrauterine administration of prostaglandin $F_{2\alpha}$ alpha and histopathological studies of gestational sac. *Contraception*, **10**, 13–23

Hingorani, V. and Ganesh, K. (1972). Induction of abortion by extra-amniotic administration of prostaglandin $F_{2\alpha}$; a preliminary report. *Contraception*, **6**, 353–359

Horwitz, D. A. (1974). Uterine rupture following attempted saline abortion with oxytocin in a grand multiparous patient. *Obstet. Gynecol. (N.Y.)*, **43**, 921–922

Igel, H., Lau, H.-U., Hengst, P. and Halle, H. (1973). Erste Erfahrungen mit dem Prostaglandin $F_{2\alpha}$ bei der künstlichen Abortusauslösung. *Zentralblatt Gynäk.*, **95**, 353–357

Järvinen, P. A., Pennanen, S. and Ylöstalo, P. (1973). Induction of abortion by intra- and extra-amniotic prostaglandin $F_{2\alpha}$ administration. *Prostaglandins*, **3**, 491–504

Jones, J. R., Perez, R. J. and Bienart, W. (1974). Intravaginal PGE_2 in early abortion. *Prostaglandins*, **7**, 149–163

Kajanoja, P., Jungner, G., Widholm, O., Karjalainen, O. and Seppälä, M. (1974). Rupture of the cervix in prostaglandin abortions. *J. Obstet. Gynaecol. Brit. Cwlth.*, **81**, 242–244

Karim, S. M. M. (1966). Identification of prostaglandins in human amniotic fluid. *J. Obstet. Gynaecol. Brit. Cwlth.*, **73**, 903–908

Karim, S. M. M. (1968). Appearance of prostaglandin $F_{2\alpha}$ in human blood during labour. *Brit. Med. J.*, **4**, 618–621

Karim, S. M. M. (1970). The use of prostaglandin E_2 in the management of missed abortion, missed labour and hydatidiform mole. *Brit. Med. J.*, **3**, 196–197

Karim, S. M. M. (1971a). Effects of oral administration of prostaglandins E_2 and $F_{2\alpha}$ on the human uterus. *J. Obstet. Gynaecol. Brit. Cwlth.*, **78**, 289–293

Karim, S. M. M. (1971b). Once-a-month vaginal administration of prostaglandins E_2 and $F_{2\alpha}$ for fertility control. *Contraception*, **3**, 173–183

Karim, S. M. M. (1971c). Prostaglandins as abortifacients. *New Eng. J. Med.*, **285**, 1534–1535

Karim, S. M. M. (1971d). The use of prostaglandins in abortion. In: Abortion, techniques and services. Proceedings of the Conference N.Y. June 3–5, 1971. *Excerpta Medica*, 68–77

Karim, S. M. M. (1971e). Action of prostaglandin in the pregnant woman. *Ann. N.Y. Acad. Sci.*, **180**, 483–498

Karim, S. M. M. (1972). Prostaglandins and human reproduction: Physiological roles and clinical uses of prostaglandin in relation to human reproduction. In: *The Prostaglandins—Progress in Research*, 71–164 (S. M. M. Karim, editor) (Lancaster: M.T.P.)

Karim, S. M. M. (1973). Intrauterine prostaglandins for outpatient termination of very early pregnancy. *Lancet*, 2, 794

Karim, S. M. M. (1974). Adverse reactions to intra-amniotic prostaglandin. *Brit. Med. J.*, 3, 347

Karim, S. M. M. and Amy, J. J. (1973). Effect of prostaglandin 16,16-dimethyl E$_2$ methyl ester on the pregnant human uterus. *Prostaglandins*, 4, 581–592

Karim, S. M. M. and Amy, J. J. (1974). Termination of pregnancy with prostaglandin E$_2$ methyl ester. *Prostaglandins*, 7, 293–302

Karim, S. M. M. and Choo, H. T. (1974). Cervical dilatation with prostaglandin analogues prior to vaginal termination of first trimester pregnancy in nulliparous patients. *Prostaglandins*, 9, 631–638

Karim, S. M. M. and Devlin, J. M. (1967). Prostaglandin content of amniotic fluid during pregnancy and labour. *J. Obstet. Gynaecol. Brit. Cwlth.*, 74, 230–234

Karim, S. M. M. and Filshie, G. M. (1970a). Therapeutic abortion using prostaglandin F$_{2\alpha}$. *Lancet*, 1, 157–159

Karim, S. M. M. and Filshie, G. M. (1970b). Use of prostaglandin E$_2$ for therapeutic abortion. *Brit. Med. J.*, 3, 198–200

Karim, S. M. M. and Filshie, G. M. (1972). The use of prostaglandin E$_2$ for therapeutic abortion. *J. Obstet. Gynaecol. Brit. Cwlth.*, 79, 1–13

Karim, S. M. M. and Hillier, K. (1970). Prostaglandins and spontaneous abortion. *J. Obstet. Gynaecol. Brit. Cwlth.*, 77, 837–839

Karim, S. M. M., Hillier, K., Somers, K. and Trussell, R. R. (1971). The effects of prostaglandins E$_2$ and F$_{2\alpha}$ administered by different routes on uterine activity and the cardiovascular system in pregnant and non-pregnant women. *J. Obstet. Gynaecol. Brit. Cwlth.*, 78, 172–179

Karim, S. M. M. and Ratnam, S. S. (1974). Midtrimester termination. *Brit. Med. J.*, 4, 161–162

Karim, S. M. M., Ratnam, S. S. and Choo, H. T. (1974a). Intrauterine administration of prostaglandin 15 (S) 15 methyl E$_2$ methyl ester in the management of patients with a hydatidiform mole. *J. Obstet. Gynaecol. Brit. Cwlth.*, 81, 650–651

Karim, S. M. M. and Sharma, S. D. (1971a). Therapeutic abortion and induction of labour by the intravaginal administration of prostaglandins E$_2$ and F$_{2\alpha}$. *J. Obstet. Gynaecol. Brit. Cwlth.*, 78, 294–300

Karim, S. M. M. and Sharma, S. D. (1971b). Second trimester abortion with single intra-amniotic injection of prostaglandins E$_2$ or F$_{2\alpha}$. *Lancet*, 2, 47–48

Karim, S. M. M. and Sharma, S. D. (1972). Termination of second trimester pregnancy with 15 methyl analogues of prostaglandins E$_2$ and F$_{2\alpha}$. *J. Obstet. Gynaecol. Brit. Cwlth.*, 79, 737–743

Karim, S. M. M., Sharma, S. D. and Filshie, G. M. (1972a). Termination of pregnancy with 15-methyl analogues of prostaglandins E$_2$ and F$_{2\alpha}$. In: *The Prostaglandins – Clinical Applications in Human Reproduction*, 307–321 (E. M. Southern, editor) (Mount Kisco, N.Y.: Futura)

Karim, S. M. M., Sharma, S. D. and Filshie, G. M. (1972b). Termination of second trimester pregnancy with intra-amniotic administration of prostaglandins E$_2$ and F$_{2\alpha}$. *The Prostaglandins – Clinical Applications in Human Reproduction*, 403–416 (E. M. Southern, editor) (Mount Kisco, N.Y.: Futura)

Karim, S. M. M., Sharma, S. D., Filshie, G. M., Salmon, J. A. and Adaikan Ganesan, P. (1973). Termination of pregnancy with prostaglandin analogs. *Adv. Biosciences*, 9, 811–830

Karim, S. M. M. and Sivasamboo, R. (1974). Termination of second trimester pregnancy with intraamniotic 15(S),15 methyl prostaglandin F$_{2\alpha}$ – A two dose schedule study. (In press)

Karim, S. M. M., Sivasamboo, R. and Ratnam, S. S. (1974b). Abortifacient action of orally administered 16,16 dimethyl prostaglandin E$_2$ and its methyl ester. *Prostaglandins*, 6, 349–354

Karim, S. M. M. and Trussell, R. R. (1971). The use of prostaglandins in obstetrics. *East African Med. J.*, 48, 1–12

Karim, S. M. M., Trussell, R. R., Patel, R. C. and Hillier, K. (1968). Response of pregnant human uterus to prostaglandin F$_{2\alpha}$ – Induction of labour. *Brit. Med. J.*, 4, 621–623

Karman, H. and Potts, M. (1972). Very early abortion using syringe as vacuum source. *Lancet*, 1, 1051–1052

Kaufman, R. G., Freeman, R. K. and Mishell, D. R. Jr (1971). Abortifacient activity of intravenously administered prostaglandins. *Contraception*, 3, 121–132

Kerenyi, T. D. (1969). Hypernatremia following intrauterine instillation of hypertonic saline solution. Report of a case and discussion. *Obstet. Gynecol. (N.Y.)*, 33, 520–527

Kerenyi, T. D., Mandelman, N. and Sherman, D. H. (1973). Five thousand consecutive saline inductions. *Amer. J. Obstet. Gynecol.*, 116, 593–600

Kinòshita, K., Wagatsuma, T., Hogaki, M. and Sakamoto, S. (1971). The induction of abortion by prostaglandin $F_{2\alpha}$. *Amer. J. Obstet. Gynecol.*, 111, 855–858

Kirshen, E. J., Naftolin, F. and Ryan, K. J. (1972). Intravenous $PGF_{2\alpha}$ for therapeutic abortion. *Amer. J. Obstet. Gynecol.*, 113, 340–344

Kirton, K. T. and Forbes, A. D. (1971). Abortifacient efficacy of prostaglandin $F_{2\alpha}$ administered intra-amniotically to rhesus monkeys. *Contraception*, 4, 31–35

Kochenour, N., Engel, T., Henry, G. and Droegemueller, W. (1972). Midtrimester abortion produced by intra-amniotic prostaglandin $F_{2\alpha}$ augmented with intravenous oxytocin. *Amer. J. Obstet. Gynecol.*, 114, 516–519

Korda, A., Shearman, R. P. and Smith, I. D. (1972). Termination of pregnancy by intrauterine prostaglandin $F_{2\alpha}$. *Aust. N.Z. J. Obstet. Gynaecol.*, 12, 166–169

Landesman, R., Kaye, R. E. and Wilson, K. H. (1973). Menstrual extraction: Review of 400 procedures at the Women's Services, New York, New York. *Contraception*, 8, 527–539

Laros, R. K., Collins, J., Penner, J. A., Hage, M. L. and Smith, S. (1973). Coagulation changes in saline-induced abortion. *Amer. J. Obstet. Gynecol.*, 116, 277–283

Lauersen, N. H. and Schulman, J. D. (1973). Oxytocin administration in mid-trimester saline abortions. *Amer. J. Obstet. Gynecol.*, 115, 420–429

Lauersen, N. H. and Wilson, K. (1973). Continuous prostaglandin $F_{2\alpha}$ infusion for middle trimester abortion. *Lancet*, 1, 1195

Lauersen, N. H. and Wilson, K. H. (1974a). Midtrimester abortion induced with a single intra-amniotic instillation of prostaglandin $F_{2\alpha}$. *Amer. J. Obstet. Gynecol.*, 118, 210–217

Lauersen, N. H. and Wilson, K. H. (1974b). Continuous extraovular administration of prostaglandin $F_{2\alpha}$ for midtrimester abortion. *Amer. J. Obstet. Gynecol.*, 120, 273–280

Lauersen, N. H. and Wilson, K. H. (1975). Mid-trimester abortion induced by serial intramuscular injections of 15(S)-15-methyl-prostaglandin $F_{2\alpha}$. *Amer. J. Obstet. Gynecol.*, 121, 273–276

Lauersen, N. H., Wilson, K. H., Beling, C. G. and Fuchs, F. (1974). Comparison of prostaglandin $F_{2\alpha}$ and hypertonic saline for induction of mid-trimester abortion. *Amer. J. Obstet. Gynecol.*, 120, 875–889

Lehmann, F., Breckwoldt, M. and Bettendorf, G. (1972a). Abort Induktion durch Prostaglandin $F_{2\alpha}$. *Geburtsh. Frauenheilk.*, 32, 477–483

Lehmann, F., Peters, F., Breckwoldt, M. and Bettendorf, G. (1972b). Plasma progesterone levels during infusion of prostaglandin $F_{2\alpha}$ in the human. *Prostaglandins*, 1, 269–277

Lehmann, F., Peters, F., Breckwoldt, M. and Bettendorf, G. (1972c). Plasma progestins during infusion of prostaglandin $F_{2\alpha}$. *Acta Endocrinol.*, **Suppl. 159**, 61.

Lehmann, F., Peters, F., Breckwoldt, M. and Bettendorf, G. (1973). Plasma progestin and plasma estrogen levels during infusion of $PGF_{2\alpha}$ in the human. *Adv. Biosciences*, 9, 679–688

Leibman, T., Saldana, L., Schulman, H., Cunningham, M. A. and Randolph, G. (1974). Midtrimester abortion with 15 (S) methyl prostaglandin $F_{2\alpha}$. *Prostaglandins*, 7, 443–448

Lemkin, S. R. and Kattlove, H. E. (1973). Maternal death due to DIC after saline abortion. *Obstet. Gynecol. (N.Y.)*, 42, 233–235

Leslie, D. C. and Laufe, L. E. (1972). The evaluation of intraamniotic prostaglandin $F_{2\alpha}$ in the management of early midtrimester pregnancy termination. In: *The Prostaglandins – Clinical Applications in Human Reproduction*, 451–455 (E. M. Southern, editor) (Mount Kisco, N.Ỹ.: Futura)

Lewis, S. C., Lal, S., Branch, B. and Beard, R. W. (1971). Outpatient termination of pregnancy. *Brit. Med. J.*, 4, 606–610

Lichtman, A. S., Brenner, P. and Mishell, D. R. (1974). Intrauterine administration of prostaglandin $F_{2\alpha}$ as an outpatient procedure for termination of early pregnancy. *Contraception*, 9, 403–408

Lindmark, G., Melander, S., Nilsson, B. A. and Zador, G. (1973). Inhibition of prostaglandin induced uterine activity in the second trimester pregnancy by β-mimetic adrenergic agents. *Prostaglandins*, 3, 481–489

Lippert, T. H., Bärtschi, R. and Lüthi, A. (1973). Therapeutic abortion by intrauterine infusion of prostaglandin $F_{2\alpha}$. *Arch. Gynäk.*, 213, 197–201

Lippert, T. H. and Modly, T. (1973). Induction of abortion by the extra-amniotic administration of prostaglandin gels. *J. Obstet. Gynaecol. Brit. Cwlth.*, 80, 1025–1027

Lischke, J. H. and Goodlin, R. C. (1972). Use of laminaria tents with saline abortion. *Lancet*, 1, 49

Liu, D. T. Y. and Hudson, I. (1974). Karman cannula and first trimester termination of pregnancy. *Amer. J. Obstet. Gynecol.*, 118, 906–909

Lowensohn, R. and Ballard, C. A. (1974). Cervicovaginal fistula: An apparent increased incidence with prostaglandin $F_{2\alpha}$. *Amer. J. Obstet. Gynecol.*, 119, 1057–1061

Lyneham, R. C., Low, P. A., McLeod, J. G., Shearman, R. P., Smith, I. D. and Korda, A. R. (1973). Convulsions and electroencephalogram abnormalities after intraamniotic prostaglandin $F_{2\alpha}$. *Lancet*, 2, 1003–1005

MacKenzie, I. Z., Embrey, M. P. and Hillier, K. (1974). Intraamniotic prostaglandin for induction of abortion: an improved regime using prostaglandin E_2. *J. Obstet. Gynaecol. Brit. Cwlth.*, 81, 554–557

MacKenzie, I. Z. and Hillier, K. (1974). Extra-amniotic administration of prostaglandins. *Lancet*, 1, 511

MacKenzie, I. Z., Hillier, K. and Embrey, M. P. (1973). Convulsions and prostaglandin induced abortion. *Lancet*, 2, 1323

MacKenzie, I. Z., Hillier, K. and Embrey, M. P. (1974). Single extra-amniotic injection of prostaglandin E_2 in viscous gel to induce midtrimester abortion. *Brit. Med. J.*, 1, 240–242

Manabe, Y. (1971). Laminaria tent for gradual and safe cervical dilation. *Amer. J. Obstet. Gynecol.*, 110, 743–745

Manabe, Y., Nakajima, A. and Griggs, J. F. (1973). Uterine contractility and placental histology in abortion by laminaria and metreurynter. *Obstet. Gynecol. (N.Y.)*, 41, 753–759

Mann, L. I., Duchin, S., Newman, M. and Weiss, R. R. (1973). Saline instillation with oxytocin administration in midtrimester abortion. *Obstet. Gynecol. (N.Y.)*, 41, 748–752

Midwinter, A., Bowen, M. and Shepherd, A. (1972). Continuous intrauterine infusion of prostaglandin E_2 for termination of pregnancy. *J. Obstet. Gynaecol. Brit. Cwlth.*, 79, 807–809

Midwinter, A., Shepherd, A. and Bowen, M. (1973). Continuous extra-amniotic prostaglandin E_2 for therapeutic termination and the effectiveness of various infusion rates and dosages. *J. Obstet. Gynaecol. Brit. Cwlth.*, 80, 371–373

Miller, A. W. F. (1973). The use of prostaglandins for missed abortion, fetal death *in utero* and hydatidiform mole. In: *Prostaglandins Symposium: The Use of Prostaglandins E_2 and $F_{2\alpha}$ in Obstetrics and Gynaecology*, 63–67 (R. G. Jacomb, editor) (Miami: Symposia Specialists)

Miller, A. W. F., Calder, A. A. and Macnaughton, M. C. (1972). Termination of pregnancy by continuous intrauterine infusion of prostaglandins. *Lancet*, 2, 5–7

Mocsary, P. and Csapo, A. I. (1973). Delayed menstruation induced by prostaglandin in pregnant patients. *Lancet*, 2, 683

Morewood, G. A. (1973). Therapeutic abortion employing the synergistic action of extra-amniotic prostaglandin E_2 and an intravenous infusion of oxytocin. *J. Obstet. Gynaecol. Brit. Cwlth.*, 80, 473–475

Naftolin, F., Kirshen, E. J. and Ryan, K. J. (1972). Therapeutic abortion utilizing local application of prostaglandin $F_{2\alpha}$. In: *The Prostaglandins – Clinical Applications in Human Reproduction*, 423–431 (E. M. Southern, editor) (Mount Kisco, N.Y.: Futura)

Naismith, W. C. M. K. and Barr, W. (1974). Simultaneous intravenous infusion of prostaglandin E_2 (PGE_2) and oxytocin in the management of intrauterine death of the fetus, missed abortion and hydatidiform mole. *J. Obstet. Gynaecol. Brit. Cwlth.*, 81, 146–149

Najak, Z., Hillier, K. and Karim, S. M. M. (1970). The action of prostaglandins on the human isolated non-pregnant cervix. *J. Obstet. Gynaecol. Brit. Cwlth.*, 77, 701–709

Newton, M. W. (1972). Laminaria tent: Relic of the past or modern medical device? *Amer. J. Obstet. Gynecol.*, 113, 442–448

Newton, J. and Collins, W. (1973). Plasma hormone changes during infusions of prostaglandins $F_{2\alpha}$ and E_2 for therapeutic abortion. *Adv. Biosciences*, 9, 689–699

Nyberg, R. (1973). Therapeutic abortion by intraamniotic administration of prostaglandin $F_{2\alpha}$. *Adv. Biosciences*, 9, 533–537

Ostergard, D. R. (1973). The cervical relaxant properties of prostaglandin E_2 in non-pregnant subjects. *Prostaglandins*, **4**, 701–702

Pace-Asciak, C., Wolfe, L. S., Gillett, P. G. and Kinch, R. A. (1972). Disappearance of prostaglandin $F_{2\alpha}$ from human amniotic fluid after intraamniotic injection. *Prostaglandins*, **1**, 469–477

Pedersen, P. H., Larsen, J. F. and Sorensen, B. (1972). Induction of labour with prostaglandin $F_{2\alpha}$ in missed abortion, fetus mortuus, and anencephalia. *Prostaglandins*, **2**, 135–141

Phillips, L. L., Mohajer-Shojai, E. and Dillon, T. F. (1974). Coagulation studies during second trimester abortions induced by $PGF_{2\alpha}$. *Amer. J. Obstet. Gynecol.*, **119**, 577–582

Pion, R. J., Hale, R. W. and Reich, L. (1972). Vaginal administration of prostaglandins and early abortion. In: *The Prostaglandins – Clinical Applications in Human Reproduction*, 367–372 (E. M. Southern, editors) (Mount Kisco, N.Y.: Futura)

Pitkanen, Y. and Rauramo, L. (1974). The efficacy of the extraovular 'prostaglandin-impact' in provoking first trimester abortion. *Prostaglandins*, **5**, 269–274

Pulkkinen, M. O., Pitkanen, Y., Ojala, A. and Hannelin, H. (1974). Decrease of utero–placental blood flow during prostaglandin $F_{2\alpha}$ induced abortion. (In press)

Roberts, G. (1974). Induction of labour and abortion by intravenous prostaglandins in pregnancies complicated by intra-uterine foetal death and hydatidiform mole. *Current Med. Research and Opinion*, **2**, 342–350

Roberts, G., Cassie, R. and Turnbull, A. C. (1971). Therapeutic abortion by intrauterine instillation of prostaglandin E_2. *J. Obstet. Gynaecol. Brit. Cwlth.*, **78**, 834–837

Roberts, G., Gomersall, R., Adams, M. and Turnbull, A. C. (1973). Therapeutic abortion by intraamniotic injection of prostaglandins. *Adv. Biosciences*, **9**, 555–560

Roth-Brandel, U. (1971). Response of the pregnant human uterus to low and high doses of prostaglandin E_1 and E_2. *Acta Obstet. Gynecol. Scand.*, **50**, 159–166

Roth-Brandel, U., Bygdeman, M. and Wiqvist, N. (1970a). A comparative study on the influence of prostaglandin E_1, oxytocin and ergometrin on the pregnant human uterus. *Acta Obstet. Gynecol. Scand.*, **49, Suppl. 5**, 1–7

Roth-Brandel, U., Bygdeman, M., Wiqvist, N. and Bergström, S. (1970b). Prostaglandins for induction of therapeutic abortion. *Lancet*, **1**, 190–191

Ruppen, M., Keller, P. J., Schmid, J. and Schreiner, W. E. (1972). Prostaglandine bei 'missed abortion' und bei 'missed labor'. *Schweiz. Z. Gynäk. Geburtsh.*, **3**, 439–442

Saldana, L., Schulman, H. and Yang, W.-H. (1973). On the mechanism of midtrimester abortions induced by the prostaglandin impact. *Prostaglandins*, **3**, 847–858

Salmon, J. A., Ghodgaonkar, R. and Telli, T. H. (1974). Comparison of the actions of the 15-methyl analogs of prostaglandins E_2 and $F_{2\alpha}$ on hormone levels after their administration for therapeutic abortion. *Prostaglandins*, **5**, 197–207

Sandberg, F., Ingelman-Sundberg, A., Ryden, G. and Joelsson, I. (1968). The absorption of tritium-labelled prostaglandin E_1 from the vagina of non-pregnant women. *Acta Obstet. Gynecol. Scand.*, **47**, 22–26

Sato, T., Ami, K. and Matsumoto, S. (1973a). The induction of abortion and menstruation by the intravaginal administration of prostaglandin $F_{2\alpha}$. *Amer. J. Obstet. Gynecol.*, **116**, 287–289

Sato, T., Ami, K., Shinada, T. and Igarashi, M. (1973b). Plasma progesterone and prostaglandin $F_{2\alpha}$ levels during the insertion of prostaglandin $F_{2\alpha}$ vaginal tablet. *Prostaglandins*, **4**, 107–113

Seppälä, M., Kajanoja, P., Widholm, O. and Vara, P. (1972). Prostaglandin-oxytocin abortion; a clinical trial on intra-amniotic prostaglandin $F_{2\alpha}$ in combination with intravenous oxytocin. *Prostaglandins*, **2**, 311–319

Seppälä, M., Renkonen, O.-V. and Vara, P. (1973). Extra-amniotic prostaglandin-oxytocin abortion; comparison with the intra-amniotic method. *Prostaglandins*, **3**, 17–28

Sharp, D. S. and Burslem, R. W. (1973). The termination of pregnancy by intravenous infusion of a synthetic prostaglandin $F_{2\alpha}$ analogue. *J. Obstet. Gynaecol. Brit. Cwlth.*, **80**, 138–141

Shearman, R., Smith, I. and Korda, A. (1972). Second trimester termination by intra-uterine prostaglandin $F_{2\alpha}$. Clinical and hormonal results with observations on induced lactation and chronoperiodicity. In: *The Prostaglandins – Clinical Applications in Human Reproduction*, 443–450 (E. M. Southern, editor) (Mount Kisco, N.Y.: Futura)

Shutt, D. A., Smith, I. D. and Shearman, R. P. (1973). Changes in estrogen levels in maternal venous plasma after intra-amniotic infusion of prostaglandin $F_{2\alpha}$ for therapeutic abortion. *Prostaglandins*, **4**, 291–299

Smith, A. M. (1974a). Adverse reactions to intra-amniotic prostaglandins. *Brit. Med. J.*, 2, 382–383

Smith, A. P. (1972). Side effects of prostaglandins. *Lancet*, 2, 653

Smith, A. P. (1973). The effects of intravenous infusion of graded doses of prostaglandins $F_{2\alpha}$ and E_2 on lung resistance in patients undergoing termination of pregnancy. *Clin. Sci.*, 44, 17–25

Smith, I. D. (1974b). Circadian timing, duration, dose and cost of prostaglandin $F_{2\alpha}$-induced termination of middle trimester pregnancy. *Chronobiologia*, 1, 41–53

Smith, I. D., Shearman, R. P. and Korda, A. R. (1972). Lactation following therapeutic abortion with prostaglandin $F_{2\alpha}$. *Nature (London)*, 240, 411–412

Smith, I. D., Shearman, R. P. and Korda, A. R. (1973). Chronoperiodicity in response to the intra-amniotic injection of prostaglandin $F_{2\alpha}$ in the human. *Nature (London)*, 241, 279–280

Smith, I. D. and Temple, D. M. (1973). The influence of analgesic drugs on the actions of prostaglandin $F_{2\alpha}$ on the human uterus *in vivo* and rabbit myometrial strips *in vitro*. *Prostaglandins*, 4, 469–477

Speroff, L., Caldwell, B. V., Brock, W. A., Anderson, G. G. and Hobbins, J. C. (1972). Hormone levels during prostaglandin $F_{2\alpha}$ infusions for therapeutic abortion. *J. Clin. Endocrinol. Metab.*, 34, 531–536

Stallworthy, J. A., Moolgaoker, A. S. and Walsh, J. J. (1971). Legal abortion: a critical assessment of its risks. *Lancet*, 2, 1245

Stander, R. W., Flessa, H. C., Glueck, H. I. and Kisker, C. T. (1971). Changes in maternal coagulation factors after intra-amniotic injection of hypertonic saline. *Obstet. Gynecol. (N.Y.)*, 37, 660–666

Stubblefield, P. G., Naftolin, F., Frigoletto, F. D. and Ryan, K. J. (1974). Pretreatment with laminaria tents before mid-trimester abortion with intra-amniotic prostaglandin $F_{2\alpha}$. *Amer. J. Obstet. Gynecol.*, 118, 284–285

Symonds, E. M., Fahmy, D., Morgan, C., Roberts, G., Gomersall, C. R. and Turnbull, A. C. (1972). Maternal plasma oestrogen and progesterone levels during therapeutic abortion induced by intra-amniotic injection of prostaglandin $F_{2\alpha}$. *J. Obstet. Gynaecol. Brit. Cwlth.*, 79, 976–980

Thiery, M., Amy, J.-J., de Hemptinne, D. and Yo Le Sian, A. (1974). Prostaglandins and convulsions. *Lancet*, 1, 218

Toppozada, M., Béguin, F., Bygdeman, M., Wide, L. and Wiqvist, N. (1973a). Postconceptional fertility control by prostaglandins. *Adv. Biosciences*, 9, 567–573

Toppozada, M., Béguin, F., Bygdeman, M. and Wiqvist, N. (1972a). Response of the mid-pregnant human uterus to systemic administration of 15(S)-15-methyl-prostaglandin $F_{2\alpha}$. *Prostaglandins*, 2, 239–249

Toppozada, M., Bygdeman, M., Papageorgiou, C. and Wiqvist, N. (1973b). Administration of 15-methyl-prostaglandin $F_{2\alpha}$ as a pre-operative means of cervical dilatation. *Prostaglandins*, 4, 371–379

Toppozada, M., Bygdeman, M. and Wiqvist, N. (1971). Induction of abortion by intra-amniotic administration of prostaglandin $F_{2\alpha}$. *Contraception*, 4, 293–301

Toppozada, M., Bygdeman, M. and Wiqvist, N. (1972b). Prostaglandin administration for induction of mid-trimester abortion in complicated pregnancies. *Lancet*, 2, 1420–1421

Toppozada, M., Bygdeman, M., and Wiqvist, N. (1973c). Systemic and local administration of prostaglandins for postconceptional fertility control. In: *Prostaglandins in Fertility Control*, Vol. 3, 108–115 (S. Bergström, editor) (Stockholm: WHO Research and Training Centre on Human Reproduction)

Tredway, D. R. and Mishell, D. R. (1973). Therapeutic abortion of early human gestation with vaginal suppositories of prostaglandin $F_{2\alpha}$. *Amer. J. Obstet. Gynecol.*, 116, 795–798

Tyack, A. J., Lambadarios, C., Parsons, R. J., Stewart, C. R. and Cooke, I. D. (1974). Plasma progesterone and oestradiol-17β changes during abortion induced by prostaglandin $F_{2\alpha}$. *J. Obstet. Gynaecol. Brit. Cwlth.*, 81, 52–56

Van der Plaetsen, L., Thiery, M., Amy, J. J. and de Hemptinne, D. (1974). Effect of prostaglandin E_2 therapy on the cerebral cortex. *Lancet*, 1, 1226

Waltman, R. and Tricomi, V. (1974). Pentazocine, mefenamic acid, and hypertonic-saline abortions. *Lancet*, 2, 468

Waltman, R., Tricomi, V. and Palav, A. V. (1972). Mid-trimester hypertonic saline-induced abortion: Effect of indomethacin on induction/abortion time. *Amer. J. Obstet. Gynecol.*, 114, 829–831

Waltman, R., Tricomi, V. and Palav, A. V. (1973). Aspirin and indomethacin: Effect on instillation/abortion time of mid-trimester hypertonic saline induced abortion. *Prostaglandins*, 3, 47–58

Weiss, A. E., Easterling, W. E. Jr, Odom, M. H., McMillan, C. W., Johnson, A. M. and Talbert, L. M. (1972)). Defibrination syndrome after intra-amniotic infusion of hypertonic saline. *Amer. J. Obstet. Gynecol.*, 113, 868–874

Wentz, A. C., Austin, K. and King, T. M. (1973a). Abortifacient efficacy of intravaginal prostaglandin $F_{2\alpha}$. *Amer. J. Obstet. Gynecol.*, 115, 27–32

Wentz, A. C., Burnett, L. S., Atienza, M. F. and King, T. M. (1973b). Experience with intra-amniotic prostaglandin $F_{2\alpha}$ for abortion. *Amer. J. Obstet. Gynecol.*, 117, 513–521

Wentz, A. C., Cushner, I. M., Austin, K. and Shams, M. (1972a). Intra-amniotic administration of prostaglandin $F_{2\alpha}$ for abortion. *Amer. J. Obstet. Gynecol.*, 113, 793–803

Wentz, A. C., Jones, G. S. and Graeber, J. (1972b). Effect of infused prostaglandin $F_{2\alpha}$ on hormonal levels during early pregnancy. *Amer. J. Obstet. Gynecol.*, 114, 908–913

Wentz, A. C. and King, T. M. (1972). Intramyometrial prostaglandin $F_{2\alpha}$. *Amer. J. Obstet. Gynecol.*, 114, 112–114

Wentz, A. C., Thompson, B. H. and King, T. M. (1973c). Posterior cervical rupture following prostaglandin-induced mid-trimester abortion. *Amer. J. Obstet. Gynecol.*, 115, 1107–1110

Wiqvist, N., Béguin, F., Bygdeman, M., Fernström, I. and Toppozada, M. (1972a). Induction of abortion by extra-amniotic prostaglandin administration. *Prostaglandins*, 1, 37–53

Wiqvist, N., Béguin, F., Bygdeman, M. and Toppozada, M. (1972b). Extra-amniotic administration of prostaglandin for induction of abortion. In: *Prostaglandins in Fertility Control*, Vol. 2, 118–128 (S. Bergström, K. Gréen and B. Samuelsson, editors) (Stockholm: WHO Research and Training Centre on Human Reproduction)

Wiqvist, N., Béguin, F., Bygdeman, M. and Toppozada, M. (1972c). Vaginal administration of prostaglandin. In: *Prostaglandins in Fertility Control*, Vol. 2, 164–169 (S. Bergström, K. Gréen and B. Samuelsson, editors) (Stockholm: WHO Research and Training Centre on Human Reproduction)

Wiqvist, N., Béguin, F., Bygdeman, M. and Toppozada, M. (1972d). Recent aspects on systemic administration of prostaglandin. In: *The Prostaglandins—Clinical Applications in Human Reproduction*, 295–306 (E. M. Southern, editor) (Mount Kisco, N.Y.: Futura)

Wiqvist, N., Béguin, F., Bygdeman, M. and Toppozada, M. (1973a). 15 (S)-15-methyl-prostaglandin $F_{2\alpha}$. Myometrial response and abortifacient efficacy. *Adv. Biosciences*, 9, 831–842

Wiqvist, N. and Bygdeman, M. (1970). Therapeutic abortion by local administration of prostaglandin. *Lancet*, 2, 716–717

Wiqvist, N., Bygdeman, M., Kwon, S. U., Mukherjee, T. and Roth-Brandel, U. (1968). Effect of prostaglandin E_1 on the midpregnant human uterus. Intravenous, intramuscular, intra-amniotic, and vaginal administration. *Amer. J. Obstet. Gynecol.*, 102, 327–332

Wiqvist, N., Bygdeman, M., Papageorgiou, C. and Toppozada, M. (1974). Intrauterine administration of prostaglandin by the extra-amniotic route. *Prostaglandins*, 6, 193–205

Wiqvist, N., Bygdeman, M. and Toppozada, M. (1971). Induction of abortion by the intravenous administration of prostaglandin $F_{2\alpha}$. A critical evaluation. *Acta Obstet. Gynecol. Scand.*, 50, 381–389

Wiqvist, N., Bygdeman, M. and Toppozada, M. (1973b). Intra-amniotic prostaglandin administration—A challenge to the currently used methods for induction of midtrimester abortion. *Contraception*, 8, 113–131

Wiqvist, N., Bygdeman, M. and Toppozada, M. (1973c). Prostaglandins in Fertility Regulation. In: *Prostaglandins in Fertility Control*, Vol. 3, 80–107 (S. Bergström, editor) (Stockholm: WHO Research and Training Centre on Human Reproduction)

Wolfe, L. S. and Pace-Asciak, C. (1972). Measurement of prostaglandin $F_{2\alpha}$ concentration in plasma during clinical evaluation in therapeutic abortion. In: *Prostaglandins in Fertility Control*, Vol. 2, 201–207 (S. Bergström, K. Gréen and B. Samuelsson, editors) (Stockholm: WHO Research and Training Centre on Human Reproduction)

Wright, C. S. W., Campbell, S. and Beazley, J. (1972). Second-trimester abortion after vaginal termination of pregnancy. *Lancet*, 1, 1278–1279

Yankee, E. W. and Bundy, G. L. (1972). (15 S)-15-methyl-prostaglandins. *J. Amer. Chem. Soc.*, 94, 3651–3652

Ylikorkala, O., Jouppila, P., Ylöstalo, P. and Jarvinen, P. A. (1974). Intrauterine injection of prostaglandin $F_{2\alpha}$ for termination of early pregnancy in out-patient. *Prostaglandins*, 7, 57–70

Ylikorkala, O. and Pennanen, S. (1973). Human placental lactogen (HPL) levels in maternal serum during abortion induced by intra- and extra-amniotic injection of prostaglandin $F_{2\alpha}$. *J. Obstet. Gynaecol. Brit. Cwlth.*, **80**, 927–931

Ylöstalo, P., Kauppila, E. and Vapaatalo, H. (1974). Complications following the intra-amniotic administration of prostaglandin $F_{2\alpha}$ for therapeutic abortion. *Acta Obstet. Gynecol. Scand.*, **53**, 279–282

Zoltan, I., Csillag, M., Zsolnai, B., Zubek, L., Moksony, I. and Matanyi, S. (1974). The termination of first trimester pregnancy by extraovular 'prostaglandin impact'. *Prostaglandins*, **6**, 211–216

4
Induction of Labour with Prostaglandins

M. THIERY and J.-J. AMY

Abbreviations

ECG : electrocardiogram
FHR : fetal heart rate
HCG : human chorionic gonadotrophin
HCS : human chorionic somato-mammotrophin
     (=human placental lactogen)
IUD : intrauterine fetal death
i.v. : intravenous, intravenously
PG : prostaglandin
pH_a : actual pH of umbilical-artery blood
pH_s : actual pH of scalp blood
pH_v : actual pH of umbilical-vein blood

4.1 INTRODUCTION

Long before the prostaglandins were recognised as a distinct group of biologically active substances, there were hints that some unknown compounds capable of inducing uterine activity existed. Pregnant Eskimo women ingested fat from the paws of polar bears to enhance sluggish uterine activity (Schotman, 1974) and for the same purpose, oral ingestion of seminal fluid was practised by some African tribes (Harley, 1941). In Belgium, it was common practice in some strata of the population to indulge in intercourse at the onset of labour, in order to hasten its progress. Conversely, coitus was considered harmful during pregnancy, because of the threat of triggering labour prematurely (Pystynen and Nummi, 1974). Since semen is one of the richest natural sources of prostaglandins and as the vaginal and oral administration of prostaglandins causes the uterus to contract, the above-mentioned beliefs could have a sound physiological basis. It is worth remembering, however, that factors other than deposition of semen into the vagina are involved and that orgasm in the female is of particular importance in this connection (Masters and Johnson, 1966; Goodlin, 1969; Goodlin et al., 1971). Wiqvist et al. (1968) and Karim (1972, page 141) were unable to stimulate uterine activity at mid-pregnancy or at term by vaginal instillation of seminal fluid. It is probable that the amount of prostaglandin present in semen deposited during intercourse is not sufficient to stimulate the uterus. Another possibility is that these prostaglandins are to some degree inactivated in the vagina (Karim, 1972, pp. 141–142). Higher than normal amounts of prostaglandins in semen, or repeated coitus, or an undue sensitivity of the myometrium to prostaglandins could of course stimulate the uterus and induce premature labour. This is more likely to happen in the third trimester as a result of increasing sensitivity of the myometrium to prostaglandins with progression of pregnancy.

In 1968, Karim et al. first reported on the successful use of purified prostaglandin $F_{2\alpha}$ ($PGF_{2\alpha}$) for the induction of labour at term. Numerous clinical trials with prostaglandins of the groups E and F, given by various routes, have since confirmed their value as oxytocic agents. Some of the naturally occurring prostaglandins are now commercially available for termination of early and late pregnancy. In 1972, the Committee on Safety of Medicines of the British Government approved the sale of PGE_2 and $PGF_{2\alpha}$ for labour induction. One year later, $PGF_{2\alpha}$ was made available in the USA for interruption of second trimester pregnancy by intra-amniotic instillation.

Since publication of the first edition of this book (1972), numerous reports on the induction of labour with prostaglandins have appeared. A review of all published material is hardly possible, particularly because of the dissimilarity of protocols and the lack of generally accepted definitions (e.g. 'success' or 'failure' of induction). Relevant information is often missing; for instance many investigators fail to make a clear distinction between cases electively induced and cases of 'therapeutic induction'. However, elective inductions, by definition performed at term (38–42 full menstrual weeks) in uncomplicated pregnancies, form the only acceptable material for evaluation of the fetal and neonatal effects of an oxytocic. Therapeutic inductions, on the other hand, are performed because of a complication of pregnancy which by itself may be detrimental to mother or fetus, or may alter the effects of the prostaglandins to them. Finally, some investigators have published progress reports at short intervals and it has not always been possible to accurately define the number of patients treated.

Classification of the data is a problem too because several factors must be taken into consideration, such as length of gestation, indication for the induction, type of prostaglandin used, dose and route of administration. We have attempted to do this in the present chapter which we hope, for a short time to come, may serve as a ready source of reference to investigators. Labour induction at term (Section 4.2) and before term are discussed separately. In the latter event, the indication necessitating termination of pregnancy and the relative resistance of the preterm uterus to classical techniques of labour induction, may affect the outcome of the induction trial. Consequently, a section is devoted to the induction of labour in complicated pregnancies (Section 4.3). Acceleration of labour (Section 4.4) and the use of prostaglandins for the active management of the third stage of labour (Section 4.5) are also discussed under separate headings. A final section (Section 4.6) is devoted to the comparison of prostaglandins with oxytocin for the induction of labour.

4.2 INDUCTION OF LABOUR AT TERM

4.2.1 Intravenous route

The stimulatory action of a prostaglandin (PGE_1) on the gravid myometrium *in vitro* was first reported by Bygdeman in 1964. Karim (1966) and Karim and Devlin (1967), finding elevated levels of prostaglandins in amniotic fluid collected during labour, suggested that these compounds could play a physiological role in the initiation of uterine activity. Soon thereafter, Karim *et al.* (1968) published the first report on the successful induction of labour at term by means of intravenously infused $PGF_{2\alpha}$. This initial paper, which prompted other investigators to conduct comparable trials with this compound (Embrey, 1969; Roberts, 1970), was soon followed by a more extensive report from Uganda confirming that continuous fixed-dose infusion of $3\mu g\ min^{-1}\ PGF_{2\alpha}$ produced uterine contractions similar to those characterising normal labour (Karim *et al.*, 1969). Then came the first reports on labour induction at term by intravenous infusion of PGE_2 (Embrey, 1969; Beazley *et al.*, 1970; Karim *et al.*, 1970). These early clinical investigations with $PGF_{2\alpha}$ and PGE_2 set the stage for a large number of trials designed to answer the basic questions of safety and effectiveness of these drugs. Comparative studies with oxytocin, however, could only be tackled by using standardised and adequately designed protocols. As early as 1971, Anderson *et al.* (1971) and Karim (1971b) reported preliminary results of double-blind comparative studies conducted with $PGF_{2\alpha}$, PGE_2 and oxytocin. Anderson and colleagues suggested the incorporation of Bishop's inducibility score (Bishop, 1964) into research protocols to enhance intergroup comparability and the use of constant dose levels infused during fixed periods of time. Gillespie (1971) stressed the need to increase rapidly the infusion rate of PG in order to obtain effective uterine contractions. He thus introduced the drug-titration method currently used for labour induction with oxytocin (Turnbull and Anderson, 1968) into the field of PG research. Most of these improvements in protocol design have been adopted and have proven immensely successful. Sadly enough, a large-scale international double-blind comparative trial planned by the Upjohn Company had to be interrupted prematurely because of shelf instability of PGE_2. The temporary withdrawal of this compound explains the delay in the investigation of PGE_2 for labour induction which occurred in many countries.

Simultaneously, the Karolinska group (Bygdeman *et al.*, 1970; Roth-Brandel *et al.*, 1970; Roth-Brandel and Adams, 1970; Roth-Brandel, 1971) concentrated on studying the response of the pregnant uterus *in vivo* to bolus intravenous injections or short lasting infusions of prostaglandins. These carefully conducted experiments led the Swedish authors to question whether—as postulated by Karim and others—the uterine contractions produced by these drugs could be considered physiological. Their statements were the basis of a controversy which has since been largely resolved by the conduct of extensive labour induction trials. Four naturally occurring PGs (E_1, E_2, $F_{1\alpha}$ and $F_{2\alpha}$) —(but no analogues)—have been studied for the induction of labour at term by the i.v. route. Investigations were mainly restricted to $PGF_{2\alpha}$ and PGE_2. With these compounds results of such a large number of trials have accumulated since publication of the first edition of this book that it is not possible to cover this material completely. Therefore, to assess effectiveness and maternal safety of labour induction at term with $PGF_{2\alpha}$ and PGE_2 we have concentrated on the larger clinical studies. The same approach is followed for the comparison of intravenous prostaglandins and oxytocin for the induction of labour.

4.2.1.1 Prostaglandin $F_{2\alpha}$

A thorough review of this subject was published by Anderson in 1973.

4.2.1.1.1 *Individual reports. In vitro*, $PGF_{2\alpha}$ (0.05–0.1 μg ml^{-1} bath solution) has a stimulant action ('spasmogenic effect') on fundal myometrial strips from the term human uterus (Embrey and Morrison, 1968). This compound, when given by i.v. infusion, also stimulates the term pregnant uterus *in vivo*, the threshold dose being of the order of 5 μg min^{-1} (Karim *et al.*, 1968, 1969).

In their initial study Karim *et al.* (1968) reported successful induction of labour in 10 women at or about term (34–44 weeks) to whom a fixed dose of 0.05 μg kg^{-1} min^{-1} $PGF_{2\alpha}$ (equivalent to 3.0 μg min^{-1} for a woman of 60 kg) was infused. Uterine activity was monitored by external tocography. In all cases uterine contractions, which started after a latent period of 15–20 min, were comparable to those observed in normal spontaneous labour. The average induction–delivery interval was 6 hours 46 min. In the eight living fetuses (there were two cases of intrauterine death) the fetal heart rate (FHR), recorded every 10 min, remained normal and the infants were in good condition at birth. The third stage of labour was uncomplicated. Vital signs remained within normal limits. In a more extensive clinical trial reported by the same group and applying the same dose schedule, labour was successfully induced in 29 of 35 subjects (Karim *et al.*, 1969).

In England, Embrey (1969) attempted induction of labour at term with i.v. infusions of $PGF_{2\alpha}$ of short duration (18–44 min) at the dose level of 2–8 μg min^{-1}. The procedure succeeded in one out of four women. Roberts (1970) and Roberts and Turnbull (1971) reported on seven women at or near term (38–43 weeks) induced by combined amniotomy and i.v. infusion of 3–6 μg min^{-1} PGF$_{2\alpha}$. The induction–delivery interval was less than 14 hours in each of the successful cases. Induction failed in one patient whose cervix was only 2 cm dilated after 18 hours of infusion; the supply of prostaglandin being exhausted, uterine activity was successfully augmented by i.v. oxytocin. All infants were normal at birth. Uterine hypertonus was not observed. However, venous erythema over the course of the infused vein was a constant feature. These authors suggested that the lack of antidiuresis associated with the use of PGF$_{2\alpha}$ was an advantage over oxytocin for the induction of labour.

Kinoshita *et al.* (1971), combining PGF$_{2\alpha}$ with amniotomy, successfully induced 30/30 women at or near term. Dose levels were titrated and ranged from 0.04 to 0.18 μg kg^{-1} min^{-1} (equivalent to 2.4–10.8 μg min^{-1} for a subject of 60 kg). The method appeared safe for both mother and child. Although uterine hypertonus was not registered, the pattern of myometrial activity produced by the PG was different from that of oxytocin.

Karim (1971b) next reported on two studies, in the first of which induction of labour was attempted in 100 patients (14 nulliparas and 86 parous patients) by infusing 5–10 μg min^{-1} PGF$_{2\alpha}$. The procedure was successful in 93 women; two of these were delivered by Caesarean section. The seven patients in whom induction had failed were successfully induced or stimulated with PGE$_2$. The average time to delivery was 17 hours and 10 hours 30 min for the nulliparous and parous groups respectively. The second study compared in a double-blind fashion the effectiveness of PGF$_{2\alpha}$, PGE$_2$ and oxytocin. Only 67% of the inductions attempted with PGF$_{2\alpha}$ succeeded, giving a failure rate almost five times as high as that of the previous study. This discrepancy may be due to differences in patient selection and in protocol design. All women in the double-blind study had intact membranes, whereas the first study included cases with ruptured membranes. Secondly, the duration of infusion was fixed to 12$\frac{1}{2}$ hours in the double-blind trial, while this was not the case in the previous study.

Anderson and collaborators (Anderson *et al.*, 1971; Anderson *et al.*, 1972a, b) studied in a double-blind fashion PGF$_{2\alpha}$, PGE$_2$ and oxytocin given for induction of labour to 169 parous patients. Strict criteria were used for patient selection and the Bishop score of each subject was noted for comparative purposes. In their final protocol (148 women), dose levels ranged from 2.5 to 40 μg min^{-1} for PGF$_{2\alpha}$, from 0.3 to 4.8 μg min^{-1} for PGE$_2$ and from 1 to 16 mU min^{-1} for oxytocin. Labour was monitored externally until the patients were in good progressive labour; amniotomy was then performed. The successful induction rate was 81% for PGF$_{2\alpha}$, 83% for PGE$_2$ and 84% for oxytocin. All patients with a Bishop score of 7 or greater delivered no matter which drug they received. There was no difference in efficacy between the various oxytocics for inducing subjects with lower scores. Neither was there a significant difference between the mean induction–delivery intervals of the various groups. Nine episodes of uterine hypertonus were recorded, all of which in patients receiving prostaglandins (seven patients: PGF$_{2\alpha}$ and two: PGE$_{2\alpha}$ and the authors felt that the safety margin of PGF$_{2\alpha}$, in terms of uterine response, was not as wide as that for oxytocin. These studies of Anderson and his group have formed the basis of an international double-blind comparative trial of labour induction by intravenous prostaglandins or oxytocin.

Witting *et al.* (1972) and Laros *et al.* (1973) studied the response of the uterus at term to the infusion of $PGF_{2\alpha}$ maintained during four hours at one of six dose levels ranging from 0.5 to 16 μg min^{-1}. Thirty patients had intact membranes; the other 30 had spontaneously or artificially ruptured membranes. Whereas an infusion rate of 2 μg min^{-1} or less was often ineffective in adequately stimulating uterine activity, a rate of 4 μg min^{-1} usually promoted clinical progress and delivery. At higher infusion rates, hypersystole and hypertonus were occasionally noted. The authors felt that a constant infusion of about 4 μg min^{-1} constituted a reliable method of induction of labour with $PGF_{2\alpha}$. From this study, it also appeared that amniotomy markedly increased the probability of success of the attempted induction.

Ring (1972) attempted induction of labour with intravenous $PGF_{2\alpha}$ in 42 patients. The initial dose of 2.5 μg min^{-1} was increased to 5.0 and then to 10 μg min^{-1} where necessary. Amniotomy was delayed. Thirty-eight of the 42 patients delivered within 24 hours. Apgar scores and fetal and neonatal pH values fell within normal ranges.

From 1971 onwards, several double-blind studies have been reported. Rangarajan *et al.* (1971) compared $PGF_{2\alpha}$ in a range of 7.5–20 μg min^{-1} with oxytocin in 40 patients with similar inducibility features. $PGF_{2\alpha}$ was less effective (80% success) than oxytocin (95%). The occurrence of prolonged contractions in 40% of the patients and two instances of fetal bradycardia in the prostaglandin group, prompted the authors to question the safety of the drug. Elias (1972) compared intravenous $PGF_{2\alpha}$ and PGE_2 in 30 patients at term, with intact membranes. Infusion rates of $PGF_{2\alpha}$ ranged from 2.5 to 40 μg min^{-1}, the rate being doubled at intervals, where necessary. All patients were successfully induced and the drugs appeared equally efficacious. However, fetal bradycardia and acidosis (scalp pH of 6.90) were noted following an episode of uterine hypertonus occurring in a patient receiving 40 μg min^{-1} $PGF_{2\alpha}$. Vakhariya and Sherman (1972) compared the effect of $PGF_{2\alpha}$ and oxytocin in 100 subjects at 36–43 weeks' gestation and found both drugs comparable in terms of efficacy and safety. They did note seven cases of hypertonus, among patients given $PGF_{2\alpha}$, but this did not affect the fetal outcome. Applying the same protocol to a series of 222 patients, Spellacy *et al.* (1973) reached different conclusions. Although both drugs proved equally effective, there was a significant increase in maternal side-effects and uterine hypertonus and Caesarean section for fetal bradycardia was more often required in patients given $PGF_{2\alpha}$. Rosa *et al.* (1972), Thiery *et al.* (1972) and Vroman *et al.* (1972) confirmed that uterine hypertonus could be observed during induction of labour with i.v. $PGF_{2\alpha}$, but it has since been demonstrated that the procedure is entirely safe to the fetus, if hypertonus is avoided (Thiery *et al.*, 1973a).

A co-operative double-blind study comparing i.v. oxytocin and $PGF_{2\alpha}$ in a group of 80 patients at term was reported by Hogaki (1972). In women with intact membranes, $PGF_{2\alpha}$ appeared more efficacious for the induction of labour. Moreover, uterine contractility patterns induced by $PGF_{2\alpha}$ were similar to those of normal labour and no significant difference in the incidence of fetal bradycardia was detected.

Brown *et al.* (1973) attempted to induce labour at term in 32 patients by combining i.v. $PGF_{2\alpha}$ and low amniotomy. Results were compared with paired controls matched for prospects of inducibility. Preset infusion levels (ranging from 2.5 to 7.5 μg min^{-1}) and time intervals were used to escalate the PG dose. The procedure was unsuccessful in 12.5% of the patients treated with $PGF_{2\alpha}$ while there were no failures with oxytocin. The mean induction–delivery interval (for successful cases) was 9 hours 15 min and 7 hours 33 min for $PGF_{2\alpha}$ and oxytocin, respectively. Thus, administered in low doses, $PGF_{2\alpha}$ proved less effective than oxytocin. Besides, side-effects were more prominent and necessitated discontinuation of the infusion in several patients.

Naismith *et al.* (1973) studied three groups of patients (10 with $PGF_{2\alpha}$ and PGE_2 each, and 20 with oxytocin) matched for inducibility features. Drug doses were doubled at intervals until regular contractions were monitored (external tocography) at which time low amniotomy was performed. Dose levels ranged from 3 to 340 mU min^{-1} for oxytocin, from 2.5 to 80.0 μg min^{-1} for PGE_2 and from 0.25 to 8.0 μg min^{-1} for PGE_2. Oxytocin proved more efficacious (producing 19/20 vaginal deliveries) than the PGs. Indeed, in five of the 20 patients to whom a PG was administered (no distinction is made by the authors between E_2 and $F_{2\alpha}$) the cervix failed to dilate properly; when oxytocin was substituted, all five patients progressed to vaginal delivery. Side-effects were not severe, and Apgar scores showed no significant intergroup differences. This small-scale trial in which patients were carefully matched for individual inducibility features and in which comparable dose schedules were applied, would suggest the superior effectiveness of oxytocin over PGs when infused to women with intact membranes.

Caballero *et al.* (1974) attempted to induce labour with $PGF_{2\alpha}$ in 100 patients at term. The initial dose level of 2.5 μg min^{-1} was increased by 2.5 μg min^{-1} every 15–30 min until good contractility was obtained or a maximum dose level of 25 μg min^{-1} had been reached. In the earlier cases external tocography was used and amniotomy was delayed; later, early amniotomy and intra-amniotic tocography were generally combined. According to these authors uterine activity produced by $PGF_{2\alpha}$ generally differed from that characterising spontaneous on oxytocin-induced labour. Indeed, contractions produced by the PG showed a tendency towards dysrhythmia, the mean amplitude and duration were greater and the interval between contractions tended to be longer. The success (induction producing vaginal delivery) rate was 87% and the mean induction–delivery interval was 5 hours 56 min. Although in 23 women receiving 25 μg min^{-1} $PGF_{2\alpha}$ patterns of uterine hyperstimulation were recorded, all infants had five-minute Apgar scores of 8 or more. Gastrointestinal side-effects occurred in 27% of the patients.

To another group of 100 patients Caballero *et al.* (1974) administered i.v. $PGF_{2\alpha}$ (maximum 12.5 μg min^{-1}) combined with buccal deamino–oxytocin (ODA, 50 IU/hour) until the end of the third stage of labour. The total mean dose of ODA was 200 IU (range 50–500 IU). Ninety-eight of the 100 women delivered in a mean of 4 hours 21 min. Thus, by combining early amniotomy, buccal ODA and an i.v. infusion of $PGF_{2\alpha}$, the efficacy of the induction was increased, the mean total dose of $PGF_{2\alpha}$ decreased (from 7.02 to 2.47 mg) and the incidence of gastrointestinal side-effects lowered (from 27% to 8%). Gain in effectiveness and in maternal acceptability of the method were, however, offset by a somewhat less favourable perinatal outcome: late deceleration patterns occurred in 10%, fetal bradycardia in 2%, low one-minute Apgar scores in 12% and low five-minute scores in 4% of the cases.

Using Turnbull's (1974) Cardiff Automatic Oxytocin Infusion System for the induction of labour at term with $PGF_{2\alpha}$, Johnson and Newton (1974) obtained vaginal delivery in all 20 patients induced. The average induction-delivery interval was 7 hours 40 min. The pump was set to increase the dose level from 0.3 to 9.6 μg min^{-1} over $1\frac{1}{4}$ hours. In no case did this dose have to be exceeded. There was one instance of uterine hypertonus in the first stage of labour and the automatic infusion pump switched itself off whereafter the hypertonus resolved. According to this small preliminary trial this type of apparatus appears effective and safe.

4.2.1.1.2 *Larger studies.* Thirteen studies which included more than 25 cases in each study have been collated to analyse the efficacy and safety of induction of labour at term with i.v. $PGF_{2\alpha}$. They total over 800 women. Essential data are tabulated (Table 4.1). When comparing these clinical trials differences in protocol design (selection criteria, inducibility features, dose regimen) must be taken into account.

Indication. In about half of the cases the procedure was elective, in the remainder it was therapeutically indicated.

Parity. Whereas investigators have generally limited themselves to studying women of a parity of five or less, Karim (1971b) included patients of higher parity. Parity ratio also differs; most authors attempted induction in groups of patients exclusively composed of multiparas (Anderson *et al.*, 1972b; Vroman *et al.*, 1972) or at least carrying an excess of such patients (Karim, 1971b; Kinoshita *et al.*, 1971; Hogaki, 1972b; Ring, 1972; Witting *et al.*, 1972; Caballero *et al.*, 1974).

State of membranes. Several investigators have included patients with prematurely ruptured membranes (Karim, 1971b; Hogaki, 1972; Ring, 1972; Witting *et al.*, 1973). The time at which amniotomy was performed varies widely, some investigators rupturing the membranes 30–60 min before (Kinoshita *et al.*, 1971; Thiery *et al.*, 1973a) or at the start of the infusion (Brown *et al.*, 1973), whereas most groups preferred to wait until labour was well established and progressing (Karim, 1971; Anderson *et al.*, 1972b; Ring, 1972; Vroman *et al.*, 1972).

Drug infusion. As far as we are aware, all investigators have made use of a pump to infuse the drug at a constant dose level, this level being adjusted manually. A fully automatic device with built-in warning system (Cardiff Automatic Oxytocin Infusion System, Turnbull, 1974) especially conceived for infusing oxytocin has recently been used to induce labour with $PGF_{2\alpha}$ (Johnson and Newton, 1974).

Dose regimens show a wide range. To simplify, these can be classified into two main categories, each presenting individual variations.

1. Constant or fixed dose infusion. In a given patient the dose level, which is rather small ($\leqslant 16$ μg min^{-1} $PGF_{2\alpha}$), is kept constant throughout the infusion (Karim, 1971b; Witting *et al.*, 1973).

2. Escalated (escalating dose) infusions are characterised by stepwise increase of the dose level. The duration of the infusion at a given (fixed) dose level, although unequal for various groups of investigators, is also generally

Table 4.1 Induction of labour at term with intravenous PGF$_{2\alpha}$

Reference	Indi-cation	No. of cases NP	MP	Total	Gestat. age (weeks)	Type	Range of levels ($\mu g\ min^{-1}$)	Amnio-tomy	Success rate (%)	Induction-delivery interval (h:min)	Total dose (mg)	Uterine hyper-stimulation %
Karim, 1971b	–	14	86	100	term	F	5–10	D	93	10:30 (mean MP) 17:00 (mean NP)		
Karim, 1971b	–			100	term	F	2.5–10		67			
Anderson et al., 1972b	T(76%)	0	91	91	term	E	2.5–40	D	81	<08:38 (mean)		7(H+P)
Kinoshita et al., 1971	EI(63%)	5	25	30	35–42	E	2.4–11	C	100	01:00–10:30 mean 4:00 (NP) & 3:35 (MP)	0.2–43.0	0
Witting et al., 1972; Laros et al., 1973	EI	7	53	60	term	F	1–16	D	86	05:15 (mean)		16(H+Hy)
Vakhariya and Sherman, 1972	EI			50	term	E	2–40	D	94	05:15 (mean)		16
Spellacy & Gall, 1972; Spellacy et al., 1973	EI			115	36–43	E	2.5–40	D	76	06:29 (mean); range 0:46–17:18		24
Vroman et al., 1972	EI	0	25	25	38–42	E	2.5–40	D	100	02:20–10:00		8
Thiery et al., 1973a	EI	30	25	55	38–42	E	2–100	C	100	02:36–15:59 mean 6:47 (NP); 2:30–16:00 mean 4:49 (MP)	0.4–16.1* in NP; 0.6–25.6† in MP	6
Ring, 1972	T	18	24	42	38–43	E	2.5–10	D	90	05:33 (mean)	2.5 (mean)	2
Hogaki, 1971		9	29	40	term	E	3.0–9.6		83		1.4 (mean)	
Brown et al., 1973				32	≥37	E	2.5–7	C	87	09:15 (mean)		0
Caballero et al., 1974	EI(73%)	10	90	100	34–44	E	2.5–25	D	87	01:12–12:40 05:56 (mean)	0.8–18.8	6(H)+7(P)

Key. NP = nulliparas; MP = parous patients. Indication: EI (elective) or T (therapeutic). Type of regimen: F (fixed dose infusion) or E (escalating dose infusion). Amniotomy: C (combined) or D (delayed). Uterine hyperstimulation: hyperonus unless stated otherwise (H = hypertonus, P = polysystole, Hy = hyperstole) * (mean 4.4) † (mean 4.1) preset (Anderson *et al.*, 1972b; Vroman *et al.*, 1972; Spellacy *et al.*, 1973). Others prefer to increase dose levels at constant time intervals (mostly approximately every 30 min) until labour is well established (Ring, 1972; Vakhariya and Sherman, 1972; Thiery *et al.*, 1973a). Although the dose increment is kept constant in some studies (Kinoshita *et al.*, 1971; Hogaki, 1972; Caballero *et al.*, 1974), consecutive doses are (roughly) doubled in others (Anderson *et al.*, 1972b; Ring, 1972; Spellacy and Gall, 1972; Vakhariya and Sherman, 1972; Vroman *et al.*, 1972; Thiery *et al.*, 1973a). With few exceptions (Thiery *et al.*, 1973a), authors fixed the upper limit of the infusion level from an unusually low 7.5 μg min^{-1} (Brown *et al.* 1973) to the more currently adopted level of 40 μg min^{-1} (Anderson *et al.*, 1972b; Vakhariya and Sherman, 1972; Vroman *et al.*, 1972; Spellacy *et al.*, 1973). As a rule, the infusion level at which labour progressed was kept constant until delivery. Of course, if uterine hyperstimulation, fetal bradycardia or disturbing maternal side-effects occurred, this level was decreased or the infusion discontinued.

Results. In view of the above-mentioned divergences in protocol design it is understandable that the effectiveness of the procedure has varied. If two groups of patients are excluded (Karim's double-blind study (1971b) and the series reported by Spellacy *et al.* (1973)) reported success rates range from 81% to 100% notwithstanding that divergent criteria were applied to define success. The possible reasons for the low success rate (67%) of PGF$_{2\alpha}$ in the double-blind trial of Karim (1971b) have been outlined elsewhere (see Section 4.2.1.1.1). Spellacy's (Spellacy *et al.*, 1973) success rate of only 76% can probably be explained by (1) the criterion these authors used to define failure (labour not established within 10 hours of infusion) and (2) the high incidence of uterine hyperstimulation (24%) and fetal bradycardia (14%) which in several cases prompted the investigators either to discontinue the infusion of prostaglandin or to terminate labour by Caesarean section.

Success of labour induction can also be expressed by the time interval between drug administration and delivery. In the successful cases reported (Table 4.1), the range of induction-delivery intervals is quite large, due to differences in protocol design and inducibility factors among the various series. Mean intervals, on the other hand, are somewhat more uniform and, in many series, range between five and seven hours. Total drug doses differ enormously, which again is connected with protocol design.

The outcome of labour induction is influenced by so-called inducibility variables. Parity probably plays a major role. Karim (1971b) obtained a success rate of 98% in parous patients *v.* only 64% in the nulliparous group. Thiery *et al.* (1973a) successfully induced all of their patients, but multiparous women in their series had a much shorter mean induction–delivery interval (4 hours 49 min) than nulliparas (6 hours 47 min). Spellacy *et al.* (1973) were in fact the only investigators to explicitly state that parity was of minor importance.

Body weight is another inducibility variable. Spellacy *et al.* (1973) found that their PGF$_{2\alpha}$ failures occurred in patients who were significantly more obese. Anderson *et al.* (1972b), comparing their overall success rate (81%) with the 93% reported in Karim's early report (1971b), hypothesised that, besides genetic influences, the lower body weight characterising Ugandan women could have contributed to the latter author's favourable results. Likewise, the two reports from Japan (Kinoshita *et al.*, 1971; Hogaki *et al.*, 1972) strike us by their high success rates (100% and 83%, resp.) and the relatively small maximum dose levels used. Japanese women too are as a rule of lighter weight than Caucasian females. Grossly obese women were generally excluded from the PG studies and few investigators (Kinoshita *et al.*, 1971; Hogaki, 1972) calculated dose levels on a pharmacological basis, i.e. expressed them in $\mu g \, kg^{-1} \, min^{-1}$.

Table 4.2 Induction of labour with intravenous $PGF_{2\alpha}$ Correlation between Bishop score and ease of induction (from Anderson *et al.*, 1972b, by courtesy of Futura)

Bishop score	Success rate (%)	Induction–delivery interval (h:min)
0–4	60	08:38
5–6	85	
≥7	100	05:17

The most important inducibility variable is the state of the cervix at induction. Although one group (Witting *et al.*, 1972) concluded that the likelihood of successful induction did not depend greatly upon the pelvic score, observations of many investigators overwhelmingly point towards the contrary. Thus, Anderson *et al.* (1972b) found that both the success rate and the mean induction–delivery interval were closely related to the Bishop score (Table 4.2). Vakhariya and Sherman (1972) obtained a success rate of 88% in patients with an 'unripe' cervix *v.* 100% in those with a 'ripe' cervix. Also the mean total doses of $PGF_{2\alpha}$ needed to effect delivery (5.2 mg *v.* 2.7 mg) and the mean induction–delivery intervals (385 min *v.* 262 min) were significantly different. Spellacy *et al.* (1973) obtained 40% success in patients with a modified Bishop score of 0–3 *v.* 100% in those with scores of 10–13.

Witting *et al.* (1972) compared two series of patients matched for inducibility variables, except for the state of the membranes. Half of the members of their group had ruptured membranes at the start of labour. The success rate amounted to 25% and 83% for patients with intact and unruptured membranes, respectively.

Regimen. There still seems to be some controversy as to the value of constant *v.* escalated dose infusions. Indeed, Karim (1971b), who introduced this first regimen, obtained excellent results (success rate 93%) at low infusion levels (5–10 $\mu g \, min^{-1}$). For this two possible explanations have been quoted above. Witting *et al.* (1973), who applied a similar regimen for much shorter periods of time (limited to four hours), also reported good results: 86% were delivered vaginally (56% within the four hours the infusion lasted). In half of their patients the membranes were ruptured at the start of the infusion and this favourably influenced the outcome of this series.

On the contrary, Kinoshita *et al.* (1971) showed that stepping up the initial dose of $PGF_{2\alpha}$ (2–4 $\mu g \, min^{-1}$) by increments of 1.2–2.4 $\mu g \, min^{-1}$ at 30 min intervals was very effective (success rate 100% within $10\frac{1}{2}$ hours), even though the maximum rate was kept relatively low (11 $\mu g \, min^{-1}$). These investigators also observed that without such gradual dose increase the uterine activity in some cases slowed down within 2–4 hours and returned to pre-infusion levels. This observation as well as results published by Anderson *et al.* (1972b) suggest that an escalating dose regimen is superior to a constant dose infusion. The fact that effective dose levels vary widely among individual patients would further substantiate that some sort of drug 'titration' is a sound practice. Using this set-up, Thiery *et al.* (1973a) produced vaginal delivery in 100% of both their nulliparous and parous patients.

Dose level in itself seems also to be important. By increasing levels in consecutive protocol modifications (plus shortening the duration of infusion, at least for the high levels), Anderson *et al.* (1972b) convincingly demonstrated the positive effect of a higher dose level on effectiveness of induction. In fact, these authors switched from a constant-rate infusion to some type of escalated-dose infusion. That Karim's results (1971b) with a constant-dose infusion were still better than those of Anderson's protocol No. III has been explained by the smaller body weight of Ugandan to Caucasian women and the different inducibility features characterising both series.

Mode of delivery. The rate of operative deliveries differs widely between the studies analysed. In general, though, it seems to correspond to accepted standard distribution of unselected patients (Ring, 1972). There are exceptions, however. Thiery (1974) reported a high rate of vacuum extractions; this, however, is in accordance with a departmental policy that encourages elective extraction and that recommends therapeutic extraction whenever abnormal second-stage FHR patterns are registered. On the other hand the high Caesarean section rate (8.5%) reported by Spellacy *et al.* (1973) was entirely due to the high incidence of fetal and maternal deleterious effects they observed.

Uterine contractility. The *latent period*, from commencement of infusion to the onset of uterine contractions, ranged from 2 to 160 min (Caballero *et al.*, 1974) and is probably related to the state of the membranes. Generally, however, the latent period was less than 30 min (Karim, 1971b; Kinoshita *et al.*, 1971; Ring, 1972).

Many investigators found the pattern of uterine contractility produced by i.v. infusion of $PGF_{2\alpha}$ to be similar to that characterising normal spontaneous labour (Chimura *et al.*, 1971; Karim, 1971b; Hogaki, 1972; Ring, 1972). Vakhariya and Sherman (1972) and Vroman *et al.* (1972) were unable to differentiate monitored uterine activity produced by $PGF_{2\alpha}$ from that induced by oxytocin. Hogaki (1971), on the other hand, found that oxytocin tended to induce short uterine contractions that recurred regularly and frequently, whereas the contractility pattern produced by $PGF_{2\alpha}$ was indistinguishable from that of normal labour. Kinoshita *et al.* (1971) comparing parameters related to uterine contractility (caused by $PGF_{2\alpha}$ and oxytocin) found that PG initially tended to produce an incoordinated and irregular pattern; during the acceleration phase, however, both PG and oxytocin-induced patterns became similar. Vakhariya and Sherman (1972) found no significant difference between oxytocin- and $PGF_{2\alpha}$-induced contractions during accelerated labour. Caballero *et al.* (1974), on the contrary, reported that patterns produced by $PGF_{2\alpha}$ differed somewhat from those characterising both normal spontaneous and oxytocin-induced labour. With PG, rhythm appeared to be less stable, individual contractions were of lower amplitude but lasted longer and the interval between contractions was greater. Finally, bell-shaped contraction waves were more often produced by $PGF_{2\alpha}$ than by oxytocin. Chimura *et al.* (1971) noted occasional episodes of tachysystoly, with $PGF_{2\alpha}$.

Witting *et al.* (1972) observed that some patients had effective and progressive labours in spite of the 'inadequate' contractions recorded. This would imply that when adequate progress of labour is made, in terms of cervical dilatation, it is probably unwise to further escalate the dose level of $PGF_{2\alpha}$ whatever uterine contractility pattern recorded.

In eight of 10 studies analysed, there were instances of uterine hypertonus. Only Kinoshita *et al.* (1971) and Brown *et al.* (1973) specifically reported not to have observed this effect. The incidence of uterine hyperstimulation varies considerably and ranges from 2% (Ring, 1972) to 24% (Spellacy *et al.*, 1973). A possible explanation for this discrepancy is the divergence in definition of hypertonus (e.g. Thiery *et al.*, 1972 = baseline $\geqslant$ 12 mmHg; Anderson *et al.*, 1972b = baseline $\geqslant$ 20 mmHg) and the fact that some authors include polysystole (Anderson *et al.*, 1972b) and/or hypersystole (Witting *et al.*, 1973) within the term 'hypertonus'. Three aspects of uterine hypertonus are disturbing:

1. In some cases, the episode appeared without warning (Anderson *et al.*, 1972b).
2. Although uterine hyperstimulation was generally associated with higher dose levels (25–80 μg min^{-1}—Ring, 1972; Caballero *et al.*, 1974) it was also observed with small doses (2–10 μg min^{-1}—Vakhariya and Sherman, 1972; Witting *et al.*, 1972).
3. Hyperstimulation was sometimes due to faulty technique, e.g. the sudden release of a temporary occlusion of the infusion cannula (Thiery *et al.*, 1973a) or the inadvertent infusion of too high a dose (Ring, 1972).

The consequences hypertonus may have on the fetus still form a controversial subject. Surely, many episodes of transient hypertonus are artifacts. But in those cases where it is associated with fetal bradycardia, it may have caused fetal hypoxia and this could conceivably have long-standing effects (Derom *et al.*, 1974). Except for Spellacy *et al.* (1973: 24% hypertonus, 14% fetal bradycardia, 20% low one-minute Apgar scores, 5% low five-minute scores), investigators found that most instances of hypertonus observed with i.v. $PGF_{2\alpha}$ were not associated with FHR deceleration. Vroman *et al.* (1972) and Thiery *et al.* (1973a) detected bradycardia in about one-half of the cases of hypertonus, Vakhariya and Sherman (1972) in only one-eighth. Goethals *et al.* (1974), in a long-term follow-up study of infants born following labour induction with $PGF_{2\alpha}$—including cases in which hypertonus had been registered—failed to detect any deleterious effect of the prostaglandin on their psycho-motor development.

Ideally, for early detection of uterine hyperstimulation, intravenous administration of a prostaglandin for induction of labour should be performed under electronic monitoring supervision. In case of hypertonus, microblood sampling may aid in choosing between (1) simple reduction of the dose level of prostaglandin infused, (2) administration of a uterine relaxant, or (3) immediate delivery. Several β-stimulating adrenergic compounds, with proven uterolytic effect on $PGF_{2\alpha}$-induced contractions, can be used in this respect (Baillie *et al.*, 1972; Lindmark *et al.*, 1973; Scher and Baillie, 1973; Thiery *et al.*, 1973a; Unbehaun and Conradt, 1973). Karim and Sharma (1971c) abolished completely uterine activity by the intravenous infusion of 10% ethyl alcohol.

Maternal effects. No side-effects were reported by Karim (1971b), Anderson *et al.* (1972b), Hogaki (1972), Vakhariya and Sherman (1972) and Witting *et al.* (1973). Ring (1972) encountered venous erythema, nausea, vomiting and allergic exanthema, in order of decreasing frequency. The incidence of gastrointestinal side-effects reported in six studies varies for vomiting from 3 to 12%, for nausea (without vomiting) from 0 to 8% and for diarrhoea from 0 to 5% (Kinoshita *et al.*, 1971; Spellacy and Gall, 1972; Vroman *et al.*, 1972; Brown *et al.*, 1973; Thiery *et al.*, 1973a; Caballero *et al.*, 1974). Other side-effects mentioned occasionally include hot flushes (Spellacy and Gall, 1972: 17%), perspiration (Caballero *et al.*, 1974: 4%), drowsiness (Caballero *et al.*, 1974: 2%) and venous erythema (Brown *et al.*, 1973: 12%; Caballero *et al.*, 1974: 3%). Certainly, individual susceptibility plays a major role: some patients infused with high doses of $PGF_{2\alpha}$ (e.g. 100 μg min^{-1}, and a total of 25 mg or more) have suffered little or no side-effects (Kinoshita *et al.*, 1971; Thiery *et al.*, 1973a). At the doses used for induction of labour, intravenous $PGF_{2\alpha}$ caused no alteration of body temperature, pulse rate, blood pressure and respiratory rate (Karim *et al.*, 1968; Kinoshita *et al.*, 1971; Ring, 1972; Vroman *et al.*, 1972; Brown *et al.*, 1973; Spellacy *et al.*, 1973; Thiery *et al.*, 1973a; Caballero *et al.*, 1974). None of the investigators having reported on induction of labour with i.v. $PGF_{2\alpha}$ mentioned the occurrence of asthmatic attacks or other evidence of bronchoconstriction. Nevertheless, caution should be exerted when inducing patients with asthma or other bronchial diseases by means of prostaglandins. These drugs may indeed cause bronchoconstriction when infused in high doses (e.g. 200 μg min^{-1} $PGF_{2\alpha}$, Fishburne *et al.*, 1972b; Smith, 1973) and asthmatic attacks have been reported during termination of pregnancy with i.v. $PGF_{2\alpha}$ (Fishburne *et al.*, 1972a). Roberts *et al.* (1972) described a single case of acrocyanosis developing in the hand and the forearm of a patient infused with 5–40 μg min^{-1} $PGF_{2\alpha}$ because of intrauterine death at 25 weeks' gestation. This reaction, probably due to intense venospasm, has not been reported in patients undergoing labour induction by means of a prostaglandin.

No change in intraocular pressure was noted by Vroman *et al.* (1972). Lyneham *et al.* (1973) reported convulsive episodes in five of 320 patients undergoing second trimester abortion by intra-amniotic instillation of $PGF_{2\alpha}$ and noted significant electroencephalographic changes in four of eight subjects tested. This experience however, has not been shared by others (Craft, 1973c; MacKenzie *et al.*, 1973; Fraser and Gray, 1974; Thiery *et al.*, 1974a). Thiery *et al.* (1974a) reported not to have observed convulsive fits in 169 inductions of labour with i.v. $PGF_{2\alpha}$, despite the fact that several of the patients were known epileptics. To the best of our knowledge, no investigator has noted this complication during induction of labour with prostaglandins.

Laboratory studies conducted during infusion of $PGF_{2\alpha}$ for labour induction, including complete blood count, sedimentation rate, serum uric acid, urea, creatinine, glucose, bilirubin, alkaline phosphatase, transaminases, total protein, albumin and cholesterol, showed no significant changes from pretreatment values. No alteration in urine sugar or protein content, sediment and density were noted (Kinoshita *et al.*, 1971; Anderson *et al.*, 1972b;

Vroman, 1972; Spellacy *et al.*, 1973; Thiery *et al.*, 1973a; Caballero *et al.*, 1974; Johnson *et al.*, 1974).

Barden (1972) and Johnson *et al.* (1974) found no change attributable to prostaglandin administration in any of the following coagulation factors: platelets, platelet adhesion, platelet aggregation, prothrombin time, thrombin time, partial thromboplastin time, fibrinogen, fibrinogen degradation products, euglobulin lysis time, factors V and VIII. Blood glucose and insulin levels were also unchanged during infusion of $PGF_{2\alpha}$ for induction of labour (Spellacy *et al.*, 1971).

Anderson *et al.* (1972b) studied the effect of $PGF_{2\alpha}$, PGE_2 and oxytocin given for labour induction on plasma steroid levels. Due to a wide range of individual values, no conclusion could be drawn regarding the effect of $PGF_{2\alpha}$ on plasma progesterone. There was a suggestion that maternal plasma oestriol levels were suppressed by $PGF_{2\alpha}$, but not by oxytocin. The fetal plasma levels of dehydroepiandrosterone sulphate—the major precursor of oestriol—were unaffected in either group. The authors therefore assumed that $PGF_{2\alpha}$ interfered with the placental biosynthesis of oestriol, with maternal conjugation, or possibly with 16-hydroxylation in the fetal liver. Lemaire *et al.* (1972), studying 20 women at term undergoing induction of labour with i.v. $PGF_{2\alpha}$, found no alteration in the plasma levels of either progesterone or oestriol in these subjects (see also Chapter 3).

Thiery and Willighagen (1973) investigated the effect of $PGF_{2\alpha}$ given for labour induction on the activity and localisation of histochemically demonstrable placental enzymes and on the distribution of placental glycogen and lipids. No differences were detected with placentas recovered after normal spontaneous labour.

The incidence of postpartum haemorrhage does not exceed that found after spontaneous or oxytocin-induced labour. Reported incidences are: 0 (Kinoshita *et al.*, 1971; Ring, 1972), 2% (Anderson *et al.*, 1972b; Thiery *et al.*, 1973a), 3% (Brown *et al.*, 1973), 4% (Vakhariya and Sherman, 1972), 6% (Caballero *et al.*, 1974) and 8% (Vroman *et al.*, 1972).

No case of maternal mortality has been reported.

Fetal and neonatal effects. Spellacy *et al.* (1973) reported one neonatal death in the first day of life, due to respiratory distress, in a baby of normal birth weight.

$PGF_{2\alpha}$ and its metabolites cross the placental barrier freely (Beazley *et al.*, 1972) and direct effects of the drug on fetal and neonatal metabolism are conceivable (e.g. coagulation mechanisms, bilirubin clearance, carbohydrate metabolism, lipolysis). However, research in this area has been scarce. Anderson *et al.* (1972b) found umbilical cord blood levels of F prostaglandins not significantly higher after induction of labour with intravenous $PGF_{2\alpha}$ than with oxytocin. Dehydroepiandrosterone sulphate levels were also within the same range. De Hemptinne *et al.* (1973) described no increase in neonatal hyperbilirubinaemia following labour induction with intravenous $PGF_{2\alpha}$.

Indirect fetal and neonatal effects, which may be reflected in alterations of the FHR or of the acid-base state, could theoretically have the following causes:

1. Utero-placental blood flow may be hampered during $PGF_{2\alpha}$-induced labour either due to uterine hyperstimulation or to vasoconstriction of the utero-placental vessels (Jungmannova *et al.*, 1972; Clark *et al.*,

1973) or umbilical arteries and veins (Karim, 1967; Hillier and Karim, 1968; Altura *et al.*, 1972; Park *et al.*, 1972; Mosler *et al.*, 1973; Novy *et al.*, 1974). However, Sherman (1972), measuring fetal, amniotic and uterine temperature throughout PG-induced labour failed to detect differences in temperature gradients. He concluded that, at the doses used for induction, $PGF_{2\alpha}$ had no significant effect on utero-placental vessels and blood flow.

2. Maternal bronchoconstriction (Fishburne *et al.*, 1972a) could influence the oxygen saturation of maternal blood.

3. Finally, the affinity of haemoglobin for oxygen could be decreased by prostaglandins. Laver (1973) reported a slight decrease when PGE_2 was added to solutions of human haemoglobin. Novy (1972) noted, just before birth, a small change in the affinity of maternal haemoglobin for oxygen and speculated that this could result from high levels of circulating $PGF_{2\alpha}$. However, Collins and Jaffe (1973), investigating *in vitro* the effects of prostaglandins A_1, A_2, E_1, E_2, $F_{1\alpha}$ and $F_{2\alpha}$ on human whole blood, found no significant alterations of the oxygen–haemoglobin dissociation curve.

Table 4.3   Incidence of fetal bradycardia and low Apgar scores in labour induced with intravenous $PGF_{2\alpha}$

	Low Apgar scores (%)		Fetal bradycardia (%)
	1-min	*5-min*	
Anderson *et al.*, 1972b	—	0	—
Kinoshita *et al.*, 1971	3	0	0
Witting *et al.*, 1972	8	—	2.5*
Vakhariya and Sherman, 1972	12	0	4
Spellacy *et al.*, 1973	20	5	14
Ring, 1972	5	—	0
Brown *et al.*, 1973	0	0	—
Caballero *et al.*, 1974	8	2	17*

* Late deceleration pattern

Generally, investigators have assessed clinical state at birth by Apgar scoring. Others have supplemented these data with FHR findings but only few have investigated the acid-base equilibrium.

In most instances, the incidence of neonatal depression (Apgar scoring) was not increased over that following normal spontaneous labour (Kinoshita *et al.*, 1971; Anderson *et al.*, 1972b; Ring, 1972; Witting *et al.*, 1972; Brown *et al.*, 1973; Caballero *et al.*, 1974—Table 4.3). This is remarkable because many series included cases complicated by toxaemia, postmaturity, diabetes, etc. There are, however, notable exceptions. Vakhariya and Sherman (1972) reported a case (2%) of uterine hypertonus associated with fetal bradycardia. Spellacy *et al.* (1973) noted fetal bradycardia in 14% of their cases and were compelled to perform a Caesarean section nine times (8.5%) on account of fetal bradycardia and/or uterine hypertonus. Ring (1972) described one instance (1%) of marked fetal tachycardia following inadvertent infusion of an excessive dose of $PGF_{2\alpha}$. The same investigator determined the pH at birth (pH$_V$) and following birth (pH heel) in 38 infants and found these values to be 'satisfactory' (mean $pH_v = 7.28$). Heidenreich *et al.* (1974) reported similar results in a series of 10 infants born after induction of labour with $PGF_{2\alpha}$ for therapeutic indications. Caballero *et al.* (1974) determined the pH at birth (pH_a ?) in the infants with low Apgar scores (8%) and reported individual values ranging from 7.12 to 7.20.

Only two groups of researchers have made detailed studies of the possible influence of $PGF_{2\alpha}$ used for labour induction on the fetus and neonate. In the first study, Blackburn *et al.* (1973) compared the effects on the neonate of labour induced with i.v. $PGF_{2\alpha}$ (11 cases) or oxytocin (12 cases). Apgar scores at one and five minutes were 8 or more for all infants and showed a comparable distribution in both groups. The duration of the umbilical pulse varied widely irrespective of the drug used for induction. Physical examinations done at birth and on the third day disclosed no anomalies in the infants of either group. There were no significant differences between the two groups regarding results of clinical and laboratory investigations performed throughout the study. These included measurements of heart rate, respiratory rate, blood pressure, temperature, haemoglobin, haematocrit, white blood cell count, blood pH, pCO_2, base excess, lactate, glucose, sodium, potassium and total serum bilirubin. Wake/sleep patterns, frequency of voiding and defaecation, behaviour and feeding were similar in both groups. Roentgenograms of the chest taken within 30 min after birth, at six hours, and on the third day showed the expected radiologic appearance of gradual and complete expansion of all areas of the lungs and resorption of residual pulmonary fluid in all infants. All neonates had normal electrocardiograms. The authors concluded that $PGF_{2\alpha}$, given intravenously for induction of labour, had no effect on the fetus or the neonate that could distinguish it from oxytocin.

The second group of investigators (Vroman *et al.*, 1972; Thiery *et al.*, 1973a) evaluated the fetus and the newborn in a total of 75 cases electively induced at term with i.v. $PGF_{2\alpha}$. A number of FHR irregularities were recorded during labour. In the first stage of labour, there were seven instances (9%) of transient or variable deceleration, with normal infants at birth, and two cases (3%) of persistent bradycardia accompanying uterine hypertonus. Both these infants were severely acidotic at birth (pH_a: 6.97 and 6.98) but only one of them appeared clinically depressed (Apgar 6–7). Potentially dangerous second-stage FHR patterns (persistent or transient bradycardia) were noted in four cases (5%); three of these infants were acidotic at birth but only two appeared clinically depressed (one case mentioned above: $pH_a = 6.97$). Overall, the mean biochemical state of the fetus at the end of the first stage of labour was normal. At birth, there were 20% low Apgar scores (< 7) at one minute and 3% (two cases) low five-minute scores. The mean biochemical state at birth was normal and not different from the control groups, except for the first series of 25 cases (Vroman *et al.*, 1972) in which the mean pH_a was significantly lower than in the controls (labour induced with oxytocin). However, in the second group of 50 cases (Thiery *et al.*, 1973a) all individual pH_a values were normal, except for two. The authors concluded that, provided hyperstimulation is avoided, the scalp blood pH is normal at the end of the first stage. However, aberrant FHR patterns during the second stage—probably not related to the administration of prostaglandin—may be associated with an abnormal (clinical and/or biochemical) status at birth.

There is also one long-term follow-up study of babies born to mothers electively induced with i.v. $PGF_{2\alpha}$ on record (Goethals *et al.*, 1974). Extensive neurologic examination of the babies according to Prechtl and Beintema (1964) gave normal results on days 3–4. The follow-up study failed to reveal any abnormalities in the psychomotor development of these children up to six months of age.

4.2.1.1.3 *Conclusions.* With a few exceptions, reported success rates are satisfying, whatever the regimen employed. Fixed-rate schedules are often successful, but escalating the dose of prostaglandin may be more efficacious. However, an upper dose limit should probably be decided upon, as uterine hypertonus is mostly associated with high dose levels. None the less, in an occasional case, transgression of this rule is necessary in order to obtain adequate uterine response. Careful electronic monitoring of labour should be the policy.

At the doses required to initiate labour, maternal side-effects have been uncommon. Specific side-effects (gastrointestinal, venous erythema) are seldom bothersome and always reversible. The only fetal hazard documented appears to be connected with uterine hypertonus. If hyperstimulation is avoided, the perinatal outcome is not different from that of oxytocin-induced or normal spontaneous labour.

4.2.1.2 Prostaglandin E_2

Like $PGF_{2\alpha}$, PGE_2 has been shown to have a stimulant effect on the pregnant uterus at term but initially some controversy arose regarding its suitability for clinical obstetrics. Administering short-lasting (15–45 min) i.v. infusions of PGE_2 to three women at 36–40 weeks' gestation, Bygdeman *et al.* (1968) found the threshold dose for stimulating the uterus to be 'around 4–8 μg min^{-1}'. Because they observed frequently 'an unphysiologic elevation of tone', these investigators felt that the E prostaglandins would prove 'less suitable for induction of labour'. However, the diagram illustrating this point in their paper is far from convincing as it shows that the highest uterine tone elevation recorded amounted to only 14 mmHg and was transient in nature and that it occurred in only one of the seven experiments while infusing 4 μg min^{-1} PGE_2. In the course of the other six infusions, uterine tone never exceeded 10 mmHg.

According to Embrey (1969) who used short-lasting (27–75 min) infusions of PGE_2 (2–8 μg min^{-1}) in patients at term, the threshold dose of this compound was of the order of 2 μg min^{-1}. In the range of 2–6 μg min^{-1}, a well-marked oxytocic effect consisting in an increase in frequency and amplitude of the contractions was observed in all patients. A transient increase in tone occurred at 8 μg min^{-1} in one instance but it quickly resolved after reduction of the dose level to 6 μg min^{-1}.

Roth-Brandel and Adams (1970) administered long-lasting (maximum duration 10 hours), low dose (0.7 μg min^{-1}) constant-rate infusions of PGE_2 to 13 gravidae at term. They observed a steady increase in frequency and amplitude of the contractions and several patients were effectively induced and delivered. In only one patient was uterine hypertonus registered.

These experiments established that (1) i.v. PGE_2 had an oxytocic effect on the human term uterus; (2) the uterotonic potency of this compound was about 10 times higher than that of $PGF_{2\alpha}$ and (3) by carefully adjusting the dose level to individual myometrial sensitivity PGE_2 could probably effectively and safely induce labour at term. The latter assumption has abundantly been confirmed by clinical trials.

The first clinical reports on labour induction at term with i.v. PGE_2 originated from Great Britain (Embrey, 1969; Beazley et al., 1970) and from Uganda (Karim et al., 1970). They were followed by a number of clinical trials and comparative studies with oxytocin (which, lately, have been hampered by shelf instability of the drug). The present section will first abstract some of the individual clinical studies and then analyse the larger ones in an attempt to define the effectiveness and the safety of i.v. PGE_2. Finally, studies giving data on both prostaglandins will be used for comparing the usefulness of i.v. PGE_2 and $PGF_{2\alpha}$ for induction of labour at term.

4.2.1.2.1 *Individual reports.* Embrey (1969) reported from Oxford to have successfully induced seven out of eight women at term with short-lasting (27–75 min) i.v. infusions of PGE_2. Dose levels ranged from 2 to 8 μg min^{-1}. The latent period varied between 15 and 20 min. There was one instance of hypertonus which vanished soon after the dose was decreased from 8 to 6 μg min^{-1}. When the infusion was discontinued, the effect on uterine contractions often waned slowly; in some instances, there was no obvious decrease in uterine activity. With one exception, labour was clinically established within a few hours of PG infusion. Induction–delivery intervals in successful cases ranged from 2 to $40\frac{1}{2}$ hours. No maternal side-effects were observed. The same author reported in 1970 19 successes in 21 women at or about term (Embrey, 1970). In this investigation the infusion was continued (as far as limited drug supplies permitted) until labour was established. The effective dose level ranged from 1 to 6 μg min^{-1}; in only one case it amounted to 8 μg min^{-1}. A later progress report (Embrey, 1971) included 30 cases treated with i.v. PGE_2, but the tabulated material does not permit to make the distinction between women to whom PGE_1 was administered and those given PGE_2.

Beazley et al. (1970) reported on the use of PGE_2 with delayed amniotomy for induction of labour. Vaginal delivery was effected in 37 of 40 patients at 29–42 weeks' gestation. The initial infusion rate (0.4 μg min^{-1}) was doubled as required. These investigators suggested that drug dose 'titration' was in order because individual uterine thresholds for PGE_2 varied widely. Transient hypertonus was noted in one woman receiving 0.04 μg kg^{-1} min^{-1} (equivalent to 2.4 μg min^{-1} for a patient weighing 60 kg) but all infants were in good condition at birth. The following year, Beazley and Gillespie (1971) published the results of a double-blind trial comparing i.v. PGE_2 (146 cases) and oxytocin (146 cases) combined with early amniotomy. Success rates (authors' definition: delivery or at least 6 cm dilatation within 12 hours) were identical (73%) for both drugs. There were two fetal deaths in the PG-group, both occurring in high-risk pregnancies, but no important maternal compli- cations were observed.

Karim et al. (1970) successfully induced labour in all of 50 women at term with a continuous infusion of 0.5 μg min^{-1} PGE_2. Some needed repeat infusion the following day. The average infusion time and induction–delivery interval amounted to $5\frac{1}{2}$ and 10 hours, respectively. The uterine activity produced closely resembled that of normal spontaneous labour. Uterine hypertonus was not observed. These remarkable results were confirmed by Karim's report (1971b) on two studies in which i.v. PGE_2 was used. In the first study, 397 out of 400 patients (success rate 99%) were successfully induced. The average induction–delivery interval amounted to 12 hours in nulliparas and to seven hours in parous patients. There were two Caesarean sections because of failed induction, 13 for cephalopelvic disproportion and two because of fetal distress. In the second study, which consisted in a double-blind comparison of PGE_2, $PGF_{2\alpha}$ and oxytocin, 96 out of the 100 inductions with i.v. PGE_2 succeeded (success rate 96%). Doses ranged from 0.3 to 1.2 μg min^{-1}.

Roth-Brandel and Adams (1970), in Stockholm, attempted to induce 13 women at term by giving i.v. PGE_2 at a constant rate of 0.7 μg min^{-1} until active labour or for a maximum of 10 hours. Seven of these patients delivered vaginally as a result of PG stimulation. In one woman, the infusion had to be stopped because of uterine hyperactivity occurring after 8 hours 40 minutes of drug administration. Ninety minutes later, the membranes having ruptured spontaneously, fetal bradycardia appeared and Caesarean section was performed. The remaining five women were successfully induced the following day with i.v. oxytocin.

Roberts (1970) presented the results of therapeutic labour induction by combined amniotomy and i.v. infusion of PGE_2 (1.5–3.0 μg min^{-1}) in five women at 37–44 weeks' gestation. All subjects were delivered within $13\frac{1}{2}$ hours. Roberts and Turnbull (1971) reported successful induction of labour with i.v. PGE_2 (0.75–3.0 μg min^{-1}) in all of 18 women at 37–42 weeks' gestation. The authors, having observed uterine hypertonus in 4/18 cases, cautioned that labour should be carefully monitored.

Craft et al. (1971) compared the value of i.v. PGE_2 and oxytocin (15 cases in each group) for the induction of labour in patients with intact membranes. Rapid titration of the oxytocic drugs was used in order to trigger an early uterine response. The initial dose of PGE_2 (0.5 μg min^{-1}), infused for 30 min, was increased every 15 min until optimum uterine activity using 0.75; 1.0; 1.5; 2.0 and 3.0 to a maximum of 4.0 μg min^{-1}. Cervical dilatation was produced in all 15 women receiving PGE_2 but in five of these subjects it occurred only after the membranes had ruptured spontaneously. All patients reached full dilatation (maximum induction-full dilatation interval was $15\frac{1}{2}$ hours) and delivered vaginally in a mean time of 9 hours 55 min. Late FHR deceleration patterns were noted in six out of 15 cases, and two infants had a one-minute Apgar score lower than 5. There was one stillbirth in a case of dysmaturity complicated by intrapartum abruption. Anderson and co-authors (Anderson et al., 1972a, b) used an escalating dose schedule of i.v. PGE_2 to induce labour in six women at term. Dose levels were roughly doubled at fixed intervals (0.3 and 0.6 μg min^{-1} for half an hour each; 1.2 μg min^{-1} for one hour; 2.4 and 4.8 μg min^{-1} for four hours, each). The procedure was successful in five women (83%). With smaller doses (range 0.3–1.2 μg min^{-1}, however, their success rate was much lower, i.e. 4/9 women (Anderson et al., 1971).

In a double-blind trial, Naismith et al. (1972) compared the value of PGE_2 + oxytocin + amniotomy with that of oxytocin + amniotomy for elective induction of labour at term. Each group contained 10 nulliparous patients.

Immediately after amniotomy, an i.v. infusion of oxytocin was started. The initial rate of 0.66 mU min⁻¹ was doubled every 15 min until adequate uterine response. In all patients, an infusion of either a placebo or PGE_2 (0.5 μg min⁻¹) was started simultaneously with the oxytocin drip. In the combined PG-oxytocin group there was a significant reduction ($p < 0.025$) in the dosage of oxytocin required to produce effective uterine action, and the duration of labour was (but not significantly so: $p > 0.05$) reduced. Side-effects were not observed except for venous erythema which occurred only in the PG-oxytocin series (3/10). Two of the babies delivered after PG-oxytocin infusion had low Apgar-scores but responded well to routine resuscitation.

The same group (Naismith *et al.*, 1973) studied nulliparas (40–42 weeks) matched for inducibility features in order to compare the effectiveness of oxytocin and PGs given in escalated doses ($PGF_{2\alpha}$ and PGE_2, 10 patients each; oxytocin, 20 patients). Amniotomy was postponed until established labour and if this did not occur within 12 hrs, drug administration was discontinued and the case considered a failure. In 3/10 patients given PGE_2, oxytocin was required to produce full dilatation. All patients eventually delivered vaginally. The induction–delivery interval in successful cases ranged from four hours 10 min to $19\frac{1}{2}$ hours. The maximum dose level of PGE_2 was 8.0 μg min⁻¹. The total dose ranged from 0.6 to 3.1 mg PGE_2. In 2/10 neonates the two-minute Apgar score was low; in 1/10 the five-minute score was low. Maternal side-effects were not severe with any of the drugs but 4/10 subjects induced with PGE_2 developed pyrexia (> 37.7 °C) and had episodes of shivering. Erythema at the infusion site was noted in only one patient who received high doses of PGE_2.

Elias (1972) compared PGE_2 and $PGF_{2\alpha}$ in a double-blind trial including nulliparas and parous patients (16 and 14, respectively). Drugs were given by an escalating dose scheme. Labour was successfully induced in all patients receiving PGE_2. There were two Caesarean sections, one for disproportion and one for mentoposterior face presentation. The mean induction–delivery interval was 11 hours 48 min. The only side-effect was reversible venous erythema. In cases monitored, FHR and uterine contraction patterns remained normal. Fetal scalp pH and Apgar scores also were normal.

Another double-blind trial of low amniotomy combined with a prostaglandin (PGE_2 or $PGF_{2\alpha}$) or with oxytocin was conducted in patients at term by Brown *et al.* (1973). Ninety-four per cent of the women receiving low doses of i.v. PGE_2 delivered within 12 hours in a mean time of 8 hours 23 min. Side-effects were troublesome in a number of women and sometimes necessitated discontinuing the infusion. The infants were in satisfactory condition at birth.

Thiery *et al.* (1974d) induced 55 clinically normal women at term by combining low amniotomy with i.v. PGE_2. One patient required a Caesarean section because of cord prolapse; the remaining 54 delivered vaginally within 12 hours 33 min. Vomiting occurred in about one-fifth of the patients and was more frequent in the nulliparas, but was never severe. Electronic monitoring of labour and biochemical and clinical evaluation of the fetus and the newborn demonstrated the safety of the procedure.

Ring *et al.* (1974) reported on therapeutic labour induction with i.v. PGE_2 (0.1–2.5 μg min⁻¹) in 20 women at term. Eighty per cent of the subjects delivered within one course of induction, in a mean time of $4\frac{1}{2}$ hours.

Acid-base studies performed on the infant, before and after birth, showed no deleterious effects. However, because tocograms displayed evidence of episodic uterine hyperstimulation, electronic monitoring was felt to be mandatory.

4.2.1.2.2 *Larger studies.* Seven studies including at least 25 cases each and totalling some 800 women have been collated for assessment of the value of i.v. PGE_2 for the induction of labour at or about term (Table 4.4). Most of what has been concluded concerning the effectiveness of labour induction with i.v. $PGF_{2\alpha}$ applies to i.v. PGE_2 with the only exception of their different uterotonic potency.

Results. With one exception (Beazley and Gillespie, 1971) and regardless of the authors' definition of failure, trials with PGE_2 have been immensely successful. Successful induction (= stimulation of uterine activity accompanied by dilatation) was produced in 96–100% of the cases (Karim *et al.*, 1970; Karim, 1971b); vaginal deliveries were obtained in 93–98% of the candidates (Beazley *et al.*, 1970; Thiery *et al.*, 1974d) whereas labour was progressing within 12 hours in 94% of the patients induced by Brown *et al.* (1973) in those cases where the infusion did not need to be discontinued because of maternal side-effects.

Not only the definition of success but also the design of the protocol and the selection of the patients influenced success rates. Karim *et al.* (1970) repeated infusions on the following day, if necessary, and their series included 16% patients with ruptured membranes, features which may account in part for the investigators' extraordinary success with fixed-rate and low-dose infusions of PGE_2.

One group of investigators has reported a success rate which contrasts with the general trend (Beazley and Gillespie, 1971). The reason why only 73% of their patients were delivered or achieved 6 cm cervical dilatation within 12 hours is not entirely clear and a restrictive definition of success is not the whole answer. Indeed, Brown *et al.* (1973), also using very narrow criteria to define success, obtained excellent results. However, their protocol design varied from that of Beazley and Gillespie in that the PGE_2 infusion was combined with low amniotomy and only women at term were induced.

For PGE_2, the importance of inducibility variables has not been studied as carefully as for $PGF_{2\alpha}$ and authors have disagreed on several points. Nevertheless, it can probably be stated that parity, without influencing much the final success rate (Karim *et al.*, 1970; Karim, 1971b; Thiery *et al.*, 1974d), does show a relation with induction–delivery interval and total drug dose required to effect delivery (Karim, 1971b; Thiery *et al.*, 1974d). Maternal weight plays little or no role (Beazley and Gillespie, 1971; Gillespie, 1972).

Duration of pregnancy affected to some extent the success rate in the series reported by Beazley and Gillespie (1971: 81% in term patients *v.* 74% in prolonged pregnancies).

The state of the membranes is still more important. Combined induction makes lower PG dosages effective (Brown *et al.*, 1973; Thiery *et al.*, 1974d) and may therefore reduce the incidence of both uterine hyperstimulation and maternal side-effects (Brown *et al.*, 1973). Karim *et al.* (1971b) showed that the induction–delivery interval also depended on the prelabour pelvic inducibility score.

Table 4.4 Induction of labour at term with intravenous PGE$_2$

Reference	Indication	No. of cases			Gestational age (weeks)	Type	Range of levels (µg min⁻¹)	Amniotomy	Success rate (%)	Induction–delivery interval (h:min)	Uterine hypertonus (%)
		NP	MP	Total							
Beazley et al., 1970	T	9	31	40	29–42	F/E	0.4 0.4–5.6	D D	93	6:00–24:00 (repeat infusion)	3
Karim et al., 1970	T	9	41	50	34–44	F	0.5	D	100	01:20–31:00 (repeat infusion); 10:00 (mean)	0
Karim, 1971b	—	56	344	400	—	F	0.5	D	99	mean:7h (MP) and 12h (NP)	—
Karim, 1971b	—	—	—	100	—	E	0.3–1.2	D	96	—	—
Beazley and Gillespie, 1971	T	76	70	146	<35 to overdue	E	0.2–6.7	D	73	14% in less than 6h; only 9% in more than 12h	0
Brown et al., 1973	T	—	—	53	37+	E	0.25–0.75	C	94	08:23 (mean); 83% less than 12h	0
Thiery et al., 1974d	EI	25	30	55	38–42	E	0.1–4.0	C	98	05:45 (mean NP); 03:17 (mean MP)	5

Key See Table 4.1

Karim advocated low doses of PGE$_2$ infused at a constant rate (Karim *et al.*, 1970; Karim, 1971b) believing as Bygdeman *et al.* (1968) that the dose of 0.5 μg min^{-1} was below that which increased uterine tone. However, Beazley *et al.* (1970), experimenting with both fixed-rate and escalating regimens, found the uterine threshold for this PG to be variable. Consequently, these authors advocated a small initial dose (0.2 μg min^{-1}) to be doubled hourly until effective contractions, the optimum dose level being maintained thereafter (Beazley and Gillespie, 1971). They also found that in some patients this dose level had to be decreased during the active phase of labour in order to avoid hyperstimulation (Beazley and Gillespie, 1971), an observation which seems to make monitor supervision mandatory. Although hyperstimulation was indeed avoided, the success rate produced with this regimen was unsatisfactory. Others, however, have applied the drug titration principle with greater success (Thiery *et al.*, 1974d).

Uterine contractility patterns. Using extra-amniotic tocography, Karim *et al.* (1970) found that uterine activity started five to 30 min after the beginning of the infusion and generally in less than 15 min. The uterine response elicited by PGE$_2$ was not different from normal spontaneous labour near term. In the early stages of both PGE$_2$-induced and spontaneous labour, uterine contractions were often irregular and incoordinated, thereafter amplitude and frequency increased and contractions became more regular. Because tachysystoly and transient uterine hypertonus were also recorded during normal spontaneous labour, Karim considered these patterns as non-specific for PGE$_2$.

No signs of uterine hyperstimulation were observed in some 200 inductions reported by Beazley and Gillespie (1971) and Brown *et al.* (1973). Beazley *et al.* (1970) registered transient hypertonus in one patient (3%) with a dead fetus to whom abnormally high doses of PGE$_2$ (42 ng kg^{-1} min^{-1}) were administered. Thiery *et al.* (1974d) using intra-amniotic tocography observed three instances of uterine hypertonus (5%) and two instances of polysystole (4%). One case of transient hypertonus was associated with an episode of vomiting. In two out of the three cases, the hypertonus was associated with fetal bradycardia. The biochemical and clinical condition of the infants at birth is given in Table 4.5.

Table 4.5 Abnormal contractility patterns in patients electively induced with amniotomy and intravenous PGE$_2$: incidence and effects on fetus and newborn (From Thiery *et al.*, 1974d)

Type of abnormality	Incidence		pH$_a$	Apgar scores (1–5 min)
	Number	(%)		
Polysystole without FHR changes	1	1.8	7.27	8–9
Polysystole + uterine hypertonus	1	1.8	7.25	5–9
Transient hypertonus + transient fetal bradycardia + vomiting	1	1.8	7.19	9–9
Transient hypertonus + transient bradycardia (→ PG discontinued)	1	1.8	7.34	8–9
Total	4	7.2		

It is concluded that as a rule PGE$_2$ produces uterine contraction patterns similar to those characterising normal spontaneous labour. The reported incidence of uterine hyperstimulation varies due to differences in interpretation on the part of the investigators. Nevertheless, with the dose regimens used, both polysystole and uterine hypertonus were uncommon.

Mode of delivery. The method of delivery does not seem to be influenced by the use of PG and largely depends on departmental policy and patient material. Thiery *et al.* (1974d) report a rate of 35% elective vacuum extraction which is identical to that in non-induced patients and women electively induced with oxytocin. The Caesarean section rate varies from 0 to 7.5% and amounts to 3.8% for the total material. Only three out of 23 abdominal deliveries were performed because of fetal distress and one for cord prolapse, the latter infant being in good condition at birth.

Maternal effects. No mortality has been reported to date following i.v. administration of PGE_2 for induction of labour.

No side-effects were reported in 540 women induced with PGE_2 by Beazley *et al.* (1970) and Karim (1971b).

Vomiting, never bothersome, was reported by two groups, but with very divergent incidences (Karim *et al.*, 1970; 2%; Thiery *et al.*, 1974d: 20%). The latter group also found vomiting to be related to the parity of the patient (36% in nulliparas against 6% in parous patients). In one-fourth of the cases vomiting was associated with transient deceleration of FHR, in one-fifth with transient uterine hypertonus.

Venous erythema at the site of infusion was reported by Beazley and Gillespie (1971: mild, in occasional cases) and Brown *et al.* (1973: 6% with infusion levels not higher than 0.5 μg min^{-1}). In several patients Brown and colleagues had to discontinue the PG infusion on account of this side-effect.

Thus, the only side-effects associated with i.v. PGE_2 for induction of labour are vomiting and venous erythema.

None of the authors reporting on larger series of inductions found that the PG had altered vital functions of the mother. This is important because on account of the vasodepressor activity of this compound (demonstrated in animals) a possible effect on maternal blood pressure could be anticipated.

Other investigators demonstrated that even high doses of i.v. PGE_2 had no effect on maternal cardiovascular function. Infusion levels as high as 40 μg min^{-1} PGE_2 did not affect ECG, blood pressure or heart rate of non-pregnant and pregnant women (first half of gestation). However, a rapid i.v. injection of 100 μg or more, or a slow continuous infusion of 64 μg min^{-1} increased the heart rate and produced a fall in blood pressure in healthy male and female volunteers (Karim *et al.*, 1971 a, c). Smith (1973), investigating the influence of PGE_2 on the respiratory system, found a small increase in lung resistance in some women infused with high doses of this prostaglandin (10–20 μg min^{-1}) for interruption of pregnancy. The author expressed concern in the use of i.v. PGE_2 in patients with bronchial disease. However, neither asthmatic attacks nor other signs of bronchoconstriction have been observed during induction of labour.

Spellacy *et al.* (1971) found normal blood sugar and plasma insulin levels in women induced with i.v. PGE_2 (0.3–2.4 μg min^{-1}). The procedure was also without effect on the acid-base and lactate-pyruvate equilibria in maternal blood (Thiery *et al.*, 1974d).

The use of PGE_2 may be contraindicated in patients with sickle-cell anaemia or trait. Indeed, Willis *et al.* (1972) showed *in vitro* that PGE_2 in concentrations as low as 10 ng ml^{-1} induced sickling in erythrocytes from these subjects. Red blood cells from healthy persons were unaffected.

Lyneham *et al.* (1973) reported epileptic seizures and electroencephalogram changes in women aborted by intra-amniotic instillation of $PGF_{2\alpha}$ but this has not been confirmed by other investigators (see Section 4.2.1.1.2). Beazley *et al.* (1970) observed a single instance of postpartum eclampsia in their series of 16 patients with toxaemia of pregnancy, induced with i.v. PGE_2. To the best of our knowledge, no other convulsive episodes have been reported during or after induction of labour with this compound. In the course of 150 elective inductions at term with oral or intravenous PGE_2, Thiery *et al.* (1974a) never observed fits although several of their patients were known epileptics.

Induction of labour with i.v. PGE_2 induced no significant changes in complete blood count, sedimentation rate, serum uric acid, urea, creatinine, glucose, bilirubin, alkaline phosphatase, transaminases, total protein, albumin and cholesterol. There was also no alteration of the urine analysis (Anderson *et al.*, 1972b; Thiery *et al.*, 1974d). No significant differences in urinary ketones were detected in the course of a double-blind comparative study of i.v. PGE_2 and oxytocin (Beazley and Gillespie, 1971). Thiery and Willighagen (1973) found no microscopic or histochemical changes in the placenta following elective induction of labour with i.v. PGE_2.

The reported incidence of postpartum haemorrhage, following induction of labour with i.v. PGE_2, ranges from 0 (Karim *et al.*, 1970; Thiery *et al.*, 1974d) to 13% (Brown *et al.*, 1973).

Fetal and neonatal effects. Two cases of intrapartum death (2%) were reported by Beazley and Gillespie (1971). The first fetus died of intrauterine asphyxia (confirmed at autopsy) during induction undertaken for severe pre-eclampsia; a tight nuchal cord was detected at birth. In the second case, labour was induced because of prolonged pregnancy and previous stillbirth. The liquor was meconium-stained at amniotomy performed seven hours after commencement of infusion; $2\frac{1}{2}$ hours later the FHR slowed rapidly and ceased.

Thiery *et al.* (1974d) lost one infant at the age of 48 hrs. The child appeared normal at birth (Apgar score 9/9; $pH_a = 7.33$) but deteriorated progressively thereafter. At autopsy, hypoplasia of the left cardiac ventricle and stenosis of the ascending aorta were found.

Clinical fetal distress necessitating Caesarean section was reported in three instances by Karim and his group (Karim *et al.*, 1970; Karim, 1971b). In the first case, fetal distress which occurred three hours after stopping the infusion, was caused by the association of placenta praevia and nuchal cord. Beazley *et al.* (1970) witnessed fetal distress in 2/40 cases (2.5%); one was terminated by Caesarean section (Apgar score 4/10), the other by forceps delivery (Apgar score 7/10). The incidence of clinical fetal distress was 8% in the series of Beazley and Gillespie (1971).

Thiery and collaborators registered abnormal FHR patterns during the first and second stages of labour in 9 and 15% respectively of the cases studied (Thiery *et al.*, 1974d). However, none of the first stage abnormalities had any influence on the biochemical status of the fetus assayed at full cervical dilatation (Table 4.6).

A wide range of values was reported for the Apgar scores at one and five

Table 4.6   Abnormal FHR patterns registered in patients induced electively at term with intravenous PGE₂ (From Thiery *et al.*, 1974d)

Stage	Type of abnormality	Incidence	
		No.	*%*
1st stage of labour	Transient bradycardia (with vomiting)	2	
	Transient bradycardia (without vomiting)	1	
	Transient bradycardia (+ transient uterine hypertonus)	1	
	Dips II	1	
		5/55	9%
2nd stage of labour	Progressive bradycardia	4	
	Transient bradycardia	3	
	Dips II (+ prolonged expulsion)	1	
		8/55	15%

minutes after birth, but the data are difficult to compare as authors' definitions for a low Apgar score ranged from 7 to less than 5. In our own series, 11% of the Apgar scores were low (<7) at one minute, but all were normal at five minutes (Thiery *et al.*, 1974d).

Only two groups of researchers reported fetal acid-base studies. Beazley and Gillespie (1971) found that the pH at birth was below 7.20 in only 2% of the cases. Thiery *et al.* (1974d) noted that the scalp pH, at the end of the first stage of labour, was normal in every case. At birth, the mean values of a number of parameters related to the acid-base and lactate–pyruvate equilibria fell within normal limits. A few low individual pH$_a$ values were due to factors acting only during expulsion (abnormal FHR patterns, prolonged expulsion) and were probably not related to the use of the prostaglandin.

4.2.1.2.3 *Comparison of intravenous PGE₂ with intravenous PGF₂ₐ.* Six studies were collated for comparison of i.v. PGE₂ with i.v. PGF₂ₐ for the induction of labour at or about term. They cover a total of 232 patients induced with PGE₂ and 304 subjects induced with PGF₂ₐ (Table 4.7).

In three of the trials, patients were selected at random and studied in a double-blind fashion (Karim, 1971b; Anderson *et al.*, 1972b; Elias, 1972) but in Anderson's study, the number of women who received PGE₂ is too small for valid intergroup comparison. In the other projects, the patients were matched either for inducibility features (parity and pelvic score: Naismith *et al.*, 1973; Thiery, 1974) or for age, parity and gestational length (Brown *et al.*, 1973). Naismith *et al.* (1973) studied only nulliparas; Anderson *et al.* (1972b) only parous patients. Dose schemes took into account that PGE₂ was about 10 times more potent than PGF₂ₐ.

Results. With the dose schedules used, PGE₂ and PGF₂ₐ had comparable efficacy. Indeed, with one exception (Karim, 1971b) both the success rates and the mean induction–delivery intervals were similar with the two compounds.

Table 4.7 Comparison of intravenous PGE$_2$ with intravenous PGF$_{2\alpha}$ for induction of labour

Reference	Number of patients		Dose levels ($\mu g\ min^{-1}$)		Success rate (%)		Mean induction–delivery interval (h:min)		Uterine hypertonus	
	PGE$_2$	PGF$_{2\alpha}$	PGE$_2$	PGF$_{2\alpha}$	PGE$_2$	PGF$_{2\alpha}$	PGE$_2$	PGF$_{2\alpha}$	PGE$_2$	PGF$_{2\alpha}$
Karim, 1971b	100	100	0.3–1.2	2.5–10	96	97	—	—	—	—
Elias, 1972	14	16	0.3–5.0 (escalated dosage, delayed amniotomy)	2.5–40	100	100	11:48	10:30	0	1/16
Anderson et al., 1972b	6	91	0.3–5.0 (escalated dosage, delayed amniotomy)	2.5–40	83	81	—	—	2/6	7%
Brown et al., 1973	53	32	0.25–0.75 (escalated dosage, combined amniotomy)	2.5–7.5	94	87	08:23	09:15	—	—
Naismith et al., 1973	10	10	0.25–8.0 (escalated dosage, delayed amniotomy)	2.5–80	75	75	similar (13:23 for both groups)		—	—
Thiery, 1974	49	55	0.1–4.0 (escalated dosage, combined amniotomy)	2.5–100	98	100	similar		similar	

Contractility patterns. Uterine contraction patterns and the incidence of uterine hypertonus were similar for both drugs (Elias, 1972; Thiery, 1974).

Maternal effects. In both groups, vital signs remained normal (Roberts and Turnbull, 1971; Anderson *et al.*, 1972b; Naismith *et al.*, 1973; Thiery, 1974), and laboratory studies failed to detect any anomalies (Anderson *et al.*, 1972b; Elias, 1972; Thiery, 1974).

Controversy persists as to the incidence of side-effects with either drug. According to Naismith *et al.* (1973), diarrhoea and vomiting were more frequent with $PGF_{2\alpha}$ than with PGE_2. Pyrexia (4/10), shivering (1/10) and venous erythema (1/10) were observed with $PGF_{2\alpha}$ exclusively. Brown *et al.* (1973) found the same incidence of venous erythema (12%) for both drugs, but vomiting (3%) occurred only with $PGF_{2\alpha}$. Thiery (1974), on the other hand, reported a higher incidence of vomiting with PGE_2 (18%) than with $PGF_{2\alpha}$ (4%).

Brown *et al.* (1973) found that the mean blood loss was greater (222 ml) and that postpartum haemorrhage was more frequent (13%) after infusion of PGE_2 than after $PGF_{2\alpha}$ (172 ml, 3%).

Fetal and neonatal effects. There was no difference in the incidence of fetal bradycardia and the scalp pH at the end of the first stage of labour was the same for both PGE_2 and $PGF_{2\alpha}$ (Elias, 1972; Thiery, 1974). Neither the values of a number of parameters related to acid–base and lactate–pyruvate equilibria (Thiery, 1974), nor the clinical condition of the newborn (Apgar score— Anderson *et al.*, 1972b; Elias, 1972; Brown *et al.*, 1973; Naismith *et al.*, 1973; Thiery, 1974) showed any difference at birth, between the two groups. Neither of the drugs was found to influence bilirubin metabolism in the neonate (de Hemptinne *et al.*, 1973) or to have altered placental histology and histochemistry (Thiery and Willighagen, 1973).

4.2.1.2.4 *Conclusions.* Except for Karim (1971b), all authors agreed that PGE_2 and $PGF_{2\alpha}$ were equally effective for labour induction at term. Maternal side-effects were somewhat more frequent with $PGF_{2\alpha}$. No deleterious effect on fetus or neonate was described.

4.2.1.3 Prostaglandin $F_{1\alpha}$

Few studies on the effect of $PGF_{1\alpha}$ on the pregnant human uterus are available and the clinical experience with this compound for the induction of labour at term is limited to two patients.

Bygdeman (1964) first demonstrated *in vitro* the oxytocic effect of $PGF_{1\alpha}$, in the dose of 0.03 μg ml^{-1} of bath fluid, on strips of early pregnant myometrium. Embrey and Morrison (1968), studying upper segment uterine strips obtained at or near term, found that low doses (0.01–0.02 μg ml^{-1} bath fluid) of $PGF_{1\alpha}$ had no effect whereas at higher dosage (0.05–0.1 μg ml^{-1}) mild stimulation was observed in only one of the two uteri tested.

In vivo experiments in the second trimester of pregnancy showed that the threshold dose for $PGF_{1\alpha}$ given by bolus i.v. injection was 200–500 μg as compared to $\pm$ 100 μg for $PGF_{2\alpha}$ (Bygdeman *et al.*, 1970). Thus, under these experimental conditions, $PGF_{1\alpha}$ appeared to be 2–5 times less potent than

$PGF_{2\alpha}$. The typical response to a single i.v. dose of $PGF_{1\alpha}$ was rapid elevation of uterine tone, followed by a gradual return to the normal resting level. Although doses up to 750 μg had no influence on maternal pulse rate and blood pressure, and no side-effects were observed, the uterine hypertonicity elicited was felt to preclude use of this compound for the induction of labour.

Embrey (1969) gave $PGF_{1\alpha}$ by continuous i.v. infusion (4–6 μg min^{-1}, total duration of infusion 28 min) to one patient at term with an unfavourable cervix and intact membranes. Definite stimulation of uterine contractions was recorded by external tocography and there was no elevation of uterine tone. Three hours after the beginning of the infusion, the patient went into labour and eventually delivered spontaneously (induction–delivery interval $6\frac{1}{2}$ hours). There were no maternal side-effects and no changes in pulse rate or blood pressure. Besides Embrey, only one other team of researchers used $PGF_{1\alpha}$ for elective induction of labour at term (Caballero *et al.*, 1974). Again, this concerned only one patient, a multipara with intact membranes and a Bishop score of 8. The initial i.v. dose level of 10 μg min^{-1} was gradually increased to a maximum level of 60 μg min^{-1}, which was maintained until delivery. For reasons unstated, an i.v. drip of oxytocin was added during the last 19 min. The induction–delivery interval amounted to 2 hrs 10 min. No maternal side-effects were noted and the infant was clinically normal at birth (Apgar score 8/10).

Conclusion. $PGF_{1\alpha}$ undoubtedly is capable of inducing labour at term in patients with favourable inducibility features. Due to the lack of interest which clinical investigators have shown for this compound, correct assessment of its value must await more extensive trials.

4.2.1.4 Prostaglandin E$_1$

The effect of intravenously infused PGE_1 on the intact human uterus near term was initially investigated by Bygdeman *et al.* (1967, 1968). Four women at 34–37 weeks' gestation, undergoing amniocentesis for iso-immunisation were given a short-lasting (8–33 min) continuous i.v. infusion of PGE_1 at dose levels of 2.5–8.0 μg min^{-1} and the intrauterine pressure changes were recorded. PGE_1 appeared equally potent to PGE_2, with a threshold dose of 4–8 μg min^{-1}. Because hypertonus with transient fetal bradycardia was recorded in at least one case, the authors suggested that PGE_1, as well as PGE_2, would be less suitable for labour induction than the PGF compounds.

Embrey and Morrison (1968), studying PGE_1 *in vitro*, had found that this compound was only moderately 'spasmogenic' on strips of human myometrium obtained at term. Based on these studies, Embrey (1969) investigated the potential value of PGE_1 for induction of labour. In an initial patient at term, with favourable cervix and intact membranes, he administered a stepwise increased i.v. infusion of PGE_1 (dose levels 2.0–6.0 μg min^{-1}) for a total duration of 28 min. After a latent interval of 15 min, a definite oxytocic effect was noted. The threshold dose was of the order of 2.0 μg min^{-1}; uterine tone was unaffected. The patient delivered spontaneously after two hours, having experienced no side-effects. In 1970, Embrey reported successful induction of labour with i.v. PGE_1 (1–6 μg min^{-1}) in four additional patients at

Table 4.8   Labour induction at term with intravenous PGE$_1$

Reference	Number of cases	Parity	Gestational age (weeks)	Indication*	Amniotomy	Dose level (μg min)	Induction– delivery interval (h:min)	Success rate	Uterine hypertonus	Maternal side-effects
Embrey, 1970	4	0–1	39–40	T	delayed	1.0–6.0	02:00–13:30	4/4	0	0
Roberts and Turnbull, 1971	10	0–3	38–41	T	combined	0.75–3.0	03:05–13:00	10/10	0	venous erythema : 10
Caballero et al., 1974	25	0–6	38–42	T(5) EI(20)	delayed	0.18–2.50	01:40–10:00 (mean 05:23)	24/25	2	venous erythema=1 vomiting=7 sleepiness=2 headache=1

Key. *Indication : T (therapeutic) or EI (elective)

term. The latent period amounted to 15–30 min and no hypertonus was recorded. The same author reported on labour induction at term using i.v. PGE_1 and PGE_2 in 30 women (Embrey, 1971). Because the data were not listed according to the compound infused, no specific conclusions can be drawn for either prostaglandin.

Roth-Brandel and Adams (1970), administering i.v. PGE_1 to eight women at term (0.4–1.2 μg min^{-1}) felt that a dose level of 0.7 μg min^{-1} would probably be effective for induction of labour.

Roberts and Turnbull (1971) reported successful induction of labour using amniotomy combined with i.v. PGE_1 in 10 women at term. The PG infusion (0.75–3.0 μg min^{-1}) was started, one hour after rupturing the membranes, in subjects who did not display good myometrial activity at that time. After a latent period of 10 min, uterine stimulation was observed which resembled that seen in normal spontaneous labour. There was no hypertonus.

In the Netherlands, Favier et al. (1972) and Favier and Rietveld (1973) infused low doses of PGE_1 (0.25–0.50 μg min^{-1}) to 35 women at 24–32 weeks' gestation and found that the PG sensitised the myometrium to mechanical stimuli such as digital stretching of the cervix or instillation of saline into the extra-amniotic space. In those cases where no uterine contractions were registered, immediate myometrial activation would follow artificial rupture of the membranes. Nausea and vomiting occurred in 6/35 women and venous erythema in 4/35. However, these side-effects were observed only in patients with intrauterine death, to whom larger i.v. doses of PGE_1 were administered (up to 3.0 μg min^{-1}).

Finally, Caballero et al. (1974) reported from Madrid on a trial of labour induction with i.v. PGE_1 (0.18–1.28 μg min^{-1}) in 25 patients. Uterine activity, similar to that induced by $PGF_{2\alpha}$, was observed after a latent period of 1–109 min. Hypertonus occurred in two cases and polysystole in one.

Three clinical trials totalling 39 patients have been retained for assessment of the value of i.v. PGE_1 for induction of labour at term (Embrey, 1970; Roberts and Turnbull, 1971; Caballero et al., 1974). The data of these trials are summarised in Table 4.8 and will be briefly commented upon.

Induction was successful (good contractions and adequate progress of cervical dilatation) in 38 out of 39 patients (98%). Dose levels ranged from 0.18 to 6.0 μg min^{-1}. Although all women delivered within 14 hrs of the start of the infusion, induction–delivery intervals varied widely. In this connection, it should, however, be specified that due to the short supply of PGE_1 (Embrey, 1970) or to the inclusion of a period of observation following amniotomy (Roberts and Turnbull, 1971), the duration of the drug infusion was in fact much shorter than the induction–delivery interval would suggest. Thus, infusion times ranged from $\frac{1}{2}$ to $10\frac{1}{2}$ hours in Embrey's study (1970) and from one to seven hours in Roberts and Turnbull's series (1971).

Of the 39 patients, 35 delivered spontaneously, two by vacuum extraction and two by Caesarean section. The indication for performing the latter is not mentioned by Caballero et al. (1974). Fetal heart rate assessed by auscultation (Embrey, 1970; Roberts and Turnbull, 1971) or by electronic monitoring (Caballero et al., 1974) was normal in all cases but two in which late decelerations (type II dips) were registered (Caballero et al., 1974). However, Apgar scores at birth were normal in both neonates.

Thirty-six of the 39 infants were 'normal' at birth. One had died *in utero* four days before induction (Embrey, 1970). Of the remaining two, one had a low Apgar score (6/9) but a pH_a at birth of 7.22 (Caballero *et al.*, 1974); the other, with a low birth weight, developed respiratory distress (Roberts and Turnbull, 1971).

The procedure had no effect on maternal functions (Embrey, 1970; Roberts and Turnbull, 1971; Caballero *et al.*, 1974) nor on blood chemistry and urine analysis (Caballero *et al.*, 1974). Side-effects included vomiting (7/39), sleepiness (2/39) and headache (1/39). Venous erythema (11/39) was found in only one out of 25 women induced by Caballero *et al.* (1974) but was a constant feature in the 10 patients treated by Roberts and Turnbull (1971) who, moreover, reported the occasional occurrence of severe pain in the forearm or shoulder on the same side as but distant from the infusion site. The third stage of labour was unremarkable except in two patients whose placenta had to be removed manually (Caballero *et al.*, 1974).

Conclusion. Despite the limited clinical material available for analysis, it is obvious that i.v. PGE_1 is highly effective to induce labour at term, even in women with unfavourable cervices. PGE_1 has approximately the same oxytocic potency as PGE_2. Maternal side-effects mainly consist in nausea, vomiting and venous erythema. The occasional occurrence of uterine hyperstimulation makes monitoring of labour desirable.

4.2.2 Oral route

Given by mouth, PGE_2 and $PGF_{2\alpha}$ stimulate uterine contractions undistinguishable from those induced by an i.v. infusion of these compounds. This observation made by Karim (1971 a, b) in patients at or about term suggested that labour could be effectively induced by oral administration of PGs. Because this route is more acceptable to the patient and requires less nursing attention than an intravenous infusion, it was given an extensive trial (up to mid 1974, over 1600 gravidae were induced with oral PGE_2).

Although there is no longer any doubt concerning efficacy and acceptability of oral PGE_2 for labour induction, the place of the oral route in clinical obstetrics is still controversial. Indeed, many are of the opinion that its safety (without applying electronic surveillance) has been insufficiently proven and buccal administration of oxytocin is generally considered heresy. Gillespie (1973) stated: 'Although the success rate is high and even if the gastrointestinal side-effects can be reduced, I cannot believe that this method will be popular with obstetricians who have come to rely on the precise control of uterine activity afforded by intravenously administered oxytocic agents'. Karim and Sharma (1971a), on the other hand, consider labour induction with oral PGE_2 a major advance and many others agree that the oral route forms an interesting alternative to the i.v. route. After having gained experience with oral PGE_2 administered under electronic control, Karim and Sharma (1971a) concluded that electronic surveillance was not essential and, as a result, discontinued monitoring in their very extensive clinical trial. Craft (1973a) is of the same opinion.

To the best of our knowledge no clinical studies on labour induction by oral

administration of PGs other than PGE_2 and $PGF_{2\alpha}$ have been published. Amy et al. (1973) observed uterine stimulation without pathologic features, in pregnant patients at term to whom 100 μg of the analogue 15(R),15-methyl-PGE_2 methyl ester was administered two-hourly by mouth for suppression of gastric acidity. Karim et al. (1972) have used 15(S),15-methyl-PGE_2 methyl ester orally to induce six women at 29–36 weeks gestation with a dead fetus.

Since the first edition of this book, which mentioned but two clinical trials (Karim and Sharma, 1971a; Khew et al., 1971), reports on oral PGE_2 have been issued steadily. Because oral $PGF_{2\alpha}$ induced severe gastrointestinal side effects too frequently, the clinical trials with this PG were abandoned at an early stage.

4.2.2.1 Prostaglandin $F_{2\alpha}$

Two groups of investigators have reported clinical trials with orally administered $PGF_{2\alpha}$ for labour induction (Table 4.9). Karim and Sharma (1971a)

Table 4.9 Induction of labour with orally administered $PGF_{2\alpha}$ (therapeutic indication in all cases)

Reference	Number of cases	Gestational age (weeks)	Dose	Success rate	Mean induction–delivery interval (h:min)	Maternal side-effects
Karim and Sharma, 1971a	20	35–44	5–10 mg, two-hourly	15/20	23:30	—
Barr, 1972	50	40–42	5–15 mg, two-hourly	33/50	9:16	Gastrointestinal side-effects in 42/50, often severe

induced 20 women using a test dose of 5 mg as a draught followed by doses of 5–10 mg (according to uterine activity) at two-hourly intervals until adequate contractions were produced and the cervix dilated to 5–6 cm. The drug was then discontinued and low amniotomy performed. In 5/20 patients, uterine contractions monitored via an intra-amniotic catheter were normal and similar to those elicited by i.v. PGE_2. The success rate (no definition of success given) was 15/20, although many patients had an unfavourable cervix. The five failures were successfully delivered with oral PGE_2. Side-effects and clinical state of the infant were not mentioned but in the pilot study (Karim, 1971a) it was stated that single oral doses up to 30 mg $PGF_{2\alpha}$ did not produce any noticeable effect on the gastrointestinal tract or the cardiovascular system, a conclusion which is in contradistinction with the findings of Barr and co-workers.

Following an initial paper (Barr and Naismith, 1972), Barr issued two follow-up studies totalling 50 women (Barr, 1972, 1973a). A test dose of 5 mg (one capsule) $PGF_{2\alpha}$ was followed after 30 min by a further dose of 10 mg.

Table 4.10 Oral PGE$_2$. Protocol design

Reference	Test dose(s) (mg)	Dosage scheme				Amniotomy	Oxytocin (i.v.)	Premedication and analgesia
		Single doses (mg)	Interval (min)	Type*	Last dose			
			Subsequent doses					
Karim and Sharma, 1971a	0.5	0.5–1.5	120	S	labour established	delayed (⌀6 cm)	—	
Karim and Sharma, 1972	0.5	0.5–2.0	120	S	labour established	delayed (⌀6 cm)	—	
Filshie, 1972	0.5	0.5–2.0	120	S	labour established	delayed (at 24 h)	—	
Barr and Naismith, 1972; Barr, 1972	0.5→1.0 (30 min)	1.0–1.5	120	S	labour established	delayed (active labour)	after 12–18 h	
Barr, 1973a, b	0.5→1.0 (30 min)	1.5–2.0	120	S	labour established	early	after 12–18 h	
Craft, 1972a, b 1973a, b	0.5→0.5 (60 min)	0.5–3.0	120	S	delivery	early	after 24 h	diazepam, epidural
Elias, 1972	0.5	1.0–1.5	120	S	?	delayed (⌀4 cm)	—	
Yip et al., 1973	—	0.5	60–120	F	labour established	delayed (⌀3-4 cm)	—	

Reference								
Thiery et al., 1973b	0.5→ 0.5–1.0 (60 min)	0.5–2.0	120+	S	delivery +	1 h prior to PG	—	
Thiery et al., 1974b	0.5→ 0.5–1.0 (60 min)	0.5–2.0	120+	S	delivery +	1 h prior to PG	—	
Kelly et al., 1973	0.5	0.5–2.0	120	S	delivery	early	after 24 h	
Murnaghan et al., 1974	0.5→ 0–1.0 (30 min)	0.5–2.0	120	S	delivery	1 h prior to PG	—	
Murnaghan et al., 1974	0.5→ 0–1.0 (30 min)	0–2.0	60	S	delivery	1 h prior to PG	—	
Corson and Bolognese, 1974	—	0.5	60	F	?	delayed (φ4 cm)	—	epidural, caudal, local, general
Elder and Stone, 1974	0.5→0.5 (30 min)	0.5–2.0	120	S	delivery	early	after 18 h	
Elder and Stone, 1974	—	0.5	60	F	delivery	early	after 12 h	
Wilkin et al., 1974	—	0.5	60	F	delivery	early	after 8 h	
Fraser, 1974	—	0.5	60	F	?	early	—	
Laersen and Wilson, 1974	0.25–0.50	1.0–3.0	30	Do	labour established	delayed (φ3–5 cm)	—	epidural

*Key. F=fixed dose; S=stepwise increase, usually by constant increment; Do=doubling of single dose; φ=cervical dilatation

Depending on uterine response subsequent doses of 15 mg were administered every two hours until labour was established and the cervix was dilated to 5–6 cm. Using external tocography the authors did not observe hypertonus. Of the 50 women, 33 (66%) were successfully induced (author's definition of success: labour well-established within 12–18 hours). In case of failure, delivery was readily effected by oxytocin (which again suggest that oxytocin may act more efficiently on a PG-primed uterus). Infants were in good condition at birth. Maternal side-effects were limited to gastrointestinal disturbances which occurred in most of the women (42/50: 33 diarrhoea, as main complaint and nine vomiting). 'Ten cases were acutely miserable on account of diarrhoea amounting to virtual incontinence and by the end of our 50 cases we could not persuade one other patient to take these capsules.'

Craft (1972a) investigated $PGF_{2\alpha}$ capsules plus amniotomy for the induction of labour at term but, because of gastrointestinal side-effects and the limited success encountered, the trial was soon discontinued. As far as we know, the results of this study were never published.

Conclusion. Effectiveness, even at the high doses used by Barr, fell below expectations. Furthermore, severe gastrointestinal side-effects, especially watery diarrhoea, preclude the clinical use of oral $PGF_{2\alpha}$ for induction of labour.

4.2.2.2 Prostaglandin E_2

Karim's (1971a) initial investigations of the uterine effect of oral PGs includes two gravidae at term with a dead fetus. In both cases single oral doses of 0.5 mg PGE_2 produced uterine contractions similar to those characterising normal spontaneous labour or labour induced by means of an intravenous infusion of 0.5–1.0 μg min^{-1} PGE_2. Uterine stimulation started after 5–10 min (5–30 min according to a subsequent clinical trial, Karim and Sharma, 1971a) and the effect lasted for 2–3 hours. This study, which provided clinicians with at least a hint at effective drug dose and time interval between doses, is at the base of most clinical protocols. These protocols, however, are very divergent as to variables which may affect the outcome of induction.

4.2.2.2.1 *Protocol design and inducibility variables.* From the data in Table 4.10 it appears that the set-up of clinical trials with oral PGE_2 has followed definite evolutionary steps.

The original protocol (Karim and Sharma, 1971a) consisted in the administration of a test dose of 0.5 mg PGE_2 as a draught followed at intervals of two hours by stepwise increased doses (0.5–1.5 mg) until labour was established and the cervix dilated to 5–6 cm. Administration of the drug was then discontinued and low amniotomy performed. The size of the maintenance dose was determined on the basis of the uterine activity registered by trans-abdominal intra-amniotic tocography. As excessive uterine response was never registered, the authors confidently and with great success embarked upon a very extensive trial ($n = 764$) using the same regimen but omitting cardio-tocographic monitoring. For the same reason, others (Craft, 1972a) have stopped monitoring their patients. In the United Kingdom, Barr and Naismith

(1972) adopted a schedule comparable to that of Karim and Sharma (1971a) except that they gave two test doses 30 min apart. Thus, the characteristic features of the oldest trials with oral PGE_2 were the stepwise increase of single doses at fixed intervals and delayed amniotomy.

Karim and collaborators delayed amniotomy for fear of cord prolapse because in many Ugandan women the fetal head remains high until completion of the first stage of labour. Filshie (1972) working with the same type of patients decided to perform amniotomy on all subjects not delivered after 24 hours and was able to show that artificial rupture of the membranes increased efficacy: 93% were delivered in 36 hours as compared to 86% who did not have routine amniotomy; 98% were delivered within 48 hours *v.* 90% in whom no amniotomy was performed. Prolapse of the cord never occurred.

As in Caucasian women early low amniotomy is an infrequent cause of cord prolapse and the procedure in itself exerts a positive effect on establishing labour, Craft (1972a) decided to incorporate early amniotomy into his protocol. His success, especially in nulliparous patients, eventually made Barr (1973a, b) adopt it. However, wishing to have his patients delivered within 12–18 hours following amniotomy, Barr substituted (after that period of time had elapsed) an intravenous infusion of oxytocin for prostaglandin in half of his patients. After stopping administration of oral PGE_2, Barr (1973a, b) waited some time before starting i.v. oxytocin because of fear of potentiation. Observing that patients receiving oxytocin after discontinuation of PG therapy, generally delivered within very short periods of time, Barr suggested that the prostaglandin could have had a 'priming action'.

The beneficial effect exerted by amniotomy on uterine contractility was clearly shown by Khew *et al.* (1971) who found that the percentage of patients in established labour within two hours of the first oral dose of PGE_2 amounted to 72% with combined amniotomy and only to 19% when membranes were left intact. The corresponding figures after four hours were 100% and 38%, respectively. Whereas Craft (1972a) and several others after him performed amniotomy at the time of the initial oral dose of PGE_2, others preferred to wait one hour to verify whether labour was not initiated by amniotomy alone (Thiery 1973b, c, 1974b; Murnaghan *et al.*, 1974).

Further modifications in protocol are recent and coincide with the introduction of PG tablets. They consist in shortening the interval between (mostly fixed) single doses. Yip *et al.* (1973) first reported hourly administration of a capsule of 0.5 mg PGE_2; if after four hours regular contractions occurred the interval was lengthened to two hours. Hourly administration of one tablet (0.5 mg) PGE_2 has been given an extensive trial since (Corson and Bolognese, 1974; Elder and Stone, 1974; Fraser, 1974; Wilkin *et al.*, 1974). Lauersen and Wilson (1975) went further and cut down the interval to half an hour while doubling single doses until good uterine activity or a maximum single dose of 3.0 mg was attained. Because they observed uterine hypertonus in a woman given a larger initial dose (1.0 mg PGE_2), they presently administer a test dose of 0.25–0.50 mg.

Dose escalation has been performed either by stepwise increase (i.e. by adding a constant increment to the previous dose) or by doubling consecutive doses (Lauersen and Wilson, 1975). As stated, recently the fixed-dose principle has been applied to oral PGE_2 administration as well. Besides its simplicity, it was anticipated that this schedule would combine a lower incidence of maternal side-effects with a decreased risk of hyperstimulation of the uterine muscle.

Whereas in the oldest clinical trials drug administration was discontinued as soon as labour was well-established, it has become current practice to give the prostaglandin until delivery. Moreover, several authors mention that for fear of maternal ketosis and intra-amniotic infection, they have set a time limit for PG administration (12–18 hours) after which, unless the patient is in active labour and the cervix dilated to 6 cm, they discontinue the PG and set up an intravenous drip of oxytocin. Craft (1972a, b, 1973a, b) and Kelly et al. (1973) adhere to 24 hours, Karim and Sharma (1972) to 48 hours.

For the administration of PGE_2 by mouth three formulations have been used. Karim and Sharma (1971a) administered an aqueous solution of crystalline PGE_2. On account of the bitter taste they switched to hard gelatin capsules containing an ethanol solution of the drug (Karim and Sharma, 1972). In the United Kingdom and in Belgium a drink of an ethanol or dimethylacetamide solution of PGE_2 diluted in water was used. The first report on the use of tablets (0.5 mg PGE_2) (Thiery et al., 1974b) was soon followed by a handful of publications from the United Kingdom and the USA. Several investigators comparing different formulations, i.e. draught v. tablets (Elder and Stone, 1974; Craft, 1974; Thiery et al., 1974c) failed to find any difference in effectivity or safety.

A last point concerns the use of analgesia. Craft (1972a) was the first to use routinely premedication (diazepam 10 mg i.v.) followed by continuous epidural analgesia. Neither procedure affected the incidence of gastrointestinal side-effects (Craft 1972b, 1973b). In 20 of the 23 women induced by Corson and Bolognese (1974), a variety of analgesic procedures were used: lumbar epidural, caudal, local or general. Lauersen and Wilson (1975) report fetal bradycardia to have occurred in a patient under epidural block. However, from most papers it is impossible to derive the extent to which analgesia was resorted to and the data listed in the last column of Table 4.10 certainly are an understatement. Indeed, we suspect analgesia to be rather common in the UK and the USA, where it has grown to be a part of clinical obstetrics. In fact, the only studies which specifically mention that no other drug than the compound under study (oral PGE_2) was administered during the induction of labour, in order to keep the observation 'clean', are those from Ghent (Thiery et al., 1973b, c, 1974b).

Selection of candidates for induction (see Table 4.11) may affect both efficacy and safety of the procedure. Three variables in particular determine the ease of induction: parity, length of gestation and cervical ripeness. Other factors, of course, such as premature rupture of the membranes (18% in the series reported by Karim and Sharma, 1972), intrauterine death (usually eliminated by the authors; constitutes nonetheless 15% of the material of Elias, 1972) and twin gestation (very few cases included within an occasional series) may contribute to the success or the failure of the induction.

Parity ratios differ considerably in the reported studies. As a rule, more parous than nulliparous women are included (ratio: 1.25), but Craft (1973a, b) deliberately concentrated on nulliparas.

Induction with oral PGE_2 was generally attempted at or about term, but

Table 4.11   Oral PGE₂. Patient material, inducibility features and indication for the induction

Reference	Number of patients*			Gestational age (weeks)	Bishop score	Indication
	NP	MP	Total			
Karim and Sharma, 1971a	30	50	*80*	35–44	—	T
Karim and Sharma, 1972	±20%	±80%	*764*	—	⩽5(85%)	T
Khew *et al.*, 1971	—	—	*51*	38–42+	—	T
Barr and Naismith, 1972	1	9	*10*	40–43	0–9	T
Barr, 1972	3	47	*50*	± term	0–9	T
Barr, 1973b	23	5	*28*	39–41	many unfa-vourable	T
Barr, 1973a	30	50	*80*	38–42	—	?
Craft, 1972a, b	32	18	*50*	38–43	2–10	T
Craft, 1973a, b	50	30	*80*	38–43	2–10	T
Filshie, 1972	24	76	*100*	?	low	T
Elias, 1972			*20*	term	1–7	T
Yip *et al.*, 1973	36	21	*57*	35–44	?	T
Thiery *et al.*, 1973b, c; Thiery *et al.*, 1974b	46	51	*97*	38–42	4–9	El
Kelly *et al.*, 1974	24	25	*49*	38–41+	0–7+	T
Murnaghan *et al.*, 1974	—	—	*50*	38–42	1–10	T+El(42%)
Corson and Bolognese, 1974	4	19	*23*	38–41	6 (mean)	El
Elder and Stone, 1974	46	24	*70*	term	ripe	?
Wilkin *et al.*, 1974	13	7	*20*	term	{ ⩾4(MP) ⩾6(NP)	?
Lauersen and Wilson, 1975	21	31	*52*	36–43	0–8+	T+El(20%)

Key. See Table 4.1. * One is often uncertain as to the true total number of women induced by a group of workers (see: section 4.1). Figures that are certainly correct have been made italic

still, a number of postmature cases and of pregnancies that had to be terminated before term because of medical complications (e.g. toxaemia of pregnancy, diabetes, Rh-isoimmunisation) were inccluded.

The use of a semi-objective method for assessing cervical status has facilitated comparison of the results (cf. 4.2.1). In their first clinical trial, Karim and Sharma (1971a) used the Friedman score (Friedman *et al.*, 1966). In 1971, Anderson *et al.* introduced the Bishop score (Bishop, 1964) which has been uniformly adopted in trials of labour induction with oral PGE₂.

Finally, the indication for induction. To simplify matters, cases were

Table 4.12 Oral PGE$_2$. Efficacy of labour induction

Reference	Parity	Total dose (mg)	Induction–delivery interval (h:min)	Success Definition	Rate	Upper time limit of PG administration
Karim and Sharma, 1971a		—	03:00–20:00	good contractions+ φ5–6 cm within 48 h	79/80(99%)	48
Karim and Sharma, 1972		—	—	vaginal delivery within 48 h	90%	48
Filshie, 1972		—	—	vaginal delivery within 48 h	98/100(98%)	—
Barr, 1972		9 (max)	04:09–16:47 (m:08:48)	labour established (φ6 cm) within 12 h	32/50(64%)	12
Barr, 1973b	NP	3.5–5.0	03:30–11:13 (m:04:30)	labour established (φ6 cm) within 12 h	5/5(100%) } 57%	12
	MP	3.0–7.5; 5.2 (m)	03:52–11:55 (m:07:18)	labour established (φ6 cm) within 12 h	11/23(48%)	12
Craft, 1973a, b	NP	4.3 (m)	10:18 (m)	labour progressing satisfactorily	43/50(84%) } 89%	24
	MP	2.4 (m)	06:20 (m)	labour progressing satisfactorily	28/30(93%)	24
Elias, 1972		1.0–7.5; 3.5(m)	02:05–21:02 (m:08:07)	labour progressing satisfactorily	18/20(90%)	24
Yip et al., 1973	NP }	±3.4 (m)	—	φ6 cm within 12 h or vaginal delivery within 24 h	27/36(75%) } 80%	12
	MP }		—	φ6 cm within 12 h or vaginal delivery within ...	19/21(90%)	12

Reference		Dose (m)	Time	Outcome	Fraction (%)		n
Thiery et al., 1973b;	NP	0.3–8.5; 2.3 (m)	02:20–18:29 (m:07:14)	full dilatation within 24 h	44/46(96%)	97%	24
Thiery et al., 1974b	MP	0.5–5.5; 1.7 (m)	01:57–09:28 (m:04:45)	full dilatation within 24 h	50/51(98%)		24
Kelly et al., 1974		1.0–25.5 6.8 (m)	09:14 (m)	full dilatation within 24 h	47/49(96%)		24
Murnaghan et al., 1974		—	08:01–11.32 (m*)	labour progressing (φ6 cm) within 19 h	50/50(100%)		19
Corson and Bolognese, 1974		2.5(m)	01:35–12:13 (m:05:47)	vaginal delivery within 12 h	20/23(87%)		12
Elder and Stone, 1974	NP	4.8–5.9 (m)**	14:30–14:42 (m*)	in active labour within 12 h	60/70(86%)		12
	MP	4.3–3.6 (m)**	08:48–10:18 (m**)	in active labour within 12 h			12
Wilkin et al., 1974	NP	2.7(m)	06:57 (m)	labour progressing satisfactorily within 8 h	12/13(92%)	90%	8
	MP	2.2 (m)	04:40 (m)	labour progressing satisfactorily within 8 h	6/7(86%)		8
Lauersen and Wilson, 1975	NP	—	11·08 (m)	adequate progress of labour	98%		—
	MP	—	06·63 (m)	adequate progress of labour			—

Key: NP = nulliparas; MP = parous patients; (m) = mean; φ = cervical dilatation; * = depending on dosage schedule (flexible titration v. fixed increment); ** = depending on drug formulation (draught v. tablet) and interval between subsequent doses (2 h v. 1 h) classified in one of two categories: elective or therapeutic inductions (cf. note at bottom of Table 4.11). Trials were more often conducted with the latter type of material, the bulk consisting in: prolonged pregnancies (Khew et al., 1971: 48%; Karim and Sharma, 1972: 54%; Lauersen and Wilson, 1975: 34%; Ratnam et al., 1974: 46%); toxaemia of pregnancy (Khew et al., 1971: 38%; Karim and Sharma, 1972: 15%; Ratnam et al., 1974: 41%; Lauersen and Wilson, 1975: 19%) and maternal diabetes (Lauersen and Wilson, 1975: 10%). Only two groups of authors conducted trials in clinically normal women (Thiery et al., 1973b, c, 1974b; Corson and Bolognese, 1974). In the series of Murnaghan et al. (1974), 42% of the inductions were elective. It goes without saying that only this type of material is suitable for assessing the fetal effects of an experimental drug.

4.2.2.2.2 *Results.* Due to the lack of standardisation of protocol design and the absence of uniform criteria for defining success, it is still difficult to define precisely the effectiveness of oral PGE_2 for induction of labour at term. Besides, very few authors have attempted to compare the efficacy of oral PGE_2 with that of conventional induction methods. Available data are summarised in Table 4.12.

The criteria used for successful induction by various authors are often divergent, e.g. the time limit set for successful induction ranged from eight (Wilkin et al., 1974) to 48 hours (Karim and Sharma, 1971a, 1972). To make matters worse, authors using the same time limit often defined success differently: some, as the initiation of 'active sustained labour', others, as the production of 'full dilatation' or 'delivery'.

With one exception (Barr, 1972, 1973b), success rates ranged from 80 (Yip et al., 1973) to 100% (Murnaghan et al., 1974), with many authors reporting a rate of over 90%.

In the first 80 patients in whom Karim and Sharma (1971a) attempted labour induction with oral PGE_2, adequate uterine activity and cervical dilatation of at least 5 cm were obtained in 79 cases (99%). The only woman who did not respond to the PG (repeated doses of 0.5–1.5 mg on two consecutive days) also failed to react to i.v. oxytocin and was delivered by Caesarean section. When their protocol was applied to 764 women, the majority with unfavourable cervix, 73% of the patients delivered vaginally within 24 hours and 90% within 48 hours (Karim and Sharma, 1972). Filshie (1972) adopted Karim's protocol in 100 patients, but performed amniotomy on those who had not delivered after 24 hours. His success rates after 24, 36 and 48 hours were 78%, 93% and 98% respectively.

Barr (1972) used very strict criteria for defining success. Of 50 patients induced (47 multiparas), 32 delivered vaginally after an average of 8 hrs 48 min. In the 18 women not in established labour within 12 hrs, drug administration was discontinued and i.v. oxytocin was started. All delivered normally. Turning his attention towards nulliparas, Barr (1973a, b) altered his protocol by combining amniotomy with PG administration, but with little success. Only 11 out of 23 nulliparas were in established labour (cervical dilatation 6 cm) within 12 hrs. In the remaining 12, PGE_2 was stopped and replaced by escalating doses of i.v. oxytocin, which eventually effected delivery. There is little doubt that if Barr had prolonged PG administration, he would have achieved higher success. Although he eventually succeeded in delivering all of his nulliparous patients with this elaborate protocol (amniotomy + oral PGE_2, followed after 12 hrs by i.v. oxytocin), the classical induction technique (amniotomy and escalating infusion of oxytocin) had a shorter amniotomy–delivery interval in the hands of this investigator.

Craft first combined amniotomy with escalating doses of oral PGE_2. In his initial series (1972a) adequate uterine activity was initiated within 24 hrs in 46/50 patients (92%). In the remaining four cases, the treatment was stopped on account of desultory labour or of side-effects, and oxytocin was administered. A comparable success characterises a more extensive trial ($n = 80$), which probably includes the previously reported cases (Craft, 1973a, b). In nulliparas, success rate amounted to 86%, the mean total dose PGE_2 was 4.3 mg and the mean induction–delivery interval 10 hrs 18 min. In parous patients, the procedure was effective in 93% (mean total dose: 2.4 mg; mean induction–delivery interval: 6 hrs 20 min).

Elias (1972) was able to induce 18 of 20 patients, three of which had intrauterine death before term. One of the failed cases had a Bishop score of 1 and no contractions were produced during the 24 hrs of attempted induction. In the other failure, PGE_2 treatment had to be discontinued after 12 hrs on account of vomiting.

Thiery and collaborators reported successful induction of labour in 94 of 97 patients by a combination of amniotomy and oral PGE_2 (Thiery *et al.*, 1973b, 1974b). Three patients did not reach full dilatation within 24 hrs and were considered failures. They included one case of desultory labour, which required i.v. oxytocin; another of cephalo-pelvic disproportion, terminated by Caesarean section and a third of fetal distress, delivered by vacuum extraction started before full dilatation. Kelly *et al.* (1974) had similar results.

Yip *et al.* (1973) considered the procedure as successful when, within 12 hrs, cervical dilatation of 6 cm was reached. Using this definition and notwithstanding a Caesarean section rate of 30%, these investigators concluded to a success rate of 80%. Their number of abdominal deliveries is difficult to explain, even if one takes into account that the overall section rate in their hospital amounted to 11% and that of women induced with i.v. oxytocin to 27%.

Corson and Bolognese (1974) first described hourly administration of one tablet (0.5 mg) PGE_2 with delayed amniotomy. Within 12 hrs, vaginal delivery was effected in 20 out of 23 patients, in a mean time of 5 hrs 47 min. Two of the failed inductions were due to cpehalo-pelvic disproportion. The third case was considered unsuccessful because the time limit arbitrarily set for producing vaginal delivery had been transgressed. Friedman and Sachtleben (1974) found that hourly administration of 0.5 mg oral PGE_2 was as effective for labour induction as regimens using higher doses and that it caused gastrointestinal side-effects much less frequently.

Elder and Stone (1974) compared combined induction with two types of drug formulation. Although the protocols of both groups were dissimilar (the draught was given in escalated doses, two-hourly; tablets were administered according to a fixed schedule, i.e. 0.5 mg/hour), efficacy and safety were comparable. Success rate amounted to 31/35 for the drink and to 29/35 for the tablets. In women given the draught, failures comprised two Caesarean sections for fetal distress (normal infants, at birth), one case of drug intoler-

Table 4.13 Labour induction with oral PGE₂. Relationship between Bishop score and effectiveness (Craft, 1973a, b, by courtesy of Symposia Specialists and *Adv. Biosciences*)

Bishop score	Mean induction–delivery interval (h:min)	
	NP	MP
0–3	22:00	11:59
4–7	11:54	06:47
8+	7:07	05:37

ance (vomiting) and one case in which delivery was not produced within 12 hrs. All six failures observed with the tablet regimen were due to the latter cause.

Wilkin *et al.* (1974) also combined early amniotomy and hourly administration of 0.5 mg PGE₂, orally, and reported vaginal delivery within eight hours in 18 of their 20 patients (90%). The other two women were stimulated with i.v. oxytocin.

Lauersen and Wilson (1975) administered an initial dose of 0.5 mg PGE₂ (one tablet) which was doubled every 30 min until adequate uterine activity or a maximum single dose of 3.0 mg was attained. Once labour was established, amniotomy was performed, PGE₂ being administered further at 30–60 min intervals. Induction was successful in 51 out of 52 patients (98%) despite the fact that one-third of them had unfavourable Bishop scores (0–3). The only failure occurred in a toxaemic patient at 37 weeks, with a Bishop score of 0. The other patients with low Bishop scores (0–3) were delivered in a mean time of 12 hrs 41 min, as compared to 8 hrs 43 min for the entire series.

Inducibility features. Regardless of the protocol used, all authors agreed that parity influenced the outcome of the attempted induction. Nulliparas had lower success rates, required a larger total dose of oral PGE₂ and had longer induction–delivery intervals than multiparous patients (Karim and Sharma, 1971a; Barr, 1973b; Craft, 1973a, b; Thiery *et al.*, 1973b, 1974b; Wilkin *et al.*, 1974; Lauersen and Wilson, 1975).

Investigators generally found that the success of induction depended on the inducibility score (Bishop, 1964; Friedman *et al.*, 1966) of the individual patient (Table 4.13). Patients with low inducibility ratings had lower success rates, longer induction times and needed a higher total dose of prostaglandin (Karim and Sharma, 1971a; Barr and Naismith, 1972; Craft, 1973a, b). However, Lauersen and Wilson (1975), using a protocol wherein the initial oral dose of 0.5 mg PGE₂ was doubled (maximum 3.0 mg) half-hourly until adequate contractions, found that even women with low Bishop scores (0–3) responded favourably.

Craft (1972a) suggested that response could be improved by allowing flexibility in the dosage. This was verified by Murnaghan *et al.* (1974), who compared the effectiveness of combined induction when applying either stepwise (fixed) increments or a more flexible type of titration and found that both the induction–delivery interval (8 hrs *v.* 11½ hrs) and the duration of labour (6 hrs *v.* 9 hrs) were considerably reduced with the latter scheme.

In conclusion, oral administration of PGE_2 is an effective means of inducing labour. Failures are usually due to low inducibility scores, that necessitate prolonged administration of high doses which may result in the development of

Table 4.14   Oral PGE_2. Incidence of hypertonus (intrauterine tocography)

Reference	Number of patients monitored	Single dose producing hypertonus (mg)	Number of patients showing hypertonus	Condition of infant at birth
Karim and Sharma, 1971a	±40	0		
Thiery et al., 1973b	94	0.5	2	normal
Kelly et al., 1974	49		0	
Murnaghan et al., 1974	50		0	
Corson and Bolognese, 1974	23		0	
Elder and Stone, 1974	70		0	
Wilkin et al., 1974	20		0	
Lauersen and Wilson, 1975	52	1.0	1	normal
Fraser, 1974	?	0.5	1	depressed
Total	±398		3 (<1%)	

ketosis, nausea and vomiting. Therefore, patients with unfavourable inducibility features, especially nulliparas, are probably better induced by combining amniotomy with the titrated i.v. administration of an oxytocic.

Uterine response. Contractions are generally produced 15–30 min after the first dose of oral PGE_2 and gradually increase in frequency and intensity, as in normal labour (Karim and Sharma, 1971a; Lauersen and Wilson, 1975).

Many clinicians fear that the dosage of orally administered oxytocics may be more difficult to adjust and, therefore, more often produces uterine hyperstimulation, potentially dangerous for both mother and fetus. However, from the data published by researchers using intrauterine tocography, it appears that the overall incidence of uterine hypertonus with oral PGE_2 amounts to less than 1% (Table 4.14). Thiery et al. (1974c) observed transient hypertonus (basal tone $\geqslant$ 12 mmHg) in two patients (2%). In both women, it occurred after a small (0.5 mg) single dose of PGE_2. In one of these patients, hypertonus was accompanied by fetal bradycardia. Both infants were normal at birth. Lauersen and Wilson (1975) having encountered a similar complication in a patient given a test dose of 1.0 mg PGE_2, have suggested reducing the initial dose to 0.25 mg to assess the individual receptivity of the uterus towards PGE_2. Fraser (1974) described one case of severe hypertonus (over 60 mmHg) with marked fetal bradycardia (60/min), 80 min after the third dose of 0.5 mg PGE_2 (single doses were given at more than one hour intervals). The hypertonus produced very rapid cervical dilatation (from a dilatation of 6 cm to delivery, in 20 min). The infant was depressed at birth (Apgar score at 1 min: 5) but responded rapidly to simple resuscitation. Oxytocin may potentiate the effect of PGs and combined administration of these oxytocics may be hazardous. The PG-primed uterus is more sensitive to the influence of oxytocin (Barr, 1972). Consequently, if the administration of oral PGE_2 is discontinued to be replaced by an i.v. infusion of oxytocin, it is probably wise to delay administration of the latter in order to avoid uterine hyperstimulation (Barr, 1972, 1973a, b; Craft, 1973b).

Few other abnormal tocographic patterns have been reported by authors using internal recording techniques during oral PGE_2 induction. Incoordinated uterine action was observed by Kelly et al. (1974) in 2/49 (4%) of their patients. Wilkin et al. (1974) report prolonged contractions (3–4 min) in 1/20 (5%) of the patients induced with hourly administration of 0.5 mg PGE_2, orally, but believe that this pattern is not specific for PG. All babies were normal at birth.

Kelly et al. (1973) compared in a double-blind fashion uterine contractions produced by oral PGE_2 to those elicited by i.v. oxytocin. These authors found that the mean amplitude and frequency of contractions, the resting tone and the number of instances of incoordinate uterine action were all significantly lower in patients given oral PGE_2 than in those given i.v. oxytocin. De Hemptinne et al. (unpublished data) analysing uterine contractility during the active phase of labour in patients induced by amniotomy + oral FGE_2, amniotomy + i.v. oxytocin and amniotomy + i.v. PGs (E_2 and $F_{2\alpha}$), found no differences in mean amplitude, frequency, resting tone and uterine work.

Thiery (1974) reported on the incidence of hypertonus during spontaneous labour and that associated with various modes of induction. Hypertonus, which was more frequent in nulliparas than in parous patients, was also seen following amniotomy alone. Hypertonus was not more common with prostaglandins (given i.v. or orally) than with i.v. oxytocin (Table 4.15).

Table 4.15   Incidence of uterine hypertonus (basal tone $\geqslant$ 12 mmHg) in comparable series of patients, according to mode of induction and parity (From Thiery, 1974, by courtesy of Masson, Paris)

Parity	Spontaneous	Induced labour		
		Amniotomy	i.v. Oxytocin	PGs (oral PGE_2+ i.v. $PGF_{2\alpha}$+ i.v. PGE_2)
NP	0/25	1/23	0/11	5/99
MP	0/23	0/24	1/23	2/103
Total	0/48 (0%)	1/47 (2%)	1/34 (3%)	7/202 (3.5%)

Maternal effects. Only gastrointestinal side-effects have been regularly mentioned (Table 4.16). As a rule, nausea and vomiting occur more frequently than diarrhoea. The wide range in incidence may be due in part to differences in appreciation and in part to differences in sensitivity of the population studied. It is generally agreed that these side-effects are dose-related (Friedman and Sachtleben, 1974) but considerable variations in individual susceptibility exist. Craft (1972a) observed vomiting and diarrhoea in women given a single dose of 0.5 mg PGE_2. Thiery (1974) observed vomiting more often in nulliparas than in parous patients but was unable to establish a clear-cut

Table 4.16 Oral PGE$_2$. Incidence (%) of gastrointestinal side-effects

Reference	Nausea	Vomiting	Nausea + vomiting	Diarrhoea	Nausea + diarrhoea	Vomiting + diarrhoea	All gastrointestinal side-effects
Karim and Sharma, 1971a		2.5	6.5	3.4			
Karim and Sharma, 1972							
Barr, 1972							20
Barr, 1973b							68
Craft, 1972a						36	
Craft, 1973a, b	19	34					
Yip et al., 1973		10	3	0			
Elias, 1972							
Kelly et al., 1973		17	31	6			
Murnaghan et al., 1974	3	5	1	2	1	9	42
Corson and Bolognese, 1974							
Elder and Stone, 1974		24					
Wilkin et al., 1974		15				56	
Lauersen and Wilson, 1974							
Thiery, 1974		20		2			

Table 4.17 Incidence of vomiting (%) according to type of labour (From Thiery, 1974, by courtesy of Masson, Paris)

Type of labour	Incidence of vomiting (%)
Spontaneous labour	8
Amniotomy alone (surgical induction)	6
Combined induction: amniotomy +	
oxytocin i.v.	6
$PGF_{2\alpha}$ i.v.	4
PGE_2 i.v.	18
PGE_2 oral	20

dose-relationship. In most instances gastrointestinal complaints do not greatly affect the patient. Nevertheless, on occasion, investigators were compelled to discontinue drug administration on this account (Craft, 1972a; Elias, 1972; Elder and Stone, 1974; Friedman and Sachtleben, 1974) and in one clinic it became increasingly difficult to obtain volunteers because of fear of side-effects (Murnaghan et al., 1974). Craft (1972b) clearly established that vomiting (although in part a reaction to stress), was related to ingestion of the prostaglandin rather than to premedication or analgesia. It occurred in 5% of the patients treated by amniotomy + diazepam + epidural analgesia and in 34% of those given the same treatment plus oral PGE_2. Thiery (1974) compared the incidence of vomiting in normal spontaneous labour and various induction procedures (Table 4.17). Although patients occasionally vomit when labour is spontaneous or induced by amniotomy alone, combined induction (amniotomy plus oral or i.v. PGE_2) had significantly higher incidences. Moreover, PGE_2 (either route) produced more often vomiting than i.v. $PGF_{2\alpha}$. In this respect, induction with i.v. oxytocin and oral PGE_2 have also been compared by others. Kelly et al. (1974), Murnaghan et al. (1974) and Ratnam et al. (1974), found much lower incidences of vomiting with oxytocin.

Serious maternal complications are not reported except by Karim and Sharma (1972) who described a case of uterine rupture in a patient with previous myomectomy. The woman died of amniotic fluid embolism.

Pulse rate and blood pressure generally remain normal during induction with oral PGE_2 (Karim and Sharma, 1971a; Yip et al., 1973; Lauersen and Wilson, 1975; Murnaghan et al., 1974) but Thiery (1974) reported a transient rise in blood pressure in two normotensive multiparas induced with PGE_2 tablets (from 135/85 to 210/90, and from 110/80 to 140/95 mmHg, respectively). Lauersen and Wilson (1975), on the other hand, who found no significant decrease of the blood pressure in normotensive patients, reported a slight decrease in women with chronic hypertension and toxaemia of pregnancy. Respiratory rate and temperature were unaffected by the procedure (Thiery, 1974).

No anomalies were found during or after induction with oral PGE_2 in the following parameters: haemoglobin, haematocrit, white cell count including the differential count, platelet count, SGOT, blood urea nitrogen, serum alkaline phosphatase, and total bilirubin in venous maternal blood. Voided urine specimens were negative for protein and glucose and the sediment was normal (Thiery, 1974; Lauersen and Wilson, 1975). Acetonuria was found in 16% of patients induced with oral PGE_2 against 28% in the i.v. oxytocin group (Kelly et al., 1974).

Maternal serum levels of HCG, HCS and oestradiol, assayed in 25 clinically normal women, remained unchanged during induction at term with oral PGE_2. A slight decrease observed in the concentration of progesterone was in agreement with data collected during normal spontaneous labour (Dhont et al., 1973).

The acid-base status of 97 clinically normal women induced at term with oral PGE_2 was determined at delivery using femoral-artery blood (Thiery et al., 1973b, c, 1974b). The mean values fell within normal limits. The range of the individual values was larger than in comparable patients induced by the i.v. route with either oxytocin or a prostaglandin. The incidence of reported hypotonic postpartum haemorrhage ranges from one (Karim and Sharma, 1972; Thiery, 1974) to seven per cent (Ratnam et al., 1974).

No data are available on long-term follow-up after labour induction with oral PGE_2. At present, five of 97 women induced with oral PGE_2 have become pregnant (Thiery, unpublished data). There were no signs of cervical incompetence and all deliveries were normal.

Fetal and neonatal effects. Most published clinical studies do not allow in depth assessment of the fetal hazards because (1) the authors' reporting is sketchy in this respect (2) the parameters used are inadequate to assess specific hazards (hypoxia), and (3) inductions were performed for therapeutic indications. Nevertheless, authors have generally concluded that the induction had no adverse effect on the fetus. Karim and Sharma (1972) reported five fresh stillbirths and seven neonatal deaths in a series of 1000 cases given PGE_2 orally for induction or stimulation of labour. Filshie (1972) had one stillbirth occurring in a case of premature rupture of the membranes. The perinatal death rate of these authors (1.3% and 1.0%, respectively) was not increased over hospital figures. There was no perinatal mortality in the series of Yip et al. (1973), Murnaghan et al. (1974) and Thiery (1974).

Apgar scores were not lowered by the use of oral PGE_2. Kelly et al. (1974) compared Apgar scores in patients induced with oral PGE_2 or i.v. oxytocin and found values similar in both groups.

No FHR abnormalities were found by Karim and Sharma (1971a), Craft (1972a, 1973a, b) and Wilkin et al. (1974).

Barr and Naismith (1972) recorded irregular uterine activity and fetal bradycardia in one of their 10 cases. These authors used external tocography which makes interpretation of their data difficult. Moreover, the same uterine reactivity pattern, as well as the fetal bradycardia, recurred when i.v. oxytocin was used; consequently, Caesarean section was performed. Barr (1972) performed a Caesarean section on two of his 50 patients because of fetal acidosis and bradycardia. Yip et al. (1973) noted fetal bradycardia in 3/57 cases but the pH in scalp blood was normal. Severe bradycardia (1/49) and late decelerations (2/49) were also observed by Kelly et al. (1974). Fraser (1974) reported a case of severe uterine hypertonus with extreme fetal bradycardia and depressed baby (one-minute Apgar score: 5).

Thiery and co-workers (Thiery et al., 1973b, c, 1974b) reported perinatal

Table 4.18 **Effectiveness of combined labour induction according to type of procedure** (From Thiery, 1974, by courtesy of Masson, Paris)

Type of induction	Mean total dose		Mean interval (h:min)		Success rate
	NP	MP	NP	MP	(%)
Amniotomy +					
i.v. oxytocin	1.6 IU	1.4 IU	04:49	04:04	100
oral PGE₂	2.3 mg	1.7 mg	07:14	04:45	97
i.v. PGE₂	0.2 mg	0.1 mg	05:45	03:17	98
i.v. PGF₂ₐ	4.4 mg	4.1 mg	06:47	04:49	100

results in 97 cases of elective induction at term by amniotomy and oral PGE_2. There was no perinatal mortality. Abnormally low (< 7) one-minute and five-minute Apgar scores were found in 2% and 1% of the neonates, respectively, a rate similar to that after normal spontaneous deliveries. Fetal bradycardia (1%) and late deceleration FHR patterns (1%) had the same frequency as in spontaneous labour. Recorded second-stage anomalies were: transient bradycardia (7%), progressive bradycardia (3%) and persistent bradycardia (2%). The mean pH at full dilatation was 7.34 in nulliparas, 7.36 in parous patients. At birth, mean acid-base and lactate–pyruvate values were normal. It is concluded that orally administered PGE_2 did not hamper the oxygen supply to the fetal tissues. Finally, oral PGE_2 therapy in the mother did not induce neonatal hyperbilirubinaemia (de Hemptinne et al., 1973).

4.2.2.2.3 *Comparison of oral PGE₂ with intravenous oxytocin.* Khew et al. (1971) conducted a double-blind trial comparing oral PGE_2 ($n = 51$) and i.v. oxytocin ($n = 49$) for the induction of labour. The success rate of the procedure was 92% with either method when membranes were intact, while it was 92% with PGE_2 and 100% with oxytocin when membranes were artificially ruptured, concomitantly.

Kelly et al. (1973) found no significant difference between two groups of cases matched for inducibility features (length of gestation, parity and Bishop score). In one group labour was induced by amniotomy and oral PGE_2, in the other by amniotomy and i.v. oxytocin. PGE_2 was successful in 47/49 patients in a mean time of 9 hrs 14 min, oxytocin in 46/49 in a mean of 9 hrs 51 min.

Ratnam et al. (1974) attempted therapeutic induction of labour in 207 women, randomly assigned to receive either i.v. oxytocin ($n = 100$) or oral PGE_2 ($n = 107$). In half the subjects of each group, the forewaters were ruptured immediately preceding administration of the oxytocic; in the others, the membranes were left intact. Labour was established within six hours in all women in whom amniotomy had been performed, but only in 55% of those on PGE_2 and 80% of those on oxytocin, when the membranes were left intact. Eventually, nine patients (17%) on oral PGE_2 and five patients (10%) on i.v. oxytocin failed to go into labour when the membranes were left intact. Once labour was established, the time taken to achieve vaginal delivery was not significantly different whether PGE_2 or oxytocin was used. Five patients receiving oral PGE_2 and one patient receiving i.v. oxytocin required Caesarean section for failed induction of labour. None of the differences between i.v. oxytocin and oral PGE$_2$ were statistically significant and the authors concluded that the two methods of induction were equally effective.

Thiery (1974) found comparable rates of success (97–100%) and similar mean induction–delivery intervals in patients induced by amniotomy and either i.v. oxytocin or oral PGE$_2$ (Table 4.18). The importance of supplementing low amniotomy by oral PGE$_2$ has been shown by Craft (1973a, b) who found that the mean time to delivery for parous patients induced by amniotomy and oral PGE$_2$ (6 hrs 20 min) was significantly shorter ($p < 0.001$) than that of women induced by means of amniotomy alone (12 hrs 22 min).

Table 4.19 Comparison of effectiveness of oral PGE$_2$ and buccal oxytocin (From Craft, 1973a, by courtesy of Symposia Specialists)

Type of induction	Success rate	Mean induction–delivery interval $\pm$ SEM (h:min)
Amniotomy + oral PGE$_2$	26/28 (93%)	06:20>0.29
Amniotomy + buccal oxytocin	23/25 (92%)	04:38>0.20

Craft (1973a) also compared oral PGE$_2$ and buccal oxytocin for inducing labour in association with amniotomy in multiparas. Escalating dose schedules were used to promote early uterine activity (Table 4.19). Both groups had a similar failure rate. Effective uterine activity occurred at the same time with both agents. However, the induction–delivery interval was significantly ($p < 0.01$) shorter in women receiving buccal oxytocin.

4.2.3 Other routes

For the induction of labour with prostaglandins, other delivery routes have been given but small-scale clinical trials.

4.2.3.1 Intra-amniotic route

Intra-amniotic injection of PGs has no place in the induction of labour (Gillespie, 1973). However, in a few cases of death *in utero* it has been used with success (Karim, 1972a, page 94).

Caballero *et al.* (1974) used intra-amniotic PGF$_{2\alpha}$ (12.5–25 mg) and PGE$_2$ (1–2 mg) in 19 cases of intrauterine death after 27 weeks' gestation. After a lag time of two to 95 minutes, the uterus started to contract (external tocography) and in all cases the fetus was delivered from one hr 21 min to 30 hrs 15 min after the PG injection. There were two postpartum haemorrhages, not related to an alteration of the coagulation mechanism. Maternal side-effects were trivial (nausea, vomitus, headache) and limited to only a few women. There occurred, however, one serious complication, i.e. uterine rupture following intra-amniotic instillation of 2 mg PGE$_2$.

4.2.3.2 Extra-amniotic route

For termination of mid-trimester pregnancies, local routes of administration are more effective and generate fewer side-effects than delivery systems which depend on systemic absorption of PGs. Labour induction requires only one-tenth of the dose needed for interruption of early pregnancy. The intravenous and oral routes therefore have proved effective, causing—except for hypertonus—only trivial side-effects. Nevertheless, Calder *et al.* (1974b) have extended the technique of continuous extra-amniotic infusion—originally devised for second trimester abortion—to therapeutic induction of labour at term in 40 women.

A urethral catheter, placed transcervically into the extra-amniotic space, served for instillation of the prostaglandin solution as well as for continuous recording of the intrauterine pressure. PGE_2 was administered at the rate of 20 μg/hour, initially, and the dose level was increased by 10 μg/hour every 15 min (maximum: 150 μg/hour) until labour was established. Low amniotomy was then performed and prostaglandin administration was continued via the same route. Before amniotomy, the FHR was registered externally, thereafter by means of a scalp electrode.

Four of the 40 patients had to be delivered by Caesarean section, one because of fetal bradycardia, the second because of slow cervical dilatation despite adequate contractions (cervical dystocia?) and the two others because of cephalopelvic disproportion. For the remaining 36 women the mean induction–delivery interval was 10 hrs 7 min for those with an unfavourable cervix (Bishop score 2–5) and 8 hrs 2 min for patients with a favourable cervix (Bishop score 6–8). For both groups as a whole, this interval was 9 hrs 3 min. The mean total dose of PGE_2 used was 550 μg for the 40 patients. Occasional transient episodes of uterine hypertonus, not associated with evidence of fetal distress, were noted. According to the authors, there was no increased incidence of fetal distress and the Apgar scores were satisfactory. The only side-effect noted was vomiting, in 'a few' patients.

The authors did not include a control group and it is difficult to judge the value of this route of administration, for induction of labour. At any rate the procedure seems to be effective, especially if one takes into account that approximately half of the women induced had an unfavourable cervix. Whether maternal side-effects (vomiting) were lower than with i.v. infusion of PGE_2 is hard to tell. Quite remarkable is the excellent clinical state of the infants at birth as judged by the Apgar scores. All of these fetuses were potentially at risk; indeed, indication for the induction was pre-eclampsia and hypertension in 21 cases, postmaturity in 11 and intrauterine growth retardation in four. The mothers were sedated routinely. In a few initial cases, not included in this study, the procedure had to be abandoned because of inadvertent rupture of the membranes at insertion of the catheter and bleeding, possibly from the placental site.

Miller and Mack (1974) attempted therapeutic induction of labour by continuous extra-amniotic administration of 90–180 μg/hour PGE_2 in 69 patients at 26–41 weeks' gestation. Forty-eight women had unfavourable induction prospects (Bishop score $\leqslant$ 5), yet labour was successfully induced in all cases. The Foley catheter (balloon inflated to 30–50 ml) was usually expelled at 3–4 cm cervical dilatation. Amniotomy was then performed, if the membranes had not ruptured spontaneously. The mean time of infusion of PGE_2 was $6\frac{1}{2}$ hrs and the mean dose 0.9 mg. After extrusion of the catheter, an i.v. infusion of oxytocin was started if uterine activity was not satisfactory. Twelve (17%) patients required Caesarean section: four for fetal distress, one for incoordinate uterine action and the remainder for cephalo-pelvic disproportion. Three infants were lost during labour or shortly after birth, but none of these demises could be attributed to the prostaglandin. The first case concerned a stillbirth following induction at 28 weeks' maturity of a patient with fulminating pre-eclampsia. The other two perinatal deaths (at 38–39 weeks' gestation) were due to intrapartum asphyxia which occurred more than nine hours after the administration of PGE_2 was discontinued and while the patients were receiving oxytocin. Uterine hypertonus was observed in only one instance following accidental injection of a bolus of PGE_2 during connection of the catheter to the pump. No other side-effects were recorded.

Continuous extra-amniotic infusion (by pump) of $PGF_{2\alpha}$ has been used for labour induction only by Kühnle and Gade (1974) who succeeded in five out of six women at 25–41 weeks' gestation with a dead fetus. This technique deserves further investigation, particularly in regard to its fetal effects.

4.2.3.3 Intravaginal and rectal routes

Wiqvist *et al.* (1968) observed no uterine stimulation following vaginal administration of 200–1000 μg PGE_1 to patients in the second trimester of pregnancy. In retrospect, the dose instilled by these authors was probably too small. The uterotonic effects of vaginally (and rectally) administered prostaglandins have been demonstrated in both non-pregnant (Sandberg *et al.*, 1967) and pregnant patients (Karim and Sharma, 1971b). Small amounts of these drugs reach the general circulation (10–20% of PGE_1 according to Sandberg *et al.*, 1967) and are thought to be responsible for the oxytocic activity exerted. That there is no direct stimulatory effect on the uterus by way of the cervical canal was shown by Kirton (1972) who covered the cervix with collodion before administering prostaglandin vaginally to rhesus monkeys.

Two different groups of workers have successfully induced labour by vaginal (Karim and Sharma, 1971b; Henzl *et al.*, 1973) or rectal (Karim and Sharma, 1971b) administration of PGE_2 and $PGF_{2\alpha}$. These routes compare favourably to the intravenous infusion of prostaglandins, producing fewer side-effects (Karim and Sharma, 1971b) and rather short induction–delivery intervals. Compared to the classical delivery systems (i.v. and oral), however, the vaginal and rectal routes seem less acceptable to the patient, hence, probably, the lack of sustained enthusiasm on the part of the clinician.

Karim and Sharma (1971b) induced labour in 10 women at or about term using lactose tablets containing 2 mg PGE_2 or 5 mg $PGF_{2\alpha}$ (five patients with each regimen). The pessaries were inserted into the posterior vaginal fornix every two hours until labour was established (cervix dilated to 5–6 cm, adequate myometrial activity) at which stage low amniotomy was performed. In case the membranes ruptured spontaneously at an earlier stage, the medication was further administered by rectal route. In all these women normal uterine contractions were monitored. All patients were delivered vaginally, the mean induction–delivery interval being 8 hrs 20 min for the PGE_2 group and 14 hrs for the $PGF_{2\alpha}$ group. There were no maternal side-effects attributable to the drug and all neonates were in good condition. Henzl et al. (1973) succeeded in producing expulsion of a dead fetus in four women by intravaginal insertion of suppositories containing 4 mg of PGE_2 each. Also in this clinical trial, maternal side-effects were absent. Similarly, Southern (personal communication, 1974) could terminate 70 of 72 second and third trimester pregnancies with intrauterine death by 2–3-hourly administration of a 20 mg PGE_2 suppository. But with these higher doses, vomiting occurred in 44% and diarrhoea in 33% of the subjects.

4.2.3.4 Unexplored routes

For induction of abortion intramuscular and subcutaneous injections (as well as intermittent i.v. injections) of natural PGs have been found either ineffective or generating too many maternal side-effects. To the best of our knowledge neither of these approaches nor the intraperitoneal route have been tried for labour induction.

4.3 INDUCTION OF LABOUR IN COMPLICATED PREGNANCIES

For induction of labour at term, prostaglandins E_2 and $F_{2\alpha}$ are equally effective, but not superior to oxytocin and they may cause uterine hyperstimulation more frequently. Before term, the myometrium is less sensitive to the action of oxytocin and it requires for adequate activation larger doses of the hormone than at term. This may lead to complications including severe cutaneous vasoconstriction, arterial hypertension and acute water intoxication with convulsions (Liggins, 1962). In some cases (e.g. intrauterine death), the uterus proves refractory even to large amounts of oxytocin. Prostaglandins, which are capable of stimulating the myometrium and of interrupting pregnancy at any stage, are here at a distinct advantage. Detailed studies of the maternal and fetal effects of prostaglandins administered to toxaemic and diabetic patients are still lacking. Yet, it is already evident, at this stage, that these are the agents of choice for terminating pregnancy complicated by intrauterine death.

4.3.1 Intrauterine fetal death (IUD)

Mors in utero or intrauterine death (IUD) idefined as fetal demise occurring from 28 weeks' gestation onwards. In most cases, delivery occurs spontaneously within 2–3 weeks; if not, one speaks of 'missed labour' or 'retained dead fetus'.

Besides the psychological burden it imposes upon the mother, this condition may lead, in the long run, to a severe consumption coagulopathy (Hodgkinson et al., 1954). It is presently accepted that these cases should be actively managed and that labour should be induced once the diagnosis of fetal death is confirmed and hypofibrinogenaemia is ruled out (fibrinogen $\geqslant$ 200 mg %). In the event of hypofibrinogenaemia, this anomaly should first be corrected. Because of the danger of trauma and infection, and of the risk of escape of thromboplastin-rich material from the amniotic cavity into the maternal vascular bed, a strictly medical approach should be preferred to surgical treatment.

Intravenous oxytocin, given alone, often proves insufficient for inducing labour in case of IUD. Moreover, the massive doses required to effect delivery, through their antidiuretic effect, may cause acute water intoxication and convulsions (Liggins, 1962). The combination of amniotomy with oxytocin therapy increases the success rate and shortens the induction–delivery interval (Ursell, 1972), but it carries the risk of adding sepsis or amniotic fluid embolism to the patient's problems (Peterson and Taylor, 1970). Intra-amniotic instillation of hypertonic saline has occasionally caused hyper-natraemia and brain damage (Wagatsuma, 1965; Cameron and Dayan, 1966), whereas there is an increased risk of intrauterine infection when hypertonic glucose is used. Hysterotomy or Caesarean section leave the patient with a scarred uterus and are unacceptable for this indication. Prostaglandins, which are capable of stimulating the uterus throughout gestation and which lack the antidiuretic effect of oxytocin, have provided clinicians with a simple, safe and effective means of terminating pregnancy complicated by IUD (Karim, 1970).

Data from 12 papers dealing with induction of labour with PGs in women with IUD, have been classified in Table 4.20 according to route of administration and type of compound. The total number of cases should amount to about 135, the 15 cases reported by Karim in 1970 having been included most probably in a later report (Karim and Trussell, 1971). All authors refrained from performing amniotomy at the start of the induction, for fear of causing infection. Naismith and Barr (1974) were the only investigators to combine systematically administration of a PG and of oxytocin. Other authors did not use oxytocin except for sporadic cases where labour needed to be accelerated (Miller, 1973: one case; Embrey *et al.*, 1974: two cases).

4.3.1.1 Intravenous prostaglandins for IUD

The PG was infused either at a constant dose-level (Karim, 1970) or, in a lesser number of patients, by titrating the drug to stimulate the uterus adequately (Ring, 1972; Ruppen *et al.*, 1972). Uterine activity was comparable to that of normal labour (Karim, 1970; Filshie, 1971; Karim and Trussell, 1971; Hickl *et al.*, 1973). The first uterine contractions occurred 15–45 min from the start of the infusion (Filshie, 1971; Ring, 1972; Ruppen *et al.*, 1972). Eighty-six of 89 women with IUD (97%) were successfully induced by i.v. infusion of PGE_2 or $PGF_{2\alpha}$, all within $29\frac{1}{2}$ hrs. Reported dose levels ranged from 1.5 to 5.0 μg min^{-1} for PGE_2 and from 25 to 100 μg min^{-1} for $PGF_{2\alpha}$. Mean induction–delivery intervals varied between $8\frac{1}{2}$ and $12\frac{1}{2}$ hrs for PGE_2, and between $6\frac{1}{2}$ and $8\frac{1}{2}$ hrs for $PGF_{2\alpha}$. Roberts (1974, not included in Table 4.20) successfully induced labour and delivery in 18 of 20 cases of IUD in the third trimester by i.v. administration of 1.5–6 μg min^{-1} PGE_1, 2.5–20 μg min^{-1}

Table 4.20   Induction of labour with prostaglandins in cases of intrauterine death

Reference	No. of cases	Duration of IUD	PG	Dose level (range) (µg min)	Dosage Total dose (mg) Range	Dosage Total dose (mg) Mean	Induction-delivery interval (h:min) Range	Induction-delivery interval (h:min) Mean	No. of successes
Intravenous prostaglandin									
Karim, 1970	15	28–84 days	E_2	0.5–2.0			03:30–29:30	12:10	14/15
Karim and Trussell, 1971	33	28–84 days	E_2	0.5–2.0				12:30	31/33
Filshie, 1971	7	1–28 days	E_2	0.5–2.5			07:30–11:30	08:30	7/7
Miller, 1973	7	7–10 days	E_2	2.5–5.0	2.1–10.0	5.0	05:35–25:20	08:30	7/7
Pedersen et al., 1972	6	3–21 days	$F_{2\alpha}$	62–90 (max. dose level)		36.0	04:16:50	08:23	6/6
Ruppen et al., 1972	3	7–28 days	$F_{2\alpha}$	25–100		35.8		06:26	3/3
Hickl, et al., 1973	5	—	$F_{2\alpha}$	25–100	3.8–50.0		05:20–12:30		5/5
Ring, 1972	13		$F_{2\alpha}$	25–100		25.2		7:00	13/13
									89 (97%)

i.v. prostaglandin + oxytocin									
Naismith and Barr, 1974	17		E_2 (+oxy-tocin)	1.0–4.5 (max.)	0.09–1.60	0.72	02:35–21:00	07:42	17/17 (100%)
Intra-amniotic PG									
Karim, 1972 (page 111)	6	7–35 days	E_2 $F_{2\alpha}$	*single injection* of 5 mg and PGE_2 or 25 mg $PGF_{2\alpha}$				09:00	6/6
Frumar et al., 1974	3	—	$F_{2\alpha}$	initial dose 45 mg, + 25 mg at 6 and 18 hours if required			10:00–21:30		3/3
Caballero et al., 1974	14	7–70 days	$F_{2\alpha}$	*single dose* of 12.5 or 25 mg			01:21–27:10	10:30	14/14
	5	7–42 days	E_2	*single dose* of 1.0 or 2.0 mg			03:05–30:15	18:42	5/5 28/28 (100%)
Extra-amniotic PG									
Embrey et al., 1974	1	7 days	$F_{2\alpha}$	max. dose rate 600 μg h^{-1}; total dose 3.5 mg			12:00	—	1/1
	11	7–28 days	E_2	max. dose rate 60–240 μg h l; total dose 0.2–1.1 mg			02:30–11:12	07:06	11/11 12/12 (100%)

$PGF_{2\alpha}$, or 0.25–4 μg min^{-1} PGE_2. The two cases that failed to respond adequately to the prostaglandin eventually delivered after i.v. oxytocin augmentation of labour. As pointed out by Karim et al. (1971b), cases of prolonged retention of the dead fetus are more difficult to induce and require i.v. infusion of PG over longer periods of time.

Gastrointestinal disturbances were somewhat more frequent with $PGF_{2\alpha}$ than with PGE_2, but never were troublesome except in patients treated by Hickl et al. (1973) who all experienced rather severe nausea and vomiting. Other side-effects included pyrexia (Ruppen et al., 1972; Miller, 1973; Roberts, 1974) and venous erythema (Hickl et al. 1973; Roberts, 1974), in occasional subjects. Blood loss was within normal limits (Karim, 1970; Karim and Trussell, 1971; Pedersen et al., 1972; Ruppen et al., 1972; Hickl et al., 1973).

One case of hypofibrinogenaemia (110 mg %) and haemorrhage occurring during labour induced by i.v. PGE_2 was reported by Filshie (1971). Fetal death had occurred one month before treatment, but no coagulation studies were performed upon admission. It is very likely that the PG was not linked to the coagulopathy, which should have been diagnosed and treated before the induction of labour.

No alteration in vital signs (except for body temperature: Ruppen et al., 1972; Miller, 1973) nor in routine laboratory examinations (complete blood count; clotting factors; serum creatinine, urea, bilirubin, SGOT, SGPT, alkaline phosphatase, electrolytes, glucose; urine analysis—Ruppen et al., 1972; Hickl et al., 1973) was detected.

Hickl et al. (1973) reported the interesting observation that, although i.v. $PGF_{2\alpha}$ (gradually increased to a dose level of 100 μg min^{-1}) produced regular contractions within two hours, cervical dilatation did not take place until after injection of 10 ml bupivacaine 0.5% for paracervical block. Confirmation of a facilitating effect of paracervical block upon PG-induced labour certainly warrants a more extensive study.

4.3.1.2 Intravenous prostaglandins + oxytocin for IUD

Naismith and Barr (1974) induced 17 women with IUD by simultaneous i.v. infusion of PGE_2 (at a constant rate of 1 μg min^{-1}) and oxytocin, in escalated doses. All patients delivered within 21 hrs, in a mean time of 7 hrs 42 min. The mean total dose of PGE_2 amounted to 0.72 mg. For oxytocin, the maximum dose rate ranged from 16 to 1024 mU min^{-1} (mean: 249 mU min^{-1}) and the total dose infused from 2.2 to 137 IU (mean : 53 IU). There was no gastrointestinal upset. Pyrexia (> 37.7 °C) was noted in two patients, one of which also had shivering and venous erythema. Manual removal of the placenta was required in two cases.

Although simultaneous administration of oxytocin and a prostaglandin is effective without causing disturbing gastrointestinal side-effects, the infusion of doses of oxytocin such as given by Naismith and Barr may cause water retention. The oxytocic compounds should therefore be administered in electrolytic solutions (e.g. Ringer's lactate), the fluid intake and output should be recorded and, if necessary, the serum electrolytes should be determined at intervals.

4.3.1.3 Intra-amniotic prostaglandins for IUD

PGE_2 and $PGF_{2\alpha}$ solutions have been injected (single or repeated doses) at abdominal amniocentesis performed upon women with IUD by Karim (1972, page 111), Caballero et al. (1974) and Frumar et al. (1974). All 28 subjects tested delivered within 30 hrs 15 min. Gastrointestinal side-effects were mild and rare. In the series reported by Caballero and co-workers, postpartum haemorrhage occurred twice and there was one case of uterine rupture following intra-amniotic instillation of a single dose of 2 mg PGE_2.

The technique has the advantage of being simple, but it has two major drawbacks. First, it requires invasion of the amniotic cavity, with the risk of causing infection or leakage of thromboplastin-rich material into the maternal circulation. Second, the altered fetal membranes may permit faster passage of the injected prostaglandin, which in turn may lead to hyperstimulation and rupture of the uterus.

4.3.1.4 Extra-amniotic prostaglandins for IUD

The extra-amniotic route was used by Embrey et al. (1974) for administration of $PGF_{2\alpha}$ (one patient) or PGE_2 (11 patients). Escalated doses of the PG solution were infused by pump via a Foley catheter, transcervically inserted. As a rule, expulsion of the Foley catheter was followed by delivery. Side-effects were less frequent than with the i.v. route and were limited to mild vomiting in an occasional patient. Pyrexia was never observed and no third stage complications occurred.

Kühnle and Gade (1974), using an identical technique for administration of $PGF_{2\alpha}$, were able to deliver within six hours five of six women with IUD at 25 to 41 weeks. In the remaining patient, extraction of the fetus had to be performed at 5 cm cervical dilatation on account of psychological decompensation.

4.3.1.5 Oral prostaglandins for IUD

Karim et al. (1972) administered orally 20–40 μg of prostaglandin 15(S), 15-methyl-PGE_2 methyl ester to six women with IUD. The dose was repeated at 6–8 hrs intervals, if necessary. Hypertonus (20 mmHg) occurred for a duration of about 10 min in two cases, but there were no other side-effects. All patients delivered within 25 hrs (range: 12–25 hrs).

4.3.1.6 Intravaginal prostaglandins for IUD

Southern (personal communication) terminated 70 of 72 (97.2%) second and third trimester pregnancies with IUD by administering 20 mg PGE_2 intravaginally, 2–3 hourly. The only two failures were due to insufficient therapy. The mean induction–delivery interval was longer ($14\frac{1}{2}$ hrs) when the fetus had been retained for over three weeks, than when fetal demise had occurred less than three weeks before (seven hours). Vomiting occurred in 44% of the subjects, diarrhoea in 33% and temperature elevation of more than 1.1 °C in 30%.

Conclusions. Prostaglandins have been highly successful for inducing labour in cases of IUD. Effective dosages were comprised between those usually required for induction of labour at term and those needed for interruption of early pregnancy. The intra-amniotic injection of prostaglandin, or the combination of high doses of i.v. oxytocin with i.v. prostaglandin for induction of labour in women with IUD hold potential risks for the patients and i.v. administration of prostaglandin alone should be preferred. The extra-amniotic route has also given excellent results but further studies should confirm that it does not entail a higher risk of intrauterine infection.

4.3.2 Induction before term

Prostaglandins are as effective as oxytocin for induction of labour in patients with favourable induction prospects. On the other hand, patients with tightly closed, uneffaced cervices often are relatively resistant to the action of oxytocin. This is particularly so in case delivery is indicated long before term, e.g. in case of diabetes or severe pre-eclampsia (Calder and Embrey, 1973). Prostaglandins could find here a wide field of application.

4.3.2.1 Premature rupture of the membranes

Barden (1972) administered escalated doses of $PGF_{2\alpha}$, intravenously, to 10 women at 28–34 weeks' gestation with ruptured membranes and not in labour. Bishop scores ranged from 2–11 (mean 5). The initial dose level of 2.5 μg min^{-1} was doubled every 60 min until adequate uterine activity or a maximum dose level of 20 μg min^{-1}. One instance of uterine hypertonus was registered. Eight of the 10 subjects delivered vaginally in a mean time of 4 hrs 24 min; Caesarean section was performed in the two others, in one because of fetal distress (variable and late FHR decelerations), in the second because of failure of progress of labour. The one-minute Apgar score was low (< 7) in six of the 10 infants. Birth weights ranged from 1800 to 2300 g. Four of the babies developed normally, four others had respiratory distress but eventually recovered; the remaining two died in the neonatal period. There was no maternal morbidity. The authors of this study felt that the poor perinatal outcome could be attributed to the nature of the cases induced and that it was due mainly to prematurity. However, large controlled trials comparing prostaglandins with oxytocin for the induction of labour before term will be required before a possible deleterious effect of these compounds on the premature infant can be ruled out.

4.3.2.2 Gross fetal malformations

Induction of labour is often difficult when on account of anencephaly (Chef *et al.*, 1974) or of other fetal anomalies delivery before term is deemed necessary.

Fifteen cases of labour induced by a prostaglandin because of anencephaly have been collected. $PGF_{2\alpha}$ was infused intravenously to four subjects (Pedersen et al., 1972; maximum dose level 50–90 μg min^{-1}) and was given intra-amniotically to another four (Thiery et al., 1973d; Chef et al., 1974; Frumar et al., 1974; single dose of 50 mg or repeated doses of 25–45 mg). PGE_2 was administered by continuous extra-amniotic infusion in six (Embrey et al., 1974: total dose: 0.5–0.8 mg; Miller and Mack, 1974) and by intra-amniotic instillation in one (Amy, unpublished data; 2 × 5 mg). All cases but three were in the early third trimester (28–34 weeks) and all were successfully induced. In six cases, i.v. oxytocin augmentation was necessary and two of these, treated by intra-amniotic $PGF_{2\alpha}$, had very long induction–abortion intervals (47 and 54 hours respectively). Gastrointestinal side-effects were observed in some of the patients given $PGF_{2\alpha}$, but never were severe.

Only one case of termination of pregnancy by intra-amniotic injection of $PGF_{2\alpha}$, given because of a chromosomal anomaly (monosomy 45 XY) is on record, but this gestation was interrupted at 22 weeks (Frumar et al., 1974).

4.3.2.3 High risk pregnancies

In pregnancies at risk (e.g. postmaturity, diabetes, essential hypertension, pre-eclamptic toxaemia) the problem of how to deliver safely the viable fetus remains unsolved. Even in spontaneous labour, uterine activity may further jeopardise placental function, already impaired in most of these cases. Abnormal fetal maturity of course adds to the perinatal hazard.

Brosens et al. (1974a, b) felt that the use of prostaglandins might be contraindicated in case of pre-eclamptic toxaemia or chronic hypertension complicating pregnancy for fear of augmenting the existing fetal hypoxia. These authors contended that the vasoconstrictive effect of prostaglandins on the myometrial segments of the uteroplacental (spiral) vessels (Moghissi and Murray, 1970) could be exaggerated because of the structural changes encountered in pre-eclampsia (Robertson et al., 1967; Brosens et al., 1972). The validity of this hypothesis has not been substantiated so far.

Experimental intra-arterial infusion of 1–100 μg min^{-1} $PGF_{2\alpha}$ to pregnant bitches (Clark et al., 1973) caused no rise in uterine perfusion pressure indicating that, even at high doses, it did not increase utero-placental vascular tone. However, $PGF_{2\alpha}$ also failed to increase uterine activity in the dogs, suggesting an entirely different response to prostaglandin administration in this species, which precluded extrapolation of the findings to man.

Theoretically, $PGF_{2\alpha}$ has at least one advantage over oxytocin for the induction of labour in women with cardiac or renal disease, or with pre-eclampsia: unlike oxytocin, it has no antidiuretic action (Roberts et al., 1970). But a vast body of data from well-designed, preferably matched studies will have to be collected to determine which of the two oxytocic compounds is safer for induction of labour in cases at risk.

Tchilingurian (1972) induced labour with i.v. $PGF_{2\alpha}$ in 10 pregnancies at risk, mostly because of toxaemia of pregnancy. By cautiously titrating the dose, no uterine hypertonus was caused and there were no side-effects in the fetus. The same author also conducted, under monitor control, a double-blind study comparing i.v. $PGF_{2\alpha}$ and i.v. oxytocin in 14 pregnancies at risk, mostly past term. No differences were found between the two groups. In the $PGF_{2\alpha}$ group, all seven patients delivered vaginally and the infants were normal at birth (one-minute Apgar scores 7–9). During labour, the only abnormality registered consisted in one episode of severe FHR deceleration due to a tight nuchal cord.

Schmid *et al.* (1972) compared the fetal and maternal effects of escalated doses of i.v. oxytocin and i.v. $PGF_{2\alpha}$ given for induction of labour in a series of 50 pregnancies of 40 weeks + 9–17 days duration. The success rate was comparable for both methods. Transient uterine hyperstimulation was observed in two patients receiving $PGF_{2\alpha}$, but uterine activity returned to normal within five minutes of stopping the infusion. All infants born after induction by $PGF_{2\alpha}$ were normal (Apgar score $\geqslant 8$). A later study conducted by Schmid *et al.* in 1974, wherein i.v. PGE_2 and $PGF_{2\alpha}$ were compared with oxytocin, gave similar results. The authors concluded that prolonged pregnancy did not contraindicate the use of PGs but that constant monitoring of labour was mandatory. Keller *et al.* (1972), studying placental function in patients induced by Schmid *et al.* (1972), found serum levels of HCG, HCS, progesterone and heat-stable alkaline phosphatase to be no different during induction of labour with $PGF_{2\alpha}$ from those seen in labour following amniotomy alone. It can be argued, however, that pregnancies at 40 weeks + 9–17 days are not truly postmature and that the above mentioned studies referred in fact to uncomplicated cases.

Jacomb and Hinchley (1974) reviewed the results of labour induction with i.v. $PGF_{2\alpha}$ or PGE_2 in 283 cases of pre-eclamptic toxaemia or hypertension. The mean one- and five-minutes Apgar scores in this series were 8.15 and 9.4, respectively. Of the four infants with scores under 5 at five minutes, two had been delivered by mid-cavity forceps for fetal distress in the second stage of labour. All infants developed normally during the first week of life.

Calder *et al.* (1974a) compared in a double-blind fashion the combination of amniotomy with either i.v. PGE_2 or oxytocin in a series of 23 patients at 36–38 weeks with moderate to severe pre-eclampsia. Labour was monitored electronically in all cases. One patient receiving oxytocin required emergency Caesarean section for fetal distress; two others, one in each group, were delivered abdominally for failure to progress in labour. The remainder delivered vaginally, with no evidence of increased incidence of fetal distress in the PG group. The mean one-minute Apgar score was 7.0 after induction with oxytocin as compared to 8.1 after PGE_2. No neonatal deaths occurred. An additional 18 nulliparas at 36–38 weeks' gestation with hypertension in pregnancy were induced by continuous extra-amniotic infusion of PGE_2. These patients were clinically assessed as unfavourable for induction. In two cases, fetal distress developed which required Caesarean section; the remainder delivered vaginally. The mean Apgar score at one minute was 8.0. The authors concluded that real benefit could be derived from the use of prostaglandins for inducing labour in pregnancies complicated by hypertension or pre-eclampsia; they considered the greatest danger to utero–placental blood flow to be uterine hyperstimulation and recommended electronic supervision of labour, whatever the oxytocic agent used.

Lauersen and Wilson (1974) successfully induced 52 women by oral administration of PGE_2 tablets. The indication for induction was postmaturity in 19 cases, toxaemia of pregnancy in 10, chronic hypertension in four and diabetes in five. All infants were in good condition, with Apgar scores of 7 or more at one minute and 9–10 at five minutes. In women with chronic hypertension and toxaemia, a slight decrease in blood pressure often occurred during induction, a phenomenon not observed in normotensive patients.

In conclusion, data are still fragmentary and no definite conclusions can be drawn regarding the safety of prostaglandins for the fetus at risk.

4.4 ACCELERATION OF LABOUR WITH PROSTAGLANDINS

Very few trials of labour acceleration with prostaglandins have been reported and comparative studies with oxytocin are not available.

Karim and Sharma (1972) gave PGE_2 by mouth (0.5–2 mg two-hourly) for acceleration of labour in 236 women. There were 96% vaginal deliveries: 73% of the women delivered within 12 hrs and 90% within 24 hrs after the first dose of PG. Nine patients required Caesarean section: five for fetal distress and four for cephalo-pelvic disproportion. There was one fresh stillbirth (cause of death unknown) and one neonatal death (congenital malformation, syphilitic features).

For the same indication Persianinov et al. (1973) used an i.v. drip of $PGF_{2\alpha}$ in 10 women. The trial was conducted under internal cardiotocographic control. The drug improved inadequate uterine contractions by increasing their duration and intensity, but without altering their frequency. The FHR increased with an average of 20–25 beats/minute. All patients delivered vaginally, the mean total duration of labour being 17 hrs in nulliparas and $8\frac{1}{2}$ hrs in parous patients. All infants were in good condition at birth (Apgar scores at one minute: 8–9) and there was no postpartum haemorrhage. Kühnle and Gade (1974) reported on 14 women at term in whom augmentation of labour was attempted by i.v. infusion of 10–20 μg min^{-1} $PGF_{2\alpha}$. Nine patients, adequately stimulated, delivered vaginally, after a mean duration of infusion of 4 hrs 50 min (range 2–10 hrs). In the remaining five subjects, the trial was discontinued because of failure of adequate stimulation in four and venous erythema in one.

4.5 MANAGEMENT OF THE THIRD STAGE OF LABOUR

Prostaglandins might be useful for prophylaxis and treatment of hypotonic postpartum haemorrhage (Bygdeman et al., 1968) but clinicians have barely paid attention to this possible application.

Excessive bleeding from the hypotonic postpartum uterus has been mentioned as a side-effect following the use of prostaglandins for induction or augmentation of labour. Experience with i.v. oxytocin has shown that infusion of the drug must be continued after the fetus is born, to prevent haemorrhage. Therefore, these complications should not be listed as side-effects but must be attributed to improper technique (Eskes, 1972). Little mention is made in the literature of the effects of protracted infusions of PGs, but it is our clinical impression that this practice indeed reduces the frequency of uterine haemorrhage during the fourth stage of labour.

Roth-Brandel *et al.* (1970) compared the value of PGE_1 and methyl ergonovine maleate (Methergine®) for controlling the blood loss following delivery. The trial involved 188 patients, some of which served as untreated controls. The others were subdivided in three groups and received at the moment of delivery of the infant an i.v. bolus injection of either 100 μg PGE_1, or 0.2 mg Methergine®, or a combination of both. PGE_1 failed to shorten the third stage of labour or to significantly reduce the total blood loss. Methergine®, alone or in combination with PGE_1, on the other hand, reduced blood loss and probably hastened placental separation. However, Persianinov *et al.* (1973) noted a slight decrease in total blood loss (from 200 to 150 ml) when i.v. infusions of $PGF_{2\alpha}$ used for acceleration of labour were kept running after delivery.

Intracervical or intramyometrial injections of prostaglandins have not been reported for the prophylaxis and treatment of uterine hypotonia and could be worth a clinical trial. Injecting oxytocin transvaginally into the lower segment, or directly into the uterine corpus at Caesarean section used to be a classic procedure for this indication. Recently, Wentz and King (1972), demonstrated that $PGF_{2\alpha}$ injected into the myometrium did not cause tissue necrosis.

4.6 COMPARISON OF INTRAVENOUS PROSTAGLANDINS WITH OXYTOCIN FOR THE INDUCTION OF LABOUR

The present section concentrates on clinical studies comparing i.v. $PGF_{2\alpha}$, PGE_2 and oxytocin. Only larger comparative trials, including at least 20 cases in each drug group, have been taken into consideration.

4.6.1 Intravenous $PGF_{2\alpha}$ v. oxytocin

Six studies are analysed, comprising a total of 638 patients, 341 of whom received i.v. $PGF_{2\alpha}$ and 297 oxytocin (Table 4.21). The groups were comparable except for those of Spellacy *et al.* (1973), where, on the average, parity was slightly higher in patients given oxytocin and those of Hogaki (1972), where the PG-group was at some disadvantage regarding parity and state of the membranes. Basically the same dosage schedule was used by Anderson *et al.* (1972b), Vakhariya and Sherman (1972), Vroman *et al.* (1972) and Spellacy *et al.* (1973). Hogaki (1972) increased dosages hourly, using a fixed increment. Scher *et al.* (1972) administered the oxytocics in a not strictly comparable way.

Efficacy. All authors obtained similar success rates with both drugs. The ripeness of the cervix clearly influenced the ease with which the individual patient was induced. The success rate was lower, the induction–delivery interval was longer and the total dose of oxytocic was higher when the cervix was unripe (Anderson *et al.*, 1972b; Vakhariya and Sherman, 1972). However, even in 'unfavourable' cases, $PGF_{2\alpha}$ and oxytocin were of comparable efficacy, Hogaki (1972) stated that, although his overall success rate was similar with the prostaglandin and with oxytocin, patients with intact membranes progressed significantly faster with $PGF_{2\alpha}$ than with oxytocin. On the other hand,

Table 4.21   Comparison of i.v. PGF$_{2\alpha}$ and i.v. oxytocin for induction of labour

Reference	Number of patients		Success rate (%)		Induction–delivery interval (h:min)		Uterine hypertonus (%)	
	PGF$_{2\alpha}$	Oxytocin	PGF$_{2\alpha}$	Oxytocin	PGF$_{2\alpha}$	Oxytocin	PGF$_{2\alpha}$	Oxytocin
Anderson et al., 1972	91	51	61–85* (mean: 81)	57–89* (mean: 84)	8:38–5:07*	9:15–5:19*	7	0
Vakhariya and Sherman, 1972	50	50	94	96	6:25–4:22* (mean:5:15)	7:10–4:39* (mean:5:53)	16	2
Spellacy and Gall, 1972; Spellacy et al., 1973	115	107	75	66	6:26	7:05	23	8
Vroman et al., 1972	25	25	100	100	similar	similar	8	0
Hogaki, 1972	40	40	83	80	similar	similar	—	
Scher et al., 1972	20	24	70	57	not stated		not stated	

*: depending on whether the cervix was unripe or ripe

Sànchez Ramos *et al.* (1974—not included in Table 4.21) obtained similar success rates with i.v. $PGF_{2\alpha}$ (95%) and with oxytocin (100%) but the mean induction–delivery interval with the latter drug ($3\frac{1}{2}$ hours) was significantly shorter than with the former (six hours). However, a maximum dose was arbitrarily set for $PGF_{2\alpha}$ (25 μg min,[1]) and not for oxytocin.

Uterine contractility patterns. The latent period (Anderson *et al.*, 1972b; Vakhariya and Sherman, 1972) and the uterine contraction patterns elicited (Anderson *et al.*, 1972b; Scher *et al.*, 1972) were similar for both drugs. But Vakhariya and Sherman (1972) detected a trend towards elevation of the baseline and higher contraction frequency in PG-induced labour when compared to oxytocin. This confirmed the findings of other investigators who reported more frequent uterine hypertonus in patients induced with $PGF_{2\alpha}$ (see Section 4.2.1.1.2). However, neither the incidence of fetal bradycardia nor the clinical condition of the newborn was affected. Dissimilarities in uterine activity elicited by $PGF_{2\alpha}$ and oxytocin were also noted by Hogaki (1972). Oxytocin induced short contractions, recurring regularly and frequently; $PGF_{2\alpha}$ produced contractions similar to those of spontaneous labour, initially somewhat irregular and lasting longer, then progressively becoming more regular and shorter. Caballero *et al.* (1974) had also described dissimilarities (see Section 4.2.1.1.1).

Maternal effects. Neither drug altered maternal vital signs, intraocular pressure (Vroman *et al.*, 1972) or maternal acid-base and lactate–pyruvate equilibria (Thiery *et al.*, 1972). Laboratory studies revealed no adverse effect of either compound (Anderson *et al.*, 1972b; Hogaki, 1972; Vakhariya and Sherman, 1972; Vroman *et al.*, 1972). Spellacy *et al.* (1973) found a slightly higher maternal haemoglobin after induction with oxytocin. Anderson *et al.* (1972b) noted that maternal plasma oestriol levels were partially suppressed during induction with $PGF_{2\alpha}$, but not with oxytocin.

As for side-effects, hot flushes (Spellacy *et al.*, 1973) and venous erythema at the site of infusion (Scher *et al.*, 1972; Spellacy *et al.*, 1973) were more frequent with $PGF_{2\alpha}$; but the incidence of gastrointestinal side-effects was evenly distributed between the two drug groups (Scher *et al.*, 1972; Vroman *et al.*, 1972; Spellacy *et al.*, 1973). The incidence of postpartum haemorrhage was comparable for both drugs.

Fetal and neonatal effects. Only Vroman *et al.* (1972) found the incidence of fetal bradycardia in the first stage of labour to be higher with $PGF_{2\alpha}$ than with oxytocin (16% *v.* 0%). Theirs was also the only paper to report a higher frequency of low one-minute Apgar scores after $PGF_{2\alpha}$ (20% *v.* 4%) but the acid-base and the lactate–pyruvate equilibria in the infants at birth were not significantly different from those following induction with oxytocin. Neither drug had an effect on bilirubin metabolism in the neonate (de Hemptinne *et al.*, 1973) or on the distribution of glycogen, lipids and enzymes in the placenta (Thiery and Willighagen, 1973).

4.6.2 Intravenous PGE_2 *v.* oxytocin

Four reports are reviewed comparing i.v. PGE_2 with oxytocin for induction of labour. In two (Karim, 1971b; Thiery, unpublished data) groups are comparable; in the remaining two, patients were not matched for certain inducibility features (Beazley and Gillespie, 1971; Brown *et al.*, 1973). The total number of cases amounts to 687, 354 of whom were treated with PGE$_2$ and 333 with oxytocin (Table 4.22).

Table 4.22   Comparison of i.v. PGE$_2$ and oxytocin for induction of labour

Reference	Number of patients		Success rate (%)		Mean induction–delivery interval (h:min)	
	PGE$_2$	Oxytocin	PGE$_2$	Oxytocin	PGE$_2$	Oxytocin
Karim, 1971b	100	100	96	56	—	—
Beazley and Gillespie, 1971	146	146	73	73	interval>12 hrs: 9%	interval>12 hrs: 25%
Brown et al., 1973	53	53	94	100	08:23	07:31
Thiery (unpublished data)	55	34	100	100	05:45 (NP) 03:17 (MP)	04:49 (NP) 04:04 (MP)

Efficacy. All investigators except Karim (1971b), who probably used too small a dosage of oxytocin, have reported similar success rates and comparable induction–delivery intervals for both drugs. Beazley and Gillespie (1971) found that the success rate was influenced by the parity of the patient: in nulliparas, 67% of patients could be induced with PGE$_2$ and 69% with oxytocin. Success rates were higher in parous patients, but again similar for both drugs. In other studies an overall success rate of almost 100% was reached and therefore no effect of parity upon the ultimate outcome of the induction was apparent.

Thiery (unpublished data) noted that parity had a marked influence on the induction–delivery interval and on the total drug dose required for induction when PGE$_2$ was administered: parous patients delivered after a mean time of 3 hrs 17 min and a total dose of 0.1 mg PGE$_2$, as compared to 5 hrs 45 min and 0.2 mg for nulliparas. However, the role of parity was negligible in patients given oxytocin.

Also the duration of pregnancy influenced the success rate: labour was successfully induced in 84% of patients at term receiving oxytocin and in 81% of those given PGE$_2$; in cases of prolonged pregnancies, the rates were 75% and 74%, respectively (Beazley and Gillespie, 1971).

Finally, it may be interesting to note that in women successfully induced by Beazley and Gillespie (1971), the induction–delivery interval was more frequently longer than 12 hrs when use was made of oxytocin (25%) than with PGE$_2$ (9%); but again, these patients were not matched initially for certain inducibility features.

Maternal effects. Neither drug influenced maternal vital signs, routine laboratory studies (Beazley and Gillespie, 1971; Brown *et al.*, 1973; Thiery, unpublished data) or maternal acid-base and lactate–pyruvate equilibria (Thiery, unpublished data).

Venous erythema at the site of infusion was seen only in patients given PGE$_2$ (Beazley and Gillespie, 1971; Brown *et al.*, 1973). PGE$_2$ also caused emesis more frequently (18%) than oxytocin (6% Thiery, unpublished data).

Table 4.23 Comparison of i.v. administration of PGF$_{2\alpha}$, PGE$_2$ and oxytocin for labour induction

Reference	Number of patients			Success (%)			Mean induction–delivery interval (h:min)		
	PGF$_{2\alpha}$	PGE$_2$	Oxytocin	PGF$_{2\alpha}$	PGE$_2$	Oxytocin	PGF$_{2\alpha}$	PGE$_2$	Oxytocin
Karim, 1971b	100	100	100	67	96	56	—	—	—
Brown et al., 1973	32	53	85	87	94	100	09:15	08:23	07:32
Thiery (unpublished data)	55	55	34	100	100	100	6:45 (NP) 4:49 (MP)	5:45(NP) 3:17 (MP)	4:49 (NP) 4:04 (MP)

The mean measured blood loss was greater (222 ml *v.* 135 ml) and the incidence of hypotonic postpartum haemorrhage was higher (13% *v.* 2%) with i.v. PGE_2 than with oxytocin (Brown *et al.*, 1973), but no mention is made by the authors whether the infusion of PGE_2 was continued after delivery, as it should have been.

Fetal and neonatal effects. Beazley and Gillespie (1971) had two cases of intrapartum fetal death, both in patients induced with i.v. PGE_2 (see Section 4.2.1.2.2). The incidence of clinically diagnosed fetal distress (Beazley and Gillespie, 1971) and of electronically recorded fetal bradycardia (Thiery, unpublished data) was similar in both drug groups. Several investigators nevertheless had the feeling that the dosage of PGE_2 was somewhat more difficult to adjust (Gillespie *et al.*, 1971; Roberts and Turnbull, 1971; Thiery, unpublished data).

Low one-minute Apgar scores were somewhat more frequent with PGE_2 than with oxytocin in some series (Beazley and Gillespie, 1971; Brown *et al.*, 1973), but not in others (Thiery, unpublished data) and no difference was apparent five minutes after birth. Acid–base and lactate–pyruvate equilibria at the end of the first stage and at birth were comparable in both drug groups (Thiery, unpublished data).

4.6.3 Intravenous $PGF_{2\alpha}$ *v.* intravenous PGE_2 *v.* oxytocin

Three studies have been analysed for comparison of i.v. $PGF_{2\alpha}$, PGE_2 and oxytocin for induction of labour (Table 4.23). In two, the groups were comparable (Karim, 1971b; Thiery, unpublished data), but in the third study (Brown *et al.*, 1973) patients were matched only for age, parity and maturity. The total number of women amounts to 614 ($PGF_{2\alpha}$: 187; PGE_2: 208; oxytocin: 219).

Efficacy. Thiery (unpublished data) obtained similar success rates with the three oxytocic drugs whereas in Karim's double-blind study (1971b), success rates with oxytocin and with $PGF_{2\alpha}$ were markedly lower than with PGE_2. Brown *et al.* (1973) had seven failures with the prostaglandins, but none with oxytocin. The failures were due to discontinuation of the PG infusion for troublesome maternal side-effects (venous erythema, vomiting) or because of poor progress of labour after 12 hrs of drug administration. Six of the seven failures were delivered vaginally with an infusion of oxytocin, whereas the seventh patient required Caesarean section for cephalo-pelvic disproportion.

Maternal effects. Venous erythema occurred only with the prostaglandins (12%—Brown *et al.*, 1973). Brown *et al.* (1973) observed excessive vomiting in only one patient receiving $PGF_{2\alpha}$ (3%) but Thiery (unpublished data) found vomiting to be more frequent in patients induced with PGE_2 (18%) than with $PGF_{2\alpha}$ (4%) or oxytocin (6%). However, in patients affected, episodes of vomiting were infrequent and never were bothersome.

The mean total blood loss was greater and the incidence of atonic postpartum haemorrhage higher with PGE_2 (222 ml; 13%) than with $PGF_{2\alpha}$ (172 ml; 3%) or oxytocin (145 ml; 2%—Brown *et al.*, 1973) but the authors did not specify whether infusion of the oxytocic drugs was continued after delivery.

Table 4.24 Abnormal monitor findings (no. of cases) (From Thiery, 1974, by courtesy of Masson, Paris)

Stage of labour	Type of abnormality	Nulliparas		Parous patients	
		Oxytocin	PGs*	Oxytocin	PGs*
1st stage of labour	−hypertonus ± fetal bradycardia	0/11	5/99	1/23	2/103
	−transient bradycardia (alone)	0/11	2/99	0/23	0/103
	−late deceleration patterns	0/11	0/99	0/23	1/103
2nd stage of labour	−persistent bradycardia	0/11	2/96	2/23	0/97
	−progressive bradycardia	0/11	7/96	0/23	1/97
	−transient bradycardia	0/11	8/96	0/23	1/97

* PGE_2 i.v. + PGE_2 oral + $PGF_{2\alpha}$ i.v.

Uterine hyperstimulation was significantly more frequent during induction with prostaglandins than with oxytocin. (Table 4.24 includes also cases induced with PGE_2 orally.)

Fetal and neonatal effects. Brown *et al.* (1973) found low (<5) one-minute Apgar scores in 6% of cases induced with i.v. PGE_2, in none of the cases induced by i.v. oxytocin or $PGF_{2\alpha}$. Thiery (1974) found the following frequencies of low (<7) Apgar scores: 17% at one minute and 6% at five minutes with oxytocin; 16 and 2% with $PGF_{2\alpha}$; 12 and 0% with PGE_2 (cases induced with oral PGE[2] included). Abnormal FHR patterns are given in Table 4.24. The mean scalp pH at full dilatation (pHs) was similar for oxytocin (7.37), $PGF_{2\alpha}$ (7.33) and PGE_2 (7.35; inclusive cases induced with oral PGE_2) and so were all parameters of acid–base and lactate–pyruvate equilibria examined at the time of birth (Thiery, 1974).

4.7 GENERAL CONCLUSIONS

Intravenously administered natural prostaglandins appear as safe and as effective as i.v. oxytocin for the induction of labour at term. However, the superiority of these compounds has not been proven and they cause, in about 5% of cases, minor side-effects including gastrointestinal upset and venous erythema. Uterine hyperstimulation, which reportedly has occurred more frequently during administration of prostaglandins than during infusion of oxytocin, always subsides when dosage is reduced. Extensive clinical and laboratory investigations carried out on mother, fetus and neonate have failed to reveal any deleterious effect of the prostaglandin.

Oral prostaglandin E_2 is equally efficacious as i.v. oxytocin for the induction of labour at term and has reportedly caused uterine hypertonus much less frequently. Side-effects, limited to the gastrointestinal tract, have been trivial and patients' acceptance is generally excellent. This method of induction of labour has the great advantage of simplicity.

Sufficient data are still lacking for the proper evaluation of prostaglandins for the induction of labour before term, particularly in regard to their possible effects on the fetus at risk. However, prostaglandins clearly emerge as the agents of choice for termination of pregnancy complicated by intrauterine death or gross fetal malformation. Recently, the extra-amniotic method of administration of prostaglandins has been extended to therapeutic induction of labour in women with poor inducibility features and it has given very promising results.

Acknowledgements

The authors are particularly grateful to Drs M. G. Blackburn, S. L. Corson, I. Craft, J. M. Decoster, M. P. Embrey, N. H. Lauersen, R. P. Shearman and W. N. Spellacy for bibliographic assistance.

The expert secretarial assistance of Mrs J. Sagerman, Miss E. Van Overbeke and Mrs J. Pyfferoen is gratefully acknowledged.

References

Altura, B. M., Malaviya, D., Reich, C. F. and Orkin, L. R. (1972). Effects of vasoactive agents on isolated human umbilical arteries and veins. *Amer. J. Physiol.*, **222**, 345–355

Amy. J.-J., Jackson, D. M., Adaikan Ganesan, P. and Karim, S. M. M. (1973). Prostaglandin 15 (R) 15-methyl-E_2 methyl ester for suppression of gastric acidity in gravida at term. *Brit. Med. J.*, **4**, 208–211

Anderson, G. G. (1973). Induction of term labor with intravenous $PGF_{2\alpha}$: A review. *Prostaglandins*, **4**, 765–774

Anderson, G. G., Hobbins, J. C., Cordero, L. and Speroff, L. (1971). Clinical use of prostaglandins as oxytocin substances. *Ann. N.Y. Acad. Sci.*, **180**, 499–512

Anderson, G. G., Hobbins, J. C. and Speroff, L. (1972a). Intravenous prostaglandins E_2 and $F_{2\alpha}$ for the induction of term labor. *Amer. J. Obstet. Gynecol.*, **112**, 382–386

Anderson, G. G., Hobbins, J. C., Speroff, L. and Caldwell, B. V. (1972b). Intravenous prostaglandins E_2 and $F_{2\alpha}$ and Syntocinon for the induction of term labor. In: *The Prostaglandins. Clinical Applications in Human Reproduction*, 85–94 (E. M. Southern, editor) (Mount Kisco, N.Y.: Futura)

Baillie, P., Edelstein, H., Scher, J. and Edwards, J. (1972). A comparison between fenoterol (Berotec) and orciprenaline on human uterine activity induced *in vivo* by prostaglandin $F_{2\alpha}$ and oxytocin. *Med. Proc. (Johannesburg)*, **18**, 89–91

Barden, T. P. (1972). Induction of preterm labor with prostaglandin $F_{2\alpha}$ in patients with premature rupture of membranes. In: *The Prostaglandins. Clinical Applications in Human Reproduction*, 193–205 (E. M. Southern, editor) (Mount Kisco, N.Y.: Futura)

Barr, W. (1972). Induction of labor by prostaglandins E_2. In: *The Prostaglandins. Clinical Applications in Human Reproduction*, 219–222 (E. M. Southern, editor) (Mount Kisco, N.Y.: Futura)

Barr, W. (1973a). La somministrazione delle prostaglandine nella induzione del parto. *Simposio Internationale sugli Aspetti Clinici delle Prostaglandine, Milano* (Abstract)

Barr, W. (1973b). Oral prostaglandin E_2 in the induction of labour. In: *The use of prostaglandins E_2 and F_2 alpha in Obstetrics and Gynaecology*, 21–24 (R. G. Jacomb and R. E. Hardy, editors) (Miami: Symposia Specialists)

Barr, W. and Naismith, W. C. M. K. (1972). Oral prostaglandins in the induction of labour. *Brit. Med. J.*, **2**, 188–191

Beazley, J. M., Brummer, H. C. and Kurjak, A. (1972). Distribution of 9-H^3-prostaglandin $F_{2\alpha}$ in pregnant and non-pregnant subjects. *J. Obstet. Gynaecol. Brit. Cwlth.*, **79**, 800–803

Beazley, J. M., Dewhurst, C. J. and Gillespie, A. (1970). The induction of labour with prostaglandin E_2. *J. Obstet. Gynaecol. Brit. Cwlth.*, **77**, 193–199

Beazley, J. M., and Gillespie, A. (1971). Double-blind trial of prostaglandin E_2 and oxytocin in induction of labour. *Lancet*, **1**, 152–155

Bishop, E. H. (1964). Pelvic scoring for elective induction. *Obstet. Gynecol. (N.Y.)*, **24**, 266–268

Blackburn, M. G., Mancusi-Ungaro, H. R., Orzalesi, M. M., Hobbins J. C. and Anderson, G. G. (1973). Effects on the neonate of the induction of labour with prostaglandin $F_{2\alpha}$ and oxytocin. *Amer. J. Obstet. Gynecol.*, 116, 847–853

Brosens, I., Dixon, H. G. and Robertson, W. B. (1974a). Prostaglandins and induction of labour. *Lancet*, 1, 808–809

Brosens, I., Dixon, H. G. and Robertson, W. B. (1974b). Prostaglandins and pre-eclampsia. *Lancet*, 2, 413–414

Brosens, I., Robertson, W. B. and Dixon, H. G. (1972). The role of the spiral arteries in the pathogenesis of preeclampsia. In: *Obstetric and Gynecological Annual*, 177–191 (R. M. Wynn, editor) (New York: Appleton-Century-Crofts)

Brown, A. A., Hamlett, J. D., Hibbard, B. M. and Howe, P. D. (1973). Induction of labour by amniotomy and intravenous infusions of oxytocic drugs—A comparison between prostaglandins and oxytocin. *J. Obstet. Gynaecol. Brit. Cwlth.*, 80, 111–115

Bygdeman, M. (1964). The effect of different prostaglandins on the human myometrium *in vitro*. *Acta Physiol. Scand.*, 63, Suppl. 242, 1–78

Bygdeman, M., Kwon, S. U., Mukherjee, T., Roth-Brandel, U. and Wiqvist, N. (1970). The effect of the prostaglandin F compounds on the contractility of the pregnant human uterus. *Amer. J. Obstet. Gynecol.*, 106, 567–572

Bygdeman, M., Kwon, S. U., Mukherjee, T. and Wiqvist, N. (1968). Effect of intravenous infusion of prostaglandin E_1 and E_2 on motility of the pregnant human uterus. *Amer. J. Obstet. Gynecol.*, 102, 317–326

Bygdeman, M., Kwon, S. U. and Wiqvist, N. (1967). The effect of PGE on the human pregnant myometrium *in vivo*. In: *Prostaglandins, Nobel Symposium 2*, 93–96 (S. Bergström and B. Samuelsson, editors) (Stockholm: Almqvist and Wiksell)

Caballero. A., Garcia-Albertos, F., Corredera, J., Alonso Magan, J. L., Guerra, J. M. and Gandara, A. (1974). Déclenchement du travail à l'aide des prostaglandines E_1, E_2, $F_{1\alpha}$ et $F_{2\alpha}$. *Rev. Franç. Gynécol. Obstét.*, 69, 75–95

Calder, A. A., Bonnar, J., Sheppard, B., Embrey, M. P. and Turnbull, A. C. (1974a). Prostaglandins and pre-eclampsia. *Lancet*, 2, 49

Calder, A. A. and Embrey, M. P. (1973). Prostaglandins and the unfavourable cervix. *Lancet*, 2, 1322–1323

Calder, A. A., Embrey, M. P. and Hillier, K. (1974b). Extra-amniotic prostaglandin E_2 for the induction of labour at term. *J. Obstet. Gynaecol. Brit. Cwlth.*, 81, 39–46

Cameron, J. M. and Dayan, A. D. (1966). Association of brain damage with therapeutic abortion induced by amniotic fluid replacement. Report of 2 cases. *Brit. Med. J.*, 1, 1010–1013

Chef, R., Thiery, M., Van Kets, H., Yo Le Sian, A., de Hemptinne, D. and Vrijens, M. (1974). Anencéphalie: diagnostic ultrasonique précoce et interruption. *J. Gynécol. Obstét. Biol. Reprod. (Paris)*, 3, 93–104

Chimura, T., Hiroi, M. and Yamuki, T. (1971). Uterine contractility during labor induced by prostaglandin F_2-alpha. *Obstet. Gynecol. (Tokyo)*, 38, 787–792

Clark, K. E., Ryan, M. J. and Brody, M. J. (1973). Effects of prostaglandins E_1 and $F_{2\alpha}$ on uterine hemodynamics and motility. *Adv. Biosciences*, 9, 779–782

Collins, J. A., and Jaffe, B. M. (1973). Effects of prostaglandins on the affinity of hemoglobin for oxygen in human whole blood *in vitro*. *Prostaglandins*, 3, 59–66

Corson, S. L. and Bolognese, R. J. (1974). Oral prostaglandin E_2 for induction of labor. *J. Reprod. Med.*, 12, 167–168

Craft, I. (1972a). Amniotomy and oral prostaglandin E_2 titration for induction of labour. *Brit. Med. J.*, 2, 191–194

Craft, I. (1972b). Labour induction with oral prostaglandin E_2. In: *The Prostaglandins. Clinical Applications in Human Reproduction*, 226–232 (E. M. Southern, editor) (Mount Kisco, N.Y.: Futura)

Craft, I. L. (1973a). Oral prostaglandin E_2 and amniotomy for induction of labor. In: *The Use of Prostaglandins E_2 and F_2 alpha in Obstetrics and Gynaecology*, 25–34 (R. C. Jacomb and R. E. Hardy, editors) (Miami: Symposia Specialists)

Craft, I. L. (1973b). Oral prostaglandin E_2 and amniotomy for induction of labor. *Adv. Biosciences*, 9, 593–598

Craft, I. L. (1973c). Prostaglandins and convulsions. *Lancet*, 2, 1389

Craft, I. L. (1974). Oral prostaglandins for induction of labour. *South Afr. Med. J.* (In press)

Craft, I. L., Cullum, A. R., May, D. T. L., Noble, A. D. and Thomas, D. J. (1971).

Prostaglandin E_2 compared with oxytocin for the induction of labour. *Brit. Med. J.*, 3, 276–279

Derom, R., Thiery, M., Dhont, M., Kimzeke, G., De Coster, W. and Hooft, C. (1974). Long-term follow-up study of antenatal hypoxia. A preliminary note. *4th Europ. Congress Perinatal Med., Prague*, August 1974, Abstract III-1/7, L 974

Dhont, M., Thiery, M., Lepoutre, L., Vermeulen, A. and Vandekerckhove, D. (1973). Maternal serum levels of human chorionic gonadotropin (HCG), human chorionic somato-mammotropin (HCS), progesterone (P) and estradiol (E) before and during labor induced at term by orally administered prostaglandin E_2. *IRCS (International Research Communications System)*, 73–76, 15–18–9

Elder, M. G. and Stone, M. (1974). Induction of labour by low amniotomy and oral administration of a solution compared to a tablet of prostaglandin E_2. *Prostaglandins*, 6, 427–432

Elias, J. A. (1972). Experience with prostaglandins E_2 and $F_{2\alpha}$ for induction of labor. In: *The Prostaglandins. Clinical Applications in Human Reproduction*, 121–128 (E. M. Southern, editor) (Mount Kisco, N.Y.: Futura)

Embrey, M. P. (1969). The effect of prostaglandins on the human pregnant uterus. *J. Obstet. Gynaecol. Brit. Cwlth.*, 76, 783–788

Embrey, M. P. (1970). Induction of labour with prostaglandins E_1 and E_2. *Brit. Med. J.*, 2, 256–258

Embrey, M. P. (1971). PGE compounds for induction of labour and abortion. *Ann. N.Y. Acad. Sci.*, 180, 518–523

Embrey, M. P., Calder, A. A. and Hillier, K. (1974). Extra amniotic prostaglandins in the management of intrauterine fetal death, anencephaly and hydatidiform mole. *J. Obstet. Gynaecol. Brit. Cwlth.*, 81, 47–51

Embrey, M. P. and Morrison, D. L. (1968). The effect of prostaglandins on human pregnant myometrium *in vitro*. *J. Obstet. Gynaecol. Brit. Cwlth.*, 75, 829–832

Eskes, T. K. A. B. (1972). Induction of labor and prostaglandins. *Europ. J. Obstet. Gynaecol.*, 2, 105–108

Favier, J., Mulder, R. H., Rietveld, W. J. and Gevers, R. H. (1972). Inleiding van de baring met prostaglandine E_1. *Nederl. T. Geneesk.*, 116, 1964–1965

Favier, J. and Rietveld, W. J. (1973). The effect of prostaglandin E_1 on the pregnant human uterus. *Amer. J. Obstet. Gynecol.*, 115, 33–36

Filshie, G. M. (1971). The use of prostaglandin E_2 in the management of intrauterine death, missed abortion and hydatidiform mole. *J. Obstet. Gynaecol. Brit. Cwlth.*, 78, 87–90

Filshie, G. M. (1972). Labor induction with oral prostaglandin E_2. In: *The Prostaglandins. Clinical Applications in Human Reproduction*, 223–226 (E. M. Southern, editor) (Mount Kisco, N.Y.: Futura)

Fishburne, J. I., Brenner, W. E., Braaksma, J. T. and Hendricks, C. H. (1972a). Bronchospasm complicating intravenous prostaglandin $F_{2\alpha}$ for therapeutic abortion. *Obstet. Gynecol. (N.Y.)*, 39, 892–896

Fishburne, J. I., Brenner, W. E., Braaksma, J. T., Staurovsky, L. G., Mueller, R. A., Hoffer, J. L. and Hendricks, C. H. (1972b). Cardiovascular and respiratory responses to intravenous infusion of prostaglandin $F_{2\alpha}$ in the pregnant woman. *Amer. J. Obstet. Gynecol.*, 114, 765–772

Fraser, I. S. (1974). Uterine hypertonus after oral prostaglandin E_2. *Lancet*, 2, 162

Fraser, I. A. and Gray, C. (1974). Prostaglandin $F_{2\alpha}$ and electro-encephalogram changes. *Lancet*, 2, 49–50

Friedman, E. A., Niswander, K. R., Bayonet-Riviera, N. P. and Sachtleben, M. R. (1966). Relation of prelabor evaluation to inducibility and the course of labor. *Obstet. Gynecol. (N.Y.)*, 28, 495–501

Friedman, E. A. and Sachtleben, M. R. (1974). Oral prostaglandin E_2 for induction of labor at term. *Obstet. Gynecol. (N.Y.)*, 43, 178–185

Frumar, A. M., Smith, I. D. and Korda, A. R. (1974). Prostaglandin $F_{2\alpha}$ for the induction of labor in pregnancies complicated by intrauterine death, anencephaly and chromosomal anomaly. *Prostaglandins*, 6, 125–135

Gillespie, A. (1971). Use of prostaglandins for induction of abortion and labor. *Ann. N.Y. Acad. Sci.*, 180, 524–527

Gillespie, A. (1972). Factors affecting the dose of prostaglandin E_2 and Syntocinon required to induce labour. *J. Obstet. Gynaecol. Brit. Cwlth.*, 79, 135–138

Gillespie, A. (1973). Prostaglandins and human labour. In: *Endocrine factors in labour*, 77–93 (A. Klopper and J. Gardner, editors) (Cambridge: University Press)

Gillespie, A., Brummer, H. C. and Chard, T. (1973). Oxytocin release by infused prostaglandin. *Brit. Med. J.*, 1, 543–544

Gillespie, A., Dewhurst, C. J. and Beazley, J. M. (1971). Prostaglandin-induced labour. *Brit. Med. J.*, 2, 222

Goethals, A., Decoster, W., Thiery, M. and Derom, R. (1974). Labor induction with prostaglandin $F_{2\alpha}$: effect on the neurologic state of the neonate and its psychomotor evolution up to the age of 6 months. *IRCS (International Research Communications System)*, 2, 1202

Goodlin, R. C. (1969). Orgasm and premature labour. *Lancet*, 2, 646

Goodlin, R. C., Keller, D. W. and Raffin, M. (1971). Orgasm during late pregnancy: possible deleterious effects. *Obstet. Gynecol. (N.Y.)*, 38, 916–920

Harley, G. W. (1941). *Native African Medicine with Special Reference to its Practice in the Mano Tribe of Liberia*, 237–238 (Cambridge, Mass.: Harvard University Press)

Heidenreich, J., van der Crabben, H., Terinde, R., and Beck, L. (1974). Klinik der Weheneinleitung mit Prostaglandin $F_{2\alpha}$. *Hamburger Prostaglandin-Gespräche*, 199–205 (Germany, Upjohn)

Hemptinne, D. de, Schuddinck, L., Thiery, M. and Martens, G. (1973). Neonatal bilirubinaemia—Effect of oxytocic compounds (oxytocin and prostaglandins) and vacuum extraction. *IRCS (International Research Communications System)*, 73–12, 10–14–3

Henzl, M. R., Arevalo-T, N., Noriega, L., Aznar, R., Ortega, E. and Segre, E. (1973). Quantitation of uterine activity after vaginal administration of prostaglandins. *Adv. Biosciences*, 9, 767–772

Hickl, E. J., Mickan, H. and Walther, D. (1973). Kombination von Prostaglandin $F_{2\alpha}$ und Paracervicalblock bei Missed Abortion und intrauterinem Fruchttod. *Klin. Wschr.*, 51, 140–141

Hillier, K. and Karim, S. M. M. (1968). Effects of prostaglandins E_1, E_2, $F_{1\alpha}$ and $F_{2\alpha}$ on isolated human umbilical and placental blood vessels. *J. Obstet. Gynaecol. Brit. Cwlth.*, 75, 667–674

Hodgkinson, C. P., Margulis, R. R. and Lazarde, J. H. (1954). Etiology and management of hypofibrinogenemia of pregnancy. *J.A.M.A.*, 154, 557–561

Hogaki, M. (1972). Effects of prostaglandins on labor induction, (abstracted by Upjohn Company). *Igaku No Ayumi*, 80, 848–857

Jacomb, R. G. and Hinchley, H. (1974). Prostaglandins and induction of labour. *Lancet*, I, 1226–1227

Johnson, A., Clark, K. and Newton, J. (1974). Blood coagulation in ten patients receiving intravenous prostaglandin $F_{2\alpha}$ for labour induction. *Prostaglandins*, 5, 475–481

Johnson, A., and Newton, J. R. (1974). Labour induction by prostaglandin $F_{2\alpha}$ using the Cardiff Infusion Apparatus. *Lancet*, 1, 1253–1254

Jungmannová, C., Havránek, F. and Hodr, J. (1972). The effect of prostaglandin $F_{2\alpha}$ on the placental vessels *in vitro*. *J. Reprod. Med.*, 9, 79–80

Karim, S. M. M. (1966). Identification of prostaglandins in human amniotic fluid. *J. Obstet. Gynaecol. Brit. Cwlth.*, 73, 903–908

Karim, S. M. M. (1967). The identification of prostaglandins in human umbilical cord. *Brit. J. Pharmacol. Chemother.*, 29, 230–237

Karim, S. M. M. (1970). Use of prostaglandin E_2 in the management of missed abortion, missed labour and hydatidiform mole. *Brit. Med. J.*, 3, 196–197

Karim, S. M. M. (1971a). Effects of oral administration of prostaglandins E_2 and $F_{2\alpha}$ on the human uterus. *J. Obstet. Gynaecol. Brit. Cwlth.*, 78, 289–293

Karim, S. M. M. (1971b). Action of prostaglandin in the pregnant woman. *Ann. N.Y. Acad. Sci.*, 180, 483–498

Karim, S. M. M. (1972). Prostaglandins and human reproduction: Physiological roles and clinical uses of prostaglandins in relation to human reproduction. In: *The Prostaglandins—Progress in Research*, 71–164 (S. M. M. Karim, editor) (Lancaster: M.T.P.)

Karim, S. M. M. and Devlin, J. (1967). Prostaglandin content of amniotic fluid during pregnancy and labour. *J. Obstet. Gynaecol. Brit. Cwlth.* 74, 230–234

Karim, S. M. M., Hillier, K., Somers, K. and Trussell, R. R. (1971a). The effects of prostaglandins E_2 and $F_{2\alpha}$ administered by different routes on uterine activity and the cardiovascular system in pregnant and non-pregnant women. *J. Obstet. Gynaecol. Brit. Cwlth.*, 78, 172–179

Karim, S. M. M., Hillier, K., Trussell, R. R., Patel, R. C. and Tamusange, S. (1970). Induction of labour with prostaglandin E₂. *J. Obstet. Gynaecol. Brit. Cwlth.*, **77**, 200–210

Karim, S. M. M., Patel, R. C., Sharma, S. D. and Trussell, R. R. (1971b). Two years experience with prostaglandin E₂ for the induction of labour. *J. Asian Fed. Obstet. Gynaecol.*, **2**, 1–6

Karim, S. M. M., and Sharma, S. D. (1971a). Oral administration of prostaglandins for the induction of labour. *Brit. Med. J.*, **1**, 260–262

Karim, S. M. M. and Sharma, S. D. (1971b). Therapeutic abortion and induction of labour by the intravaginal administration of prostaglandins E_2 and $F_{2\alpha}$. *J. Obstet. Gynaecol. Brit. Cwlth.*, **78**, 294–300

Karim, S. M. M. and Sharma, S. D. (1971c). The effect of ethyl alcohol on prostaglandins E_2 and $F_{2\alpha}$ induced uterine activity in pregnant women. *J. Obstet. Gynaecol. Brit. Cwlth.*, **78**, 251–254

Karim, S. M. M. and Sharma, S. D. (1972). Oral administration of prostaglandin E_2 for the induction and acceleration of labor. In: *The Prostaglandins. Clinical Applications in Human Reproduction*, 207–217 (E. M. Southern, editor) (Mount Kisco, N.Y.: Futura)

Karim, S. M. M., Sharma, S. D. and Filshie, G. M. (1972). Termination of pregnancy with 15 methyl analogues of prostaglandins E_2 and $F_{2\alpha}$. In: *The Prostaglandins. Clinical Applications in Human Reproduction*, 307–321 (E. M. Southen, editor) (Mount Kisco, N.Y.: Futura)

Karim, S. M. M., Somers, K., and Hillier, K. (1971c). Cardiovascular and other effects of prostaglandins E_2 and $F_{2\alpha}$ in man. *Cardiovasc. Res.*, **5**, 255–61

Karim, S. M. M. and Trussell, R. R. (1971). The use of prostaglandins in Obstetrics. *East African Med. J.*, **48**, 1–12

Karim, S. M. M., Trussell, R. R., Hillier, K. and Patel, R. C. (1969). Induction of labour with prostaglandin $F_{2\alpha}$. *J. Obstet. Gynaecol. Brit. Cwlth.*, **76**, 769–782

Karim, S. M. M., Trussell, R. R., Patel, R. C. and Hillier, K. (1968). Response of pregnant human uterus to prostaglandin $F_{2\alpha}$-induction of labour. *Brit. Med. J.*, **4**, 621–623

Keller, P. J., Ruppen, M., Gerber, C. and Schmid, J. (1972). Placental function in prostaglandin induced labour. *J. Obstet. Gynaecol. Brit. Cwlth.*, **79**, 804–806

Kelly, J., Flynn, A. M. and Bertrand, P. V. (1973). A comparison of oral prostaglandin E₂ and intravenous oxytocin in the induction of labour. *J. Obstet. Gynaecol. Brit. Cwlth.*, **80**, 923–926

Khew, K. S., Ratnam, S. S., Chen, C., Lim, T. C. and Karim, S. M. M. (1971). Induction of labour with oral prostaglandin E₂ (PGE₂). *J. Asian Fed. Obstet. Gynaecol.*, **2**, 78–79

Kinoshita, K., Wagatsuma, T., Hogaki, M., and Sakamoto, S. (1971). The induction of labor with prostaglandin $F_{2\alpha}$. *Acta Obstet. Gynaecol. Japonica*, **18**, 87–94

Kirton, K. T. (1972). The role of prostaglandins in reproduction in sub-human primates. In: *W.H.O. 3rd Conference on Prostaglandins in Fertility Control*, 208–216 (S. Bergström, K. Grëen and B. Samuelsson, editors) (Stockholm: Karolinska Institutet)

Kühnle, H. and Gade, J. (1974). Klinische Erfahrungen mit PGF₂α zum Schwangerschafts-afbruch und zur Weheneinleitung bei missed abortion, intrauterinem Fruchttod und primärer Wehenschwäche am Geburtstermin. *Hamburger Prostaglandin-Gespräche*, 209–211 (Germany, Upjohn)

Laros, R. K., Witting, W. C. and Work, B. A. (1973). Uterine activity response to constant infusion of prostaglandin $F_{2\alpha}$ in term human pregnancy. *Clin. Pharmacol. Ther.*, **14**, 140

Lauersen, N. H. and Wilson, K. H. (1975). Induction of labor with oral prostaglandin. *Obstet. Gynecol. N.Y.*, **44**, 793–801

Laver, M. B. (1972). Hormonal influence on hemoglobin-O₂ interaction. In: *Conference on the Current Status and the Future of Red Blood Cell Preservation Research* (Washington, D.C.: NAS-NCR), loc. cit. Collins and Jaffe, 1973

Lemaire, W. J., Spellacy, W. N., Shevack, A. B. and Gall, S. A. (1972). Changes in plasma estriol and progesterone during labor induced with prostaglandin $F_{2\alpha}$ or oxytocin. *Prostaglandins*, **2**, 93–101

Liggins, G. C. (1962). The treatment of missed abortion by high dosage Syntocinon intravenous infusion. *J. Obstet. Gynaecol. Brit. Cwlth.*, **69**, 277–281

Lindmark, G., Melander, S., Nilsson, B. A. and Zador, G. (1973). Inhibition of prostaglandin induced uterine activity in the second trimester of pregnancy by β-mimetic adrenergic agents. *Prostaglandins*, **3**, 481–490

Lyneham, R. C., McLeod, J. G., Smith, I. D., Low, P. A., Shearman, R. P., and Korda, A. R. (1973). Convulsions and electroencephalogram abnormalities after intraamniotic prostaglandin $F_{2\alpha}$. *Lancet*, **2**, 1003–1005

MacKenzie, I. Z., Hillier, K. and Embrey, M. P. (1973). Convulsions and prostaglandin-induced abortion. *Lancet*, 2, 1323

Masters, W. H. and Johnson, V. E. (1966). *Human Sexual Response* (Boston: Little and Brown)

Miller, A. W. F. (1973). The use of prostaglandins for missed abortion, foetal death *in utero* and hydatidiform mole. In: *The use of prostaglandins E₂ and F₂ alpha in Obstetrics and Gynaecology*, 63–67 (R. G. Jacomb and R. E. Hardy, editors) (Miami: Symposia Specialists)

Miller, A. W. F. and Mack, D. S. (1974). Induction of labour by extra-amniotic prostaglandins. *J. Obstet. Gynaecol. Brit. Cwlth.*, 81, 706–708

Moghissi, K. S. and Murray, C. P. (1970). The function of prostaglandins in reproduction. *Obstet. Gynecol. Survey*, 25, 281–296

Mosler, K. H., Czekanowski, R. and Dornhöfer, W. (1973). Comparative studies of the effect of oxytocin and prostaglandin F₂ₐ in the uterus. *Adv. Biosciences*, 9, 751–760

Murnaghan, G. A., Lamki, H., Rashid, S. and Pinkerton, J. H. M. (1974). Induction of labour with oral prostaglandin E₂. *J. Obstet. Gynaecol. Brit. Cwlth.*, 81, 141–145

Naismith, W. C. M. K. and Barr, W. (1974). Simultaneous intravenous infusion of prostaglandin E₂ (PGE₂) and oxytocin in the management of intrauterine death of the fetus, missed abortion and hydatidiform mole. *J. Obstet., Gynaecol. Brit. Cwlth.*, 81, 146–149

Naismith, W. C. M. K., Barr, W. and MacVicar, J. (1972). Induction of labour by simultaneous intravenous administration of prostaglandin E₂ and oxytocin. *Brit. Med. J.*, 4, 461–462

Naismith, W. C. M. K., Barr, W. and MacVicar, J. (1973). Comparison of intravenous prostaglandins F₂ₐ and E₂ with intravenous oxytocin in the induction of labour. *J. Obstet. Gynaecol. Brit. Cwlth.*, 80, 531–535

Novy, M. (1972). O₂ transport functions of maternal and fetal blood during human pregnancy. In: *Conference on the Current Status and the Future of Red Blood Cell Preservation Research* (Washington D.C.: NAS-NRC), loc. cit. Collins and Jaffe, 1973

Novy, M. J., Piasecki, G. and Jackson, B. T. (1974). Effect of prostaglandins E₂ and F₂ₐ on umbilical blood flow and fetal hemodynamics. *Prostaglandins*, 5, 543–555

Park, M. K., Rishor, C. and Dyer, D. C. (1972). Vasoactive actions of prostaglandins and serotonin on isolated human umbilical arteries and veins. *Canad. J. Physiol. Pharmacol.*, 50, 393–399

Pedersen, P. H., Larsen, J. F. and Sorensen, B. (1972). Induction of labour with prostaglandin F₂ₐ in missed abortion, fetus mortuus and anencephalia. *Prostaglandins*, 2, 135–141

Persianinov, L. S., Manuilova, I. A. and Chernukha, E. A. (1973). The results of using prostaglandin F₂ₐ for induction and stimulation of labor. *Adv. Biosciences*, 9, 585–592

Peterson, E. P. and Taylor, H. B. (1970). Amniotic fluid embolism. An analysis of 40 cases. *Obstet. Gynecol. (N.Y.)*, 35, 787–793

Prechtl, H. F. R. and Beintema, D. (1964). *The Neurologic Examination of the Full Term Newborn Infant.* (London: William Heineman)

Pystynen, P. and Nummi, S. (1974). Beziehung des Koitus zu Beginn der Uteruswehen und der Geburt gegen Ende der Schwangerschaft. *Zbl. Gynäk.*, 96, 430–432

Rangarajan, N. S., LaCroix, G. E. and Moghissi, K. S. (1971). Induction of labor with prostaglandin. *Obstet. Gynecol. (N.Y.)*, 38, 546–550

Ratnam, S. S., Khew, K. S., Chen, C. and Lim, T. C. (1974). Oral prostaglandin E₂ for induction of labour. *Aust. N.Z.J. Obstet. Gynaecol.*, 14, 26–30

Ring, A. (1972). Clinical experience with prostaglandin F₂ₐ for induction of labor. In: *The Prostaglandins. Clinical Applications in Human Reproduction*, 129–133 (E. M. Southern, editor) (Mount Kisco, N.Y.: Futura)

Ring, A., Völckers, J. and Semm, K. (1974). Geburtseinleitung am Termin mit Prostaglandin E₂. *Hamburger Prostaglandin-Gespräche*, 212–217 (Germany: Upjohn)

Roberts, G. (1970). Induction of labour using prostaglandins. *J. Reprod. Fertil.14*, 23, 370–371

Roberts, G. (1974). Induction of labour and abortion by intravenous prostaglandins in pregnancies complicated by intrauterine fetal death and hydatidiform mole. *Current Med. Research and Opinion*, 2, 342–350

Roberts, G., Anderson, A., McGarry, J. and Turnbull, A. C. (1970). Absence of antidiuresis during administration of prostaglandin F₂ₐ. *Brit. Med. J.*, 2, 152–154

Roberts, G., Mottram, R. F., Parry, H. and Bloom, A. (1972). Cyanosis due to intravenous prostaglandin F₂ₐ. *Lancet*, 2, 425–426

Roberts, G. and Turnbull, A. C. (1971). Uterine hypertonus during labour induced by prostaglandins. *Brit. Med. J.*, 1, 702–705

Robertson, W. B., Brosens, I. and Dixon, H. G. (1967). The pathological response of the vessels of the placental bed to hypertensive pregnancy. *J. Pathol. Bact.*, **93**, 581–592

Rosa, P., Delbovier, G., Ley, P. and Frerotte, M. (1972). Comparative efficacy of Pitocin* and prostaglandin $F_{2\alpha}$ in the induction of labor near term in the multipara. *Europ. J. Obstet. Gynaecol.*, **2**, 109–114

Roth-Brandel, U. (1971). Response of the pregnant human uterus to low and high doses of prostaglandin E_1 and E_2. *Acta Obstet. Gynecol. Scand.*, **50**, 159–166

Roth-Brandel, U. and Adams, M. (1970). An evaluation of the possible use of prostaglandin E_1, E_2 and $F_{2\alpha}$ for induction of labour. *Acta Obstet. Gynecol. Scand.*, **49, Suppl. 5**, 9–17

Roth-Brandel, U., Bygdeman, M. and Wiqvist, N. (1970). A comparative study on the influence of prostaglandin E_1, oxytocin and ergometrine on the pregnant human uterus. *Acta Obstet. Gynecol. Scand.*, **49, Suppl. 5**, 1–7

Ruppen, M., Keller, P. J., Schmid, J. and Schreiner, W. E. (1972). Prostaglandine bei 'missed abortion' und bei 'missed labor'. *Schweiz. Z. Gynäk. Geburtsh.*, **3**, 439–442

Sánchez Ramos, J. E., Santissimo Sacramento, J. L., Castrillo Garcia, M. J. and Fabré Gonzáles, E. (1974). Prostaglandina F_2 alfa y oxitocina en la induccion del parto de multiparas. Estudio comparativo. *Acta Ginec. (Madrid)*, **25**, 105–109

Sandberg, F., Ingelman-Sundberg, A., Joelsson, I. and Ryden, G. (1967). Preliminary investigation on the absorption of prostaglandin E_1 from the human vagina. In: *Prostaglandins*, **Nobel Symposium 2**, 91–96 (S. Bergström and B. Samuelsson, editors) (Stockholm: Almqvist and Wiksell)

Scher, J. and Baillie, P. (1973). The effect of a β-adrenergic agent on prostaglandin stimulated labor. *Adv. Biosciences*, **9**, 743–749

Scher, J., Davey, D. A., Baillie, P., Friend, J. and Friend, D. M. (1972). A comparison of prostaglandin $F_{2\alpha}$ and oxytocin in the induction of labour. *S. African Med. J.*, **46**, 2009–2012

Schmid, J., Baertschi, U., Ruppen, M. and Keller, P. J. (1974). Weheneinleitung bei Überbragungen mit $PGF_{2\alpha}$ und PGE_2. *Hamburger Prostaglandin-Gespräche*, 238–242 (Germany, Upjohn)

Schmid, J., Ruppen, M., Keller, P. J. and Schreiner, W. E. (1972). Geburtseinleitung mit Prostaglandin. *Schweiz. Z. Gynäk. Geburtsh.*, **3**, 443–445

Schotman, J. (1974). Prostaglandines, de sleutel tot het mysterie van de essentiële vetzuren. *Chemisch Weekblad*, **70**, (20), 4–6

Sherman, A. (1972). *The Prostaglandins. Clinical Applications in Human Reproduction*, 239 (E. M. Southern, editor) (Mount Kisco, N.Y.: Futura)

Smith, A. P. (1973). The effects of intravenous infusion of graded doses of prostaglandins $F_{2\alpha}$ and E_2 on lung resistance in patients undergoing termination of pregnancy. *Clin. Sci.*, **44**, 17–25

Spellacy, W. N., Buhi, W. C. and Holsinger, K. K. (1971). The effect of prostaglandin $F_{2\alpha}$ and E_2 on blood glucose and plasma insulin levels during pregnancy. *Amer. J. Obstet. Gynecol.*, **111**, 239–243

Spellacy, W. N. and Gall, S. A. (1972). Prostaglandin $F_{2\alpha}$ and oxytocin for term labor induction. In: *The Prostaglandins. Clinical Applications in Human Reproduction*, 107–113 (E. M. Southern, editor) (Mount Kisco, N.Y.: Futura)

Spellacy, W. N., Gall, S. A., Shevach, A. B. and Holsinger, K. K. (1973). The induction of labor at term. Comparisons between prostaglandin $F_{2\alpha}$ and oxytocin infusions. *Obstet. Gynecol. (N.Y.)*, **41**, 14–21

Tchilingurian, N. G. O. (1972). Comparison of prostaglandin $F_{2\alpha}$ and oxytocin in the induction of labor in high risk pregnant women. In: *The Prostaglandins. Clinical Applications in Human Reproduction*, 179–192 (E. M. Southern, editor) (Mount Kisco, N.Y.: Futura)

Thiery, M. (1974). Elective induction of labour at term with oxytocin and prostaglandins. Techniques and fetal and maternal effects. In: *Avortement et Parturition Provoqués*, 267–287 (M. J. Bose, R. Palmer and C. Sureau, editors) (Paris: Masson)

Thiery, M., Amy, J.-J., de Hemptinne, D. and Yo Le Sian, A. (1974a). Prostaglandins and convulsions. *Lancet*, **1**, 218

Thiery, M., de Hemptinne, D., Vanderheyden, K., Vroman, S., Derom, R., Van Kets, H. and Martens, G. (1973a). Intravenous prostaglandin $F_{2\alpha}$ and amniotomy for the elective induction of labor at term. *J. Perinat. Med.*, **1**, 268–282

Thiery, M., de Hemptinne, D., Vanderheyden, K., Yo Le Sian, A., Derom, R., Van Kets, H. and Martens, G. (1973b). Elective induction of term labor with amniotomy and oral prostaglandin E_2. *Europ. J. Obstet. Gynaecol. Reprod. Biol.*, **3**, 159–166

Thiery, M., de Hemptinne, D., Vanderheyden, K., Yo Le Sian, A., Derom, R., Van Kets, H. and Martens, G. (1973c). Het gebruik van perorale prostaglandine E₂ voor de inductie van de baring. *T. Geneesk.*, 21, 1033–1038

Thiery, M., Van Kets, H., Yo Le Sian, A., de Hemptinne, D., Vrijens, M. and Chef, R. (1973d). Early diagnosis of anencephaly. *Lancet*, 1, 599–600

Thiery, M., Vroman, S., Vanderheyden, K., de Hemptinne, D., Derom, R., Van Kets, H. and Martens, G. (1972). The fetal effects of prostaglandin $F_{2\alpha}$ applied in the elective induction of labor at term. In: *The Prostaglandins. Clinical Applications in Human Reproduction*, 135–158 (E. M. Southern, editor) (Mount Kisco, N.Y.: Futura)

Thiery, M., Yo Le Sian, A., de Hemptinne, D., Derom, R., Martens, G., Van Kets, H. and Amy, J. J. (1974b). Induction of labour with prostaglandin E₂ tablets. *J. Obstet. Gynaecol. Brit. Cwlth.*, 81, 303–306

Thiery, M., Yo Le Sian, A., de Hemptinne, D., Derom, R., Van Kets, H. and Martens, G. (1974c). Weheneinleitung durch die orale Gabe von Prostaglandin E₂, *Hamburger Prostaglandin-Gespräche*, 218–231 (Germany: Upjohn)

Thiery, M., Yo Le Sian, A., de Hemptinne, D., Derom, R., Van Kets, H., Martens, G. and Amy, J. J. (1974d). Elective Induction of Labor at Term by Amniotomy and Intravenous Prostaglandin E₂. *Europ. J. Obstet. Gynaecol. Reprod. Biol.*, 4, 209–214

Thiery, M. and Willighagen, R. G. J. (1973). Prostaglandins—Effect on the enzyme content of the human placenta. *IRCS (International Research Communications System)*, 73–79, 10–26–2

Turnbull, A. C. (1974). An automatic oxytocin infusion system for the induction of labor. In: *Avortement et Parturition Provoqués*, 257–265 (M. J. Bose, R. Palmer and C. Sureau, editors) (Paris: Masson)

Turnbull, A. C. and Anderson, A. B. M. (1968). Induction of labour. Part II: Intravenous oxytocin infusion. *J. Obstet. Gynaecol. Brit. Cwlth.*, 75, 24–31

Unbehaun, V. and Conradt, A. (1973). Metabolic effects during stimulation of uterine contractions by prostaglandin $F_{2\alpha}$ and inhibition by a β-adrenergic substance (Th-1165a). World Congress of Obstet. Gynecol., Moscow 1973, *Excerpta Medica*, Int. Congr. Ser. No. 279, 15

Ursell, W. (1972). Induction of labour following fetal death. *J. Obstet. Gynaecol. Brit. Cwlth.*, 79, 260–264

Vakhariya, V. R. and Sherman, A. I. (1972). Prostaglandin $F_{2\alpha}$ for induction of labor. *Amer. J. Obstet. Gynecol.*, 113, 212–222

Vroman, S., Thiery, M., Yo Le Sian, A., Depiere, M., Vanderheyden, K., Derom, R., Van Kets, H. and Brouckaert, J. (1972). A double blind comparative study of prostaglandin $F_{2\alpha}$ and oxytocin for the elective induction of labor. *Europ. J. Obstet. Gynaecol.*, 2, 115–123

Wagatsuma, T. (1965). Intra-amniotic injection of saline for therapeutic abortion. *Amer. J. Obstet. Gynecol.*, 93, 743–745

Wentz, A. C. and King, T. M. (1972). Intramyometrial prostaglandin $F_{2\alpha}$, *Amer. J. Obstet. Gynecol.*, 114, 112–114

Wilkin, D., Graham, F., Shields, M. and Craft, I. (1974). Selective induction of labour following administration of an oral prostaglandin E₂0.5 mg tablet hourly. *Prostaglandins*, 6, 405–411

Willis, A. L., Johnson, M., Rabinowitz, I. and Wolf, P. L. (1972). Prostaglandin E₂ may induce sickle-cell crisis. *New Eng. J. Med.*, 286, 783–784

Witting, W. C., Laros, R. K. and Work. B. A. (1973). Uterine response to prostaglandin $F_{2\alpha}$ infusion in term human pregnancy. *Obstet. Gynecol. (N.Y.)*, 42, 581–588

Witting, W. C., Work, B. A. and Laros, R. K. Jr. (1972). Uterine activity response to constant infusion of prostaglandin $F_{2\alpha}$ in term human pregnancy. In: *The Prostaglandins. Clinical Applications in Human Reproduction*, 77–84 (E. M. Southern, editor) (Mount Kisco, N.Y.: Futura)

Wiqvist, N., Bygdeman, M., Kwon, S. U., Mukherjee, T. and Roth-Brandel, U. (1968). Effect of prostaglandin E₁ on the midpregnant human uterus. *Amer. J. Obstet. Gynecol.*, 102, 327–332

Yip, S. K., Ma, H. K. and Ng, K. H. (1973). Induction of labour with oral prostaglandin E₂. *J. Obstet. Gynaecol. Brit. Cwlth.*, 80, 442–445

5
Prostaglandins and Reproduction in Sub-human Primates

K. T. KIRTON

5.1 INTRODUCTION

The first description of biological activity of prostaglandins was reported by Kurzrok and Lieb (1930) and the molecular structures nearly thirty years later by Bergström and Sjöval (1957). This more recent discovery has been followed by synthesis of pure materials which has led to widespread investigation of their biological activity. In keeping with their relatively high concentration in reproductive tissues and fluids, quite appropriately, a large amount of the current clinical interest in prostaglandins continues to be centered around their possible uses to control reproduction. This recent wave of interest in the effects of prostaglandins on reproductive processes was stimulated by a hypothesis (Pharriss, 1970) implicating $PGF_{2\alpha}$ as the uterine factor responsible for termination of corpus luteum activity in many species and by the early experiments of Karim (Karim, 1972), which implicated prostaglandins in human parturition.

In addition to an effect on ovarian steroidogenic tissue in non-pregnant animals, certain prostaglandins also terminate pregnancy when administered to a number of different species. This effect has been demonstrated at stages of gestation when the ovary is not necessary to maintain pregnancy in many species. Prostaglandins are effective abortifacient agents in primates if administered during early stages of pregnancy while the ovary is still required as a progesterone source to maintain the pregnancy, or later in gestation when the ovary is no longer required to maintain the pregnancy. This abortifacient activity, therefore, may be mediated by any of a number of mechanisms, including a direct effect on the uterus, or indirectly through the ovary or pituitary gland.

Results of studies to date implicate two generalised activities of prostaglandins; alteration of smooth muscle contractility and modulation of hormonal activity. Distribution of the intracellular enzyme system for prostaglandin synthesis is apparently very widespread, with endogenous tissue levels of the compounds reported for nearly every organ system examined. However, a physiological role of prostaglandins in normal reproductive processes has not been proven. The previously mentioned pharmacological activities undoubtedly will continue to dictate interest in their clinical development, but it should be emphasised that these studies describe pharmacologic effects of exogenously administered substances, and their normal physiological role remains to be determined. The purpose of this chapter is to summarise significant experimentation with prostaglandins in sub-human primates (see also Kirton, 1972).

5.2 EFFECTS IN NON-PREGNANT ANIMALS

5.2.1 Corpus luteum function

Prostaglandin $F_{2\alpha}$ antagonises corpus luteum function when administered *in vivo* in all subprimate species investigated to date (see Chapters 6 and 7). However, such inhibitory effects have been more difficult to demonstrate in non-pregnant primates. Subcutaneous injections of 15 mg of $PGF_{2\alpha}$ daily on cycle days 4 to 10 or days 7 to 11 postovulation (rhesus monkey) did not shorten the menstrual cycle or appreciably depress serum progestin levels. The injections were initiated prior to and continued past the time of maximal progestin secretion by the corpus luteum. In each of three additional monkeys 45 mg of $PGF_{2\alpha}$ was infused intravenously during a 24-hour period in the early to mid-luteal phase of their menstrual cycle. This treatment caused an initial increase in serum progestin levels from 3.2 ng ml^{-1} prior to the infusion to a peak concentration of 5.6 ng ml^{-1} four hours later—and a decline to preinjection levels within 12 hrs; the length of the menstrual cycle was not affected (Kirton *et al.*, 1970). These studies indicate that the non-pregnant primate corpus luteum is not as vulnerable to prostaglandin induced luteolysis as the corpus luteum of many laboratory and domestic animals. These studies have been expanded more recently, however, to include a more detailed examination of effects of prostaglandins on the sub-human primate ovary.

Prostaglandin $F_{2\alpha}$ was infused (45 mg) during the late luteal phase in non-pregnant rhesus monkeys (Kirton and Koering, 1973). Corpus luteum tissue was examined by light and electron microscopy and plasma samples obtained for progestin determinations. Prostaglandin infusion decreased plasma progestin concentrations, from 5.4 to 2.4 ng ml^{-1} and was also associated with morphologic tissue changes. Luteal tissue from treated animals was characterised by scattered patches of small cells, many of which contained lipid droplets of variable size and non-spherical shape. Auletta *et al.* (1973) infused $PGF_{2\alpha}$ via the femoral artery in patas and rhesus monkeys. The principal ovarian vein was cannulated for measurement of gesterone production and blood flow. Infusion of $PGF_{2\alpha}$ in low doses (< 50 μg min^{-1}) increased progesterone production, while infusions of 50 μg min^{-1} decreased progesterone production. HCG, administered intravenously, appeared to reverse the decrease in progesterone output. As measured in this experiment, prostaglandin treatment did not alter blood flow significantly.

Wan and co-workers (1974) also studied effects of $PGF_{2\alpha}$ on corpus luteum function in the rhesus monkey. They administered HCG postovulation through day 35 or 36, and imposed $PGF_{2\alpha}$ treatment on day 28 and 29. In 5/8 cycles luteal function was maintained up to day 35 or 36 by the HCG, but peripheral progesterone concentrations gradually declined after day 22–26 despite the continuous administration of HCG. Treatment with $PGF_{2\alpha}$ did not accelerate corpus luteum regression, when compared to the control cycles.

Shaikh and Klaiber (1974) reported effects of administering oestradiol and $PGF_{2\alpha}$ sequentially to *M. fascicularis*. Treatment was initiated on day 17 or 18 of the menstrual cycle, and consisted of oestradiol-17β alone (20 μg), $PGF_{2\alpha}$ alone (15 mg), progesterone alone (10 mg) or estradiol (20 μg) followed by $PGF_{2\alpha}$ (15 mg). Oestradiol alone depressed progesterone concentration but did not shorten the luteal phase of the menstrual cycle. Prostaglandin treatment depressed progesterone and initiated menstrual-like bleeding, which was followed by bleeding at the expected time of menstruation. Progesterone alone did not appear to alter the cycle. However, oestradiol and prostaglandin given sequentially shortened menstrual cycle length in 8/9 monkeys. Cycle lengths in all treatment groups were normal subsequent to treatment.

Effects of prostaglandins upon luteinisation of rhesus monkey granulosa cell cultures were studied by Channing (1972). Prostaglandin E_1 or E_2 stimulated progestin production and morphological luteinisation in each group of cultures at doses between 0.01 and 10 to 100 μg ml^{-1}. PGA_1 and $F_{2\alpha}$ were less effective. These prostaglandins were less effective stimulants than human LH. Addition of 10 μg ml^{-1} of $PGF_{2\alpha}$ or PGE_2 to 0.1 μg of LH inhibited the LH effect, thus indicating a luteolytic effect of $PGF_{2\alpha}$ or E_2 in this test system only when added in combination with gonadotrophin.

5.2.2 Ovulation

Recent investigations from a number of laboratories have indicated that prostaglandins E and F$_a$ are involved in the normal process of ovulation in the rat and rabbit (Armstrong *et al.*, 1974; Marsh *et al.*, 1974). Follicular fluid prostaglandin concentration increases, and the ratio of PGE:PGF changes, as ovulation approaches. Also intrafollicular injection of a prostaglandin synthesis inhibitor, Indomethacin, or of antisera to prostaglandin, inhibits ovulation. These studies indicate indirectly that prostaglandins are involved in the process of ovulation in these subprimate species (see also Chapters 6 and 7).

More recently, these studies have been extended to the primate. Batta and Brackett (1974) utilised a combined regimen of PMS, HCG and PGE$_1$ or E$_2$ to induce superovulation in *Macaca mulatta*. The authors concluded that prostaglandins of the E series complemented the PMS and HCG treatments, resulting in more consistent ovulation in this species. In their study the number of animals ovulating following the combined treatment was consistently greater than in those treated with gonadotrophin alone (17 of 18 compared to 1 of 5). These authors previously demonstrated that PGF$_{2\alpha}$ stimulated and PGE$_2$ inhibited ovarian contractility in this species. The PGF$_{2\alpha}$ stimulated contractility could be inhibited by isoproterenol, unless propranolol had been administered previously (Vitrutamasen *et al.*, 1973).

Rhesus monkey ovary, myometrium and endometrium released PGF$_{2\alpha}$ into media in an *in vitro* superfusion test system (Wilks *et al.*, 1972). Luteinising

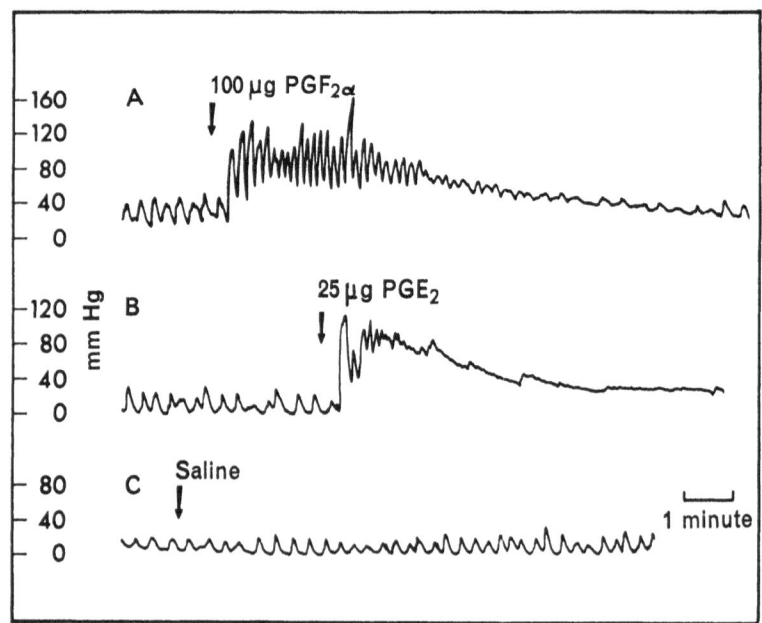

Figure 5.1 Uterine contractility induced by intravenous injection of prostaglandin E$_2$ or F$_{2\alpha}$ in a non-pregnant rhesus monkey

hormone stimulated the production of $PGF_{2\alpha}$ by ovarian tissue, but FSH and Prolactin did not. Oestradiol-17β stimulated $PGF_{2\alpha}$ synthesis by slices of myometrium but not endometrium. Progesterone had no effect.

5.2.3 Tubal and uterine motility

In addition to their effects on steroidogenic tissue, prostaglandins have been shown to alter uterine and fallopian tube motility both *in vivo* and *in vitro*. Acute intravenous injections of prostaglandins altered uterine motility of non-pregnant rhesus monkeys when injected during the luteal phase of the menstrual cycle. Prostaglandin $F_{2\alpha}$ increased uterine tone and amplitude of contractions, while PGE_2 increased tone but decreased amplitude of the contractions in this species (Figure 5.1).

Oshima and Matsumoto (1973) reported results of a study designed to measure absorption of PGE_2, given by various routes, to rhesus or Japanese monkeys. A rather slow absorption following oral administration was contrasted with the rapid disappearance following intravenous administration. A change in sensitivity of the uterus to prostaglandin was noted at various stages of the reproductive cycle as well. In general, sensitivity increased as the time of parturition approached. A decrease in sensitivity was then noted postpartum.

In an extension of earlier studies with naturally occurring primary prostaglandins and prostaglandin metabolites, Kirton and Forbes (1972) reported on the greatly increased potency of the 15 (S)-methyl analogues of PGE_2 and $PGF_{2\alpha}$. Using the pregnant uterus as a test organ, the 15 (S)-methyl analogue of both PGE_2 and $PGF_{2\alpha}$ were 8–10 times as potent as their corresponding naturally occurring precursors. Thus, alteration of the configuration at C-15 can either decrease (15-keto) or increase (15 (S)-methyl) the uterotropic potency of PGE_2 and $PGF_{2\alpha}$. Similar findings in human have been reported (see Chapter 2).

Neri and Marcus (1969) found that prostaglandin $F_{2\alpha}$ also increased fallopian tube motility of rhesus monkeys. Their work suggested these effects were altered by endogenous steroid hormones at various stages of the menstrual cycle. Such effects had been previously studied in humans (Bergström *et al.*, 1968).

Spilman *et al.* (1973) utilised a silicone balloon-ended catheter as a recording system for tubal motility in the rhesus monkey. Activity during the follicular phase of the menstrual cycle was characterised by high frequency (16/min) low amplitude (2–2.5 mmHg) contractions. The contractions decreased in frequency as the time of ovulation approached. The immediate postovulatory period was characterised by bursts of activity of relatively high amplitude (5–7.5 mmHg). The frequency and amplitude then decreased for the remainder of the cycle. Intravenous infusion of prostaglandin E_1 or E_2 (5–20 μg kg^{-1}) had little effect on oviduct motility during the follicular phase of the cycle, but depressed spontaneous motility after ovulation. $PGF_{2\alpha}$ (5–20 μg kg^{-1}) increased activity markedly after ovulation, but had only a slight stimulatory effect in the early follicular phase of the menstrual cycle.

5.3 EFFECTS IN PREGNANT ANIMALS

5.3.1 Early pregnancy termination

The original hypothesis of Pharriss (1970), suggested that $PGF_{2\alpha}$ might be luteolytic by exerting a venoconstrictor effect on the utero–ovarian vein. If prostaglandins terminate pregnancy by this mechanism, then corpus luteum function must be indispensable to maintenance of the pregnancy at the time of prostaglandin administration. Published data in rhesus monkeys (Tullner and Hertz, 1966a) and unpublished observations in humans indicate that the ovary is the indispensable source of progesterone for about the first 25–35 days of pregnancy in each of these primate species. Therefore, pharmacological interruption of pregnancy could be mediated by an effect at the ovary up to this stage of gestation.

In an experiment with rhesus monkeys (Kirton et al., 1970), $PGF_{2\alpha}$ was injected subcutaneously starting at 11–13 days after ovulation. At this early stage of pregnancy, the peripheral serum progestin concentration is increasing, presumably in response to a trophic stimulation from the implanting blastocyst (Neill et al., 1969b). This trend continues until about day 25 of pregnancy, when progestin concentrations reach a peak and then decrease abruptly, even in the presence of increased concentrations of chorionic gonadotrophin (Tullner and Hertz, 1966b). Apparently the corpus luteum of this species is no longer capable of maintaining maximal steroidogenic function after this stage of gestation. Injection of $PGF_{2\alpha}$ subcutaneously at a rate of 30 mg/animal/day for five days resulted in a rather dramatic decrease in peripheral plasma progestin levels within 24 hours after the first injection. This rapid decrease in steroid level was associated with onset of vaginal bleeding.

An increase concentration of plasma progestin indicated that at least four of the six treated animals were pregnant at the time of the first injection. Progestin levels were suppressed to non-detectable concentrations and pregnancy was terminated in all but one animal. The peripheral progestin concentration was initially depressed but again increased during the last day of treatment and pregnancy was maintained in that animal. Peripheral plasma progestin levels were also decreasing in non-treated animals at this stage of pregnancy, but the magnitude and rate of the change was significantly different from the treated animals. The decrease in progestin concentration of the non-treated animals was less precipitous and levels did not decrease to non-detectable amounts.

An ovarian source of progesterone is necessary to maintain early stages of pregnancy in both primates (Csapo et al., 1973) and subprimates species. However, a lytic effect of the uterus on the corpus luteum has not been demonstrated in primates and the factors which cause the normal demise of the corpus luteum in these species is not known. Indeed, the ovary apparently continues to cycle normally in the complete absence of the uterus in the rhesus monkey (Neil et al., 1969a) and the human (Doyle et al., 1971). Therefore, if the mechanism of prostaglandin-induced pregnancy termination in primates is by luteolysis, it does not mimic a naturally occurring uterine factor in these species. Nevertheless, the rapid depression in peripheral progestin concentration noted in the present experiment may reflect a direct effect of $PGF_{2\alpha}$ on the ovary of the treated animals.

Another possible explanation for the rapid progestin drop in the monkey experiment could be removal of the stimulus (the implanting blastocyst) for corpus luteum function, since exogenous natural E and F prostaglandins are very potent stimulants of uterine motility. Such an increased activity could be expected to interrupt pregnancy directly, by dislodging the blastocyst which would then result in a demise of the corpus luteum indirectly by removing its trophic support.

5.3.2 Late pregnancy termination

Prostaglandin E_2 and $F_{2\alpha}$ are also capable of terminating pregnancy in primates at later stages of gestation, when the ovary is no longer a required source of progesterone for maintenance of the pregnancy. Prostaglandin $F_{2\alpha}$ was effective in terminating pregnancy when administered by subcutaneous injection or intravenous infusion prior to day 30 or after day 100 of pregnancy. (Kirton et al., 1971).

Induction of rhythmical myometrial contractility of sufficient amplitude and duration to interrupt pregnancy is apparently the mechanism responsible for this effect. It is not known if this is a direct effect of prostaglandins on the myometrium, or an indirect effect initiated by prostaglandins, but mediated through another system. However, earlier reported studies indicate that the activity was caused by a direct action of prostaglandin on the myometrial cell (Paton and Daniel, 1967).

Uterine contractility was monitored by inserting an open-ended fluid-filled polyethylene catheter through the cervical canal into the uterine lumen at early stages (up to day 40) of pregnancy, or transabdominally into the amniotic sac at later stages (Caldeyro-Barcia and Poseiro, 1959). Comparison of changes in resting tone and amplitude and frequency of rhythmical contractions were used as a quantitative index of comparative potency of various compounds, sensitivity at various stages of pregnancy and effectiveness of various routes of administration.

Quantitative comparisons of uterine stimulation obtained in this way were related to the effectiveness of prostaglandins in interrupting pregnancy. The uterus was more sensitive to prostaglandin stimulation either very early in pregnancy, or during later stages. The period of relative insensitivity to prostaglandins during the mid-trimester also corresponds to a period of relative uterine quiescence during normal pregnancy in this species (Corner et al., 1963), as opposed to periods of higher endogenous activity at earlier stages of pregnancy.

Prostaglandin E_2 is about 10 times as potent a uterine stimulant in rhesus monkeys as $PGF_{2\alpha}$ when compared by a number of routes of administration. Infusion of 0.8 μg min^{-1} of PGE_2, or 8.0 μg min^{-1} of $PGF_{2\alpha}$ induced contractility of comparable strength. Higher rates of infusion were associated with increased uterine tone and a less synchronous pattern of contractility. The uterine response to a single subcutaneous injection of 15 mg of $PGF_{2\alpha}$ or 2 mg of PGE_2 is illustrated in Figure 5.1. These injections caused an initial increase in uterine tone which was then followed by a gradual initiation of rhythmic contractions and decrease in resting tone of the uterus. Synchronous contractions persisted at the maximal intensity and frequency for two to four hours after injections, then gradually decreased in frequency and amplitude.

5.4 MECHANISM OF PROSTAGLANDIN INDUCED MYOMETRIAL ACTIVITY

The mechanism whereby prostaglandins stimulate myometrial contractility has not been clearly elucidated to date. They have been strongly implicated in controlling normal blood flow in various reproductive organs (Pharriss, 1970), a mechanism which could well be involved in their uterotropic effect. Novy (1973) utilised muclide-labelled microspheres to study effects of PGE_2 induced contractility on uterine and placental blood flow. Sustained contractions decreased placental flow ($P<0.001$) and simultaneously increased myometrial flow ($P<0.02$). However, fetal umbilical blood flow was maintained during rhythmic uterine contractions. Einer-Jensen (1973) utilised 133Xe clearance to study endometrial blood flow in rhesus monkeys. Instillation of 10 μg of $PGF_{2\alpha}$ decreased blood flow to 39% of the pretreatment level ($P = 0.01$). Plasma progesterone in peripheral samples was decreased to 23% of the original pretreatment at 20 hours after the instillation.

The interrelationship between ethanol and oxytocin or prostaglandin induced uterine contractility is not entirely clear at this point. Lauersen *et al.* (1973) studied the interaction of these three agents in the pregnant baboon. They found similar patterns of uterine contractility when either oxytocin or $PGF_{2\alpha}$ were utilised. The most noticeable difference was the marked sustained stimulatory effect of the prostaglandin, which decreased by 18% one hour after discontinuance of prostaglandin as compared to a 50% decrease after oxytocin infusion. Ethanol inhibited effects of only threshold doses of oxytocin or prostaglandin. The response to higher levels of either stimulant was not diminished by ethanol. The authors concluded that 'the main effect of ethanol on uterine contractions in the baboon appears to be mediated by its central inhibitory action on oxytocin release'.

Indomethacin, an inhibitor of prostaglandin biosynthesis, prolonged normal gestation in rhesus monkeys (Novy *et al.*, 1974). The uterus was, however, still responsive to exogenous oxytocin, in the indomethacin treated animals.

In an additional study to investigate the mechanism of $PGF_{2\alpha}$ induced uterine contractility, Wilson *et al.* (1974) investigated several adrenergic drugs on PGE_2 or $PGF_{2\alpha}$ or oxytocin induced contractions. Diazoxide was the most potent inhibitor of uterine activity in this series of tests in the baboon. Neither isoproterenol nor metaproterenol had significant effects on $PGF_{2\alpha}$-induced activity, although the latter inhibited spontaneous and oxytocin induced contractions. Ritodrine also effectively reduced spontaneous contractions but did not inhibit $PGF_{2\alpha}$-induced activity.

5.5 PROSTAGLANDINS AND METABOLITES IN RHESUS MONKEY

Demers *et al.* (1974) measured $PGF_{2\alpha}$ concentrations in monkey uterine fluid collected through silicone tubing inserted into the uterine lumen. Highest values were found during the 18–20th day of the menstrual cycle. Oestrogen treatment increased the values, while progesterone had little effect.

Challis *et al.* (1974) measured the peripheral plasma $PGF_{2\alpha}$ concentration in the rhesus monkey during normal pregnancy and after administration of dexamethasone and $PGF_{2\alpha}$. Prostaglandin$_{2\alpha}$ did, but dexamethasone did not induce abortion. Plasma PGF concentration was highly variable and apparently not affected by dexamethasone treatment, nor did it change during the later stages of pregnancy before spontaneous parturition in untreated animals.

Much of the pharmacokinetics of prostaglandins was initially determined in the human (Samuelsson, 1973). However, studies conducted in sub-human primates to date indicate that they are very similar to man in this respect. Prostaglandins disappear very quickly from peripheral circulation, having a half-life of less than 30 s. This is contrasted with a much slower disappearance from amniotic fluid (5–7 hours half-life). In addition the 13, 14-dihydro-15-keto metabolite is present in higher concentrations than is the

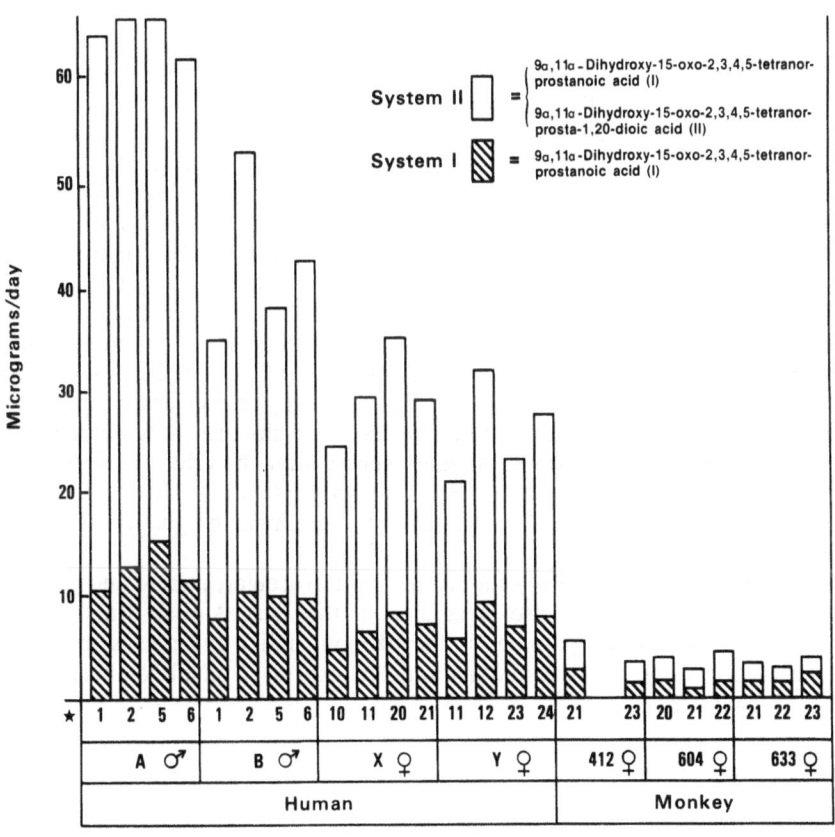

Figure 5.2 Urinary excretion of $PGF_{2\alpha}$ metabolites

parent $PGF_{2\alpha}$, thus indicating this to be a principal metabolite in the rhesus monkey as well as the human (Cornette *et al.*, 1974).

Studies have shown that cellular elements in monkey blood, probably platelets, are capable of synthesising large amounts of prostaglandin during the clotting process. However, the concentration of prostaglandin metabolite was not elevated during clotting, indicating that measurement of metabolite concentrations may more closely reflect endogenous conditions.

Measurement of $PGF_{2\alpha}$ metabolites excreted in rhesus monkey urine indicated that total synthesis is less than $30\mu g/24$ hours for this species (Cornette *et al.*, 1975). This is similar, on a body weight basis, to synthesis rates previously reported for the human (Samuelsson, 1973). However, the ratio of mono-acid to di-acid metabolite was much closer in the rhesus than values previously reported in the human (Figure 5.2).

5.6 VALUE OF SUB-HUMAN PRIMATES FOR PRECLINICAL INVESTIGATION OF PROSTAGLANDINS

The relative potency of PGE_2 and $PGF_{2\alpha}$ in producing uterine contractions in primates, is a significant departure from lower species of laboratory animals in which E_2 is a less potent pregnancy-terminating compound than $F_{2\alpha}$ (Gutknecht *et al.*, 1970). The increased potency of PGE_2 over $PGF_{2\alpha}$ in the monkey measured in terms of uterine stimulation, is similar to the potency ratio in humans when administered during the first half of pregnancy (Karim and Filshie, 1970) or near term to induce labour (Karim *et al.*, 1969). Thus; the relative potencies of these two compounds, measured in terms of initiation of myometrial contractions, are similar in the human and monkey. However, if expressed on a body weight basis, a much larger dose is required in the monkey. The relatively sensitivity of the uterus to prostaglandin-induced abortions at various stages of pregnancy is also similar in the human and rhesus monkey. A difference in basic physiological mechanism of corpus luteum maintenance is an additional area in which primates and subprimate species have been demonstrated to differ. These results then, when compared to data obtained with laboratory animals, substantiate the value of sub-human primates for preclinical investigations of prostaglandins. However, some similarities do exist, in that prostaglandins terminate pregnancy in these subprimate species also.

Ganesan and Karim (1974) studied the cardiovascular, uterine and gastro-intestinal effects of some prostaglandins in the East African Baboon (*P. Anubis*). In these three parameters the baboon, unlike the rhesus monkey, responds both qualitatively and quantitatively (expressed on a body basis) in a similar manner to man.

References

Armstrong, D. T., Grinwich, D. L., Moon, Y. S. and Zamecnik, J. (1974). Inhibition of ovulation in rabbits by intrafollicular injection of indomethacin and prostaglandin F antiserum. *Life Sci.*, **14**, 129–140

Auletta, F. J., Speroff, L. and Caldwell, B. V. (1973). Prostaglandin $F_{2\alpha}$ induced steroidogenesis and luteolysis in the primate corpus luteum. *J. Clin. Endocrinol. Metab.*, **36**, 405–407

Batta, S. K. and Brackett, B. G. (1974). Ovulation induction in rhesus monkeys by treatment with gonadotropins and prostaglandins. *Prostaglandins*, 6, 45–54

Bergstrom, S., Carlson, L. A. and Weeks, J. R. (1968). The prostaglandins: A family of biologically active lipids. *Pharmacol. Rev.*, 20, 1–48

Bergstrom, S. and Sjovall, J. (1957). The isolation of prostaglandin. *Acta Chem. Scand.*, 11, 1086

Caldeyro-Barcia, R. and Poseiro, J. J. (1959). Oxytocin and contractility of the pregnant human uterus. *Ann. N.Y. Acad Sci.*, 75, 813–830

Challis, J. R. G., Davies, I. J., Hendricks, A. G. and Ryan, K. J. (1974). Prostaglandin F in the peripheral plasma of the rhesus monkey in normal pregnancy and after the administration of dexamethasone and $PGF_{2\alpha}$. *Prostaglandins*, 6, 389–396

Channing, C. P. (1972). Stimulatory effects of prostaglandins upon luteinization of rhesus monkey granulosa cell cultures. *Prostaglandins*, 2, 331–367

Corner, G. W., Ramsey, E. M. and Stran, H. (1963). Patterns of myometrial activity in the rhesus monkey in pregnancy. *Amer. J. Obstet. Gynecol.*, 85, 179–185

Cornette, J. C., Harrison, K. L. and Kirton, K. T. (1974). Measurement of Prostaglandin $F_{2\alpha}$ metabolites by radioimmunoassay. *Prostaglandins*, 5, 155–164

Cornette, J. C., Kirton, K. T., Schneider, W. P., Sun, F. F., Johnson, R. A. and Nidy, E. G. (1975). Preparation and quantitation of urinary metabolites of prostaglandin $F_{2\alpha}$ by radioimmunoassay. *Prostaglandins*, 9, 323–338

Csapo, A. I., Pulkkinen, M. O. and Wiest, W. G. (1973). Effects of lutectomy and progesterone replacement therapy in early pregnant patients. *Amer. J. Obstet. Gynecol.*, 115, 759–765

Demers, L. M., Yoshinaga, K. and Greep, R. O. (1974). Prostaglandin F in monkey uterine fluid during the menstrual cycle and following steroid treatment. *Prostaglandins*, 5, 513–519

Doyle, L. L., Barclay, D. L., Duncan, G. W. and Kirton, K. T. (1971). Human luteal function following hysterectomy as assessed by plasma progestin. *Amer. J. Obstet. Gynecol.*, 110, 92–97

Einer-Jensen, N. (1973). Decreased endometrial blood flow and plasma progesterone level after instillation of 10 μg prostaglandin $F_{2\alpha}$ into the lumen of the uteri of rhesus monkeys. *Prostaglandins*, 45, 517–522

Ganesan, P. A. and Karim, S. M. M. (1974). Acute toxicity of prostaglandins E_2, $F_{2\alpha}$, and 15 (S), 15-methyl prostaglandin E_2 methyl ester in the baboon. *Prostaglandins*, 7, 215–221

Gutknecht, G. D., Duncan, G. W. and Wyngarden, L. J. (1970). Effect of prostaglandin $F_{2\alpha}$ on ovarian blood flow in the rabbit as measured by hydrogen desaturation. *Physiologist*, 13, 214

Karim, S. M. M. (1972). Prostaglandins and human reproduction: Physiological Roles and clinical uses of prostaglandins in relation to human reproduction. In: *Prostaglandins —Progress in Research*, 71–164 (S. M. M. Karim, editor) (Lancaster: M.T.P.)

Karim, S. M. M., Trussell, R. R., Hillier, K. and Patel, R. C. (1969). Induction of labour with prostaglandin $F_{2\alpha}$. *J. Obstet. Gynaecol. Brit. Cwlth.*, 76, 769–782

Karim, S. M. M. and Filshie, G. M. (1970). Therapeutic abortion using prostaglandin $F_{2\alpha}$, *Lancet*, I, 157–159

Kirton, K. T. (1972). Prostaglandins and Reproduction in sub-human primates. In: *Prostaglandins—Progress in Research*, 47–70 (S. M. M. Karim, editor) (Lancaster: M.T.P.)

Kirton, K. T., Pharriss, B. B. and Forbes, A. D. (1970). Luteolytic effects of prostaglandin $F_{2\alpha}$ in primates. *Proc. Soc. Exp. Biol. Med.*, 133, 314–316

Kirton, K. T., Duncan, G. W., Oesterling, T. and Forbes, A. D. (1971). Prostaglandins and reproduction in the rhesus monkey. *Ann. N.Y. Acad. Sci.*, 180, 445–455

Kirton, K. T. and Forbes, A. D. (1972). Activity of 15 (S), 15-methyl prostaglandin E_2 and $F_{2\alpha}$ as stimulants of uterine contractility. *Prostaglandins*, 1, 319–325

Kirton, K. T. and Koering, M. J. (1973). Prostaglandin $F_{2\alpha}$ and primate corpus luteum: a correlation of structure and function. *Fertility and Sterility*, 24, 926–934

Kurzrok, R. and Lieb, C. C. (1930). Biochemical studies of human semen. II. The action of semen on the human uterus. *Proc. Soc. Exp. Biol. Med.*, 28, 268–272

Lauersen, N. H., Raghavan, K. S., Wilson, K. H., Fuchs, F. and Niemann, W. H. (1973). Effects of prostaglandin $F_{2\alpha}$, oxytocin and ethanol on the uterus of the pregnant baboon. *Amer. J. Obstet. Gynecol.*, 115, 912–918

Marsh, J. M., Yang, N. S. T. and LeMaire, W. J. (1974). Prostaglandin synthesis in rabbit Graafian follicles *in vitro*. Effect of luteinizing hormone and cyclic AMP. *Prostaglandins*, 7, 269–283

Neill, J. D., Johansson, E. D. B. and Knobil, E. (1969a). Failure of hysterectomy to influence the normal pattern of cyclic progesterone secretion in the rhesus monkey. *Endocrinol.*, **84**, 464–465

Neill, J. D., Johansson, E. D. B. and Knobil, E. (1969b). Patterns of circulating progesterone concentrations during the fertile menstrual cycle and the remainder of gestation in the rhesus monkey. *Endocrinol.*, **84**, 45–48

Neri, A. and Marcus, S. L. (1969). *In vivo* study of tubal motility in the rhesus monkey during the various phases of the menstrual cycle. *Ann. N.Y. Acad. Sci. 2nd Conference on Exp. Med. and Surg. Primates*

Novy, M. J. (1973). Effect of uterine contractions on myometrial, placental and umbilical blood flow in the rhesus monkey. *Abstr. Soc. Gynecol. Invest., 20th Ann. Meet*, 28–30 March 1973 Atlanta, pp. 25

Novy, M. J., Cook, M. J. and Manaugh, L. (1974). Indomethacin block of normal onset of parturition in primates. *Amer. J. Obstet. Gynecol.*, **118**, 412–416

Oshima, K. and Matsumoto, K. (1973). Absorption of prostaglandin E_2 and uterine sensitivity of the non-pregnant and pregnant monkey *in vivo*. *Prostaglandins*, **3**, 447–455

Paton, D. M. and Daniel, E. E. (1967). On the contractile response of the isolated rat uterus to prostaglandin E_1. *Can. J. Physiol. Pharmacol.*, **45**, 795–804

Pharriss, B. B. (1970). The possible vascular regulation of luteal function. *Perspect. Biol. Med.*, **13**, 434–444

Samuelsson, B. (1973). Biosynthesis and metabolism of prostaglandins. In: *Prostaglandins 1973*, 21–41 (Paris: Inserm)

Shaikh, A. A. and Klaiber, E. L. (1974). Effects of sequential treatment with estradiol and $PGF_{2\alpha}$ on the length of the primate menstrual cycle. *Prostaglandins*, **6**, 253–262

Spilman, C. H., Forbes, A. D. and Norland, J. F. (1973). Oviduct motility during the rhesus monkey menstrual cycle: effect of prostaglandins. *Abstr. Amer. Meeting Soc. Study Reprod. in Biol. Reprod.*, **9**, 68

Tullner, W. W. and Hertz, R. (1966a). Normal gestation and chorionic gonadotropin levels in the monkey after ovariectomy in early pregnancy. *Endocrinol.*, **78**, 1076

Tullner, W. W. and Hertz, R. (1966b). Chorionic gonadotropin levels in the rhesus monkey during early pregnancy. *Endocrinol.*, **78**, 204–207

Vitrutamasen, P., Wright, K. H. and Wallach, E. E. (1973). Monkey ovarian contractility—its relationship to ovulation. *Fertility and Sterility*, **24**, 763–771

Wan, L. S., Khatamee, M., Neimann, W., Fellu, C. and Bigelow, B. (1974). The effect of prostaglandin $F_{2\alpha}$ on corpus luteum function in the rhesus monkey. *Fertility and Sterility*, **25**, 292

Wilks, J. W., Forbes, K. K. and Norland, J. F. (1972). Synthesis of prostaglandin $F_{2\alpha}$ by the ovary and uterus. *J. Reprod. Med.*, **9**, 271–276

Wilson, K. H., Lauersen, N. H., Raghavan, K. S., Fuchs, F. and Niemann, W. H. (1974). Effects of diazoxide and beta-adrenergic drugs on spontaneous and induced uterine activity in the pregnant baboon. *Amer. J. Obstet. Gynecol.*, **118**, 499–509

6
Prostaglandins and Studies Related to Reproduction in Laboratory Animals

A. P. LABHSETWAR

Abbreviations

HCG: Human chorionic gonadotrophin
GLC: Gas–liquid chromatography
LH: Luteinising hormone
PMSG: Pregnant mare serum gonadotrophin
TLC: Thin layer chromatography

6.1 INTRODUCTION

Effects of prostaglandins on the reproductive system of laboratory animals are
varied. The presence of prostaglandin-like material in many reproductive
tissues has raised the possibility concerning their physiological functions.
Although the interest in this area was rekindled by many observations
originally made on the human reproductive system (see Karim, 1972), in
recent years laboratory animals have been increasingly used. This followed the
demonstration by Pharriss and Wyngarden (1969) that $PGF_{2\alpha}$ exerts a
luteolytic effect in the rat. Because of obvious implications of their observation
to physiological control of luteal function and consequently to the regulation of
fertility in human and domestic animals, the subsequent period has witnessed a
rapid explosion of publications utilising not only rats but also other laboratory
species. It is debatable whether this flood of information often involving
repetitive experiments with conflicting results has resulted in a commensurate
increase in our understanding of the roles of prostaglandins in the reproductive
system. Nevertheless it reflects an unparallelled interest in this area. This has
resulted in numerous reviews which may be consulted for further information
(Weeks, 1972; Labhsetwar, 1974). The purpose of this chapter is to focus
attention on the effects of prostaglandins on the reproductive system with a
particular emphasis on the laboratory animals although from time to time
information on other species will be briefly included in an effort to integrate the
chapter with the rest of the book. It is assumed that the reader has a basic
familiarity with the reproductive system of the laboratory animals.

6.2 ROLE OF PROSTAGLANDINS IN LUTEAL FUNCTION

One of the most dramatic effects of prostaglandins on the reproductive system
involves their ability to reduce progesterone secretion by the corpus luteum

(luteolysis). Such an effect may or may not be accompanied by a morphological degeneration of the corpus luteum. The luteolytic effect of $PGF_{2\alpha}$ was first described in the rat (Pharriss and Wyngarden, 1969) and in the guinea-pig (Blatchley and Donovan, 1969) and later extended to other laboratory species such as the hamster (Gutknecht et al., 1971b; Labhsetwar, 1971b), the mouse (Bartke et al., 1972; Labhsetwar, 1972b) and the rabbit (Duncan and Pharriss, 1971; Keyes and Bullock, 1974). Among the laboratory animals so far studied, the hamster appears to be the most sensitive. A single subcutaneous injection of less than 25 μg of $PGF_{2\alpha}$ can induce luteolysis (Gutknecht, et al., 1971b; Labhsetwar, 1972a, b). The effect appears very prompt. In the hamster Gutknecht et al. (1971b) observed a significant drop in progesterone within 15 min and in the rat Behrman et al. (1971b) reported a similar drop by six hours after injection of $PGF_{2\alpha}$. The sensitivity of the corpus luteum to the luteolytic effects of $PGF_{2\alpha}$ varies according to its age. In the hamster and rat very young corpus luteum (less than four days old) appears to be relatively resistant unless large doses of prostaglandins are used (Gutknecht et al., 1969a; Labhsetwar, 1972a, b). The sensitivity increases around the time of implantation, i.e. days 4–6 of pregnancy and again decreases in the second half of pregnancy presumably due to placental secretion of luteotrophic hormones which apparently over-rides the luteolytic effect of exogenous prostaglandin.

Prostaglandins of the E series also exert luteolytic effects in the hamster and the rat (Nutting and Cammarata, 1969; Labhsetwar, 1972a, 1973b). In the hamster both prostaglandins E_2 and E_1 are luteolytic (Labhsetwar, 1972a, 1973b), whereas in the rat only PGE_2 proved effective; PGE_1 was found to be toxic (Labhsetwar, 1973b). In general PGE_2 is 10 times less potent than $PGF_{2\alpha}$ as a luteolytic agent. This may be due to either inherent differences in potency, conversion of PGE_2 to PGFs in vivo and/or the presence of PGF residues in the PGE samples due to incomplete separation during the process of chemical synthesis. However, it is doubtful that such a contamination alone can account for the luteolytic effects of PGEs. Synthetic analogues of PGFs and PGEs more potent than parent prostaglandins in causing luteolysis have also been described (Labhsetwar, 1974; also see Chapters 3 and 5).

6.2.1 Theories of luteolysis

Mechanisms by which prostaglandins exert luteolytic effects have been a subject of intensive research. Current theories are discussed below:

6.2.1.1 Vascular insult

Pharriss (1970) was originally motivated to explore the potential luteolytic effect of prostaglandins because of the known vasoconstrictor action of $PGF_{2\alpha}$ (DuCharme et al., 1968) and its presence in the uterine tissue of several species (Pickles, 1967). Pharriss implicated the venoconstrictor property of $PGF_{2\alpha}$ in luteolysis and postulated that $PGF_{2\alpha}$ by decreasing ovarian drainage caused vascular stasis in the ovary leading to the demise of corpora lutea (Pharriss 1970). It was found that a single intravenous injection of $PGF_{2\alpha}$ into rabbits and rats caused a sharp drop in the ovarian vein blood flow which lasted up to an hour (Pharriss *et al.*, 1970). The decrease in the ovarian blood flow was associated with a fall in the plasma progesterone but was not associated with any significant decrease in the renal blood flow (Gutknecht *et al.*, 1970). Similar observations were recently made in the rhesus monkey (Kirton *et al.*, 1972). Further evidence for this hypothesis was provided by the fact that until recently luteolytic effect of $PGF_{2\alpha}$ could not be demonstrated *in vitro*, most investigators finding a luteotrophic effect under these conditions (see page 246).

Additional evidence is, however, clearly required before the vacular insult can be accepted as a sole cause of luteolysis. It is not known if a decreased blood flow to the corpus luteum is a cause or an effect of luteolysis. It is even debatable whether there is a decreased blood flow through the ovary since others have failed to note such a decrease in the sheep (McCracken *et al.*, 1973), the hamster (Labhsetwar, 1974), the rat (Behrman *et al.*, 1971b) and the monkey (Auletta *et al.*, 1973). Even if it is accepted that failure of these investigators was due to the use of a crude rather than a sensitive technique for the measurement of blood flow, it is difficult to reconcile the fact that prostaglandins E_1 and E_2 both of which are potent vasodilators (Horton, 1969; Weeks, 1972) even with respect to the ovary (Aldridge *et al.*, 1970; McCracken, Baird and Goding, 1972a) exert luteolytic effects in rats (Labhsetwar, 1972a) hamsters (Labhsetwar, 1973b) and sheep (Aldridge *et al.*, 1970; McCracken *et al.*, 1973). As already indicated the luteolytic effect of $PGF_{2\alpha}$ in rabbits was associated with a selective decrease in the ovarian vein blood flow with no significant alterations in the renal blood flow (Gutknecht *et al.*, 1970). Yet it has been recently demonstrated that the ectopic corpus luteum in the kidney underwent luteolysis in response to $PGF_{2\alpha}$ in a manner similar to that of corpora lutea left in the ovary of the same rabbits (Keyes and Bullock, 1974). Indeed the conclusion that a decreased blood flow through the ovary or even through the corpus luteum is detrimental to the luteal function is largely intuitive. It has been recently demonstrated that the corpus luteum of the rat maintained on progesterone can be autotransplanted to an ectopic site without compromising its functions and morphological integrity (Gibori and Kraicer, 1972). Since revascularisation of the luteal tissue must take some time following transplantation, it is clear that a transient withdrawal of blood flow from the corpus luteum is not incompatible with its survival. Even the failure of many to demonstrate luteolytic effects *in vitro* cannot be taken as evidence for vascular involvement, as recently such an effect has been demonstrated in the rabbit corpora following relatively long incubation *in vitro*, i.e. six hours (O'Grady *et al.*, 1972b). It is, however, questionable if the luteolysis induced by $PGF_{2\alpha}$ *in vivo* and *in vitro* represents the same phenomenon and involves the same events since *in vivo* luteolysis can occur within an hour while *in vitro* effect apparently takes a longer time. If a decreased blood flow through the ovary and a resultant vascular stasis is critical in luteolysis, then why doesn't the same vascular stasis affect the ovarian follicles? It is known that the deleterious effects of prostaglandins are solely confined to the corpus luteum and do not extend to the follicles in guinea-pigs (Blatchley and Donovan, 1969), rabbits (Koering and Kirton, 1973) and hamsters (Labhsetwar, 1972a). A generalised vascular stasis in the ovary as postulated by

Pharriss (1970) does not account for this highly selective action of $PGF_{2\alpha}$ on the ovary.

6.2.1.2 Altered gonadotrophin secretion

The second hypothesis advanced to account for luteolytic effects of prostaglandins involves increased secretion of LH from the pituitary and perhaps alterations in the secretion of other gonadotrophins which constitute a part of the luteotrophic hormone complex (Labhsetwar, 1970, 1974). Pharriss et al. (1968) originally suggested that since pituitary LH content of spayed rats remained unchanged following treatment with $PGF_{2\alpha}$, it is unlikely that altered gonadotrophin secretion is involved in luteolysis. However, as the rats in their experiments were bilaterally spayed, the model was not sensitive enough to detect stimulatory effects of prostaglandins on the gonadotrophin secretion. Labhsetwar (1970) found that administration of antifertility doses of $PGF_{2\alpha}$ to pregnant rats for four days resulted in a significant increase in pituitary LH stores. The stimulatory effects of prostaglandins on gonadotrophin secretion have since been confirmed by a number of workers (see page 259). It has been known for some time that LH exerts a luteolytic effect in the rat (Rothchild, 1965), hamster (Greenwald, 1967a) and rabbit (Stormshak and Casida, 1965). It is thus conceivable that increased secretion of LH and/or other gonadotrophins leading to alterations in the luteotrophic hormone complex could account for luteolysis induced by prostaglandins. In effect this hypothesis implies that luteolytic effect of prostaglandins may involve the hypothalamico–pituitary complex. This does not necessarily exclude the local action of prostaglandins on the ovary in inducing luteolysis. The central action may be important under experimental conditions utilising what must be regarded as pharmacologic doses of prostaglandins. The fact that exogenous administration of hormones which are luteotrophic for a given species reverses the luteolytic effects of prostaglandins (see page 246) suggests that the central effect of prostaglandins may be important.

This hypothesis, however, was not supported by the results of Zor et al. (1972) who found that the addition of prostaglandins to the pituitary glands incubated with crude hypothalamic extracts stimulated the formation of cAMP but not the release of LH into the medium. However, at the present time the role of cAMP in the release of LH is not known and it is far from clear if their hypothalamic extract, which was only partially pure and contained other releasing factors, increased cAMP formation selectively in gonadotrophs or in other pituitary cells. Pharriss (1970) found that $PGF_{2\alpha}$ antagonised the supportive effect of prolactin on progesterone content of the ovary of hypophysecomised rats treated with gonadotrophins, (to induce formation of corpora lutea). Whether or not these induced corpora lutea are functionally comparable to normal corpora is not known. Recently, attempts have been made to apply this hypothesis to mice (Marley, 1972), guinea-pigs (Blatchley and Donovan, 1972) and sheep (Chamley and Christie, 1973), but have not been successful. This is not surprising as LH is not known to be luteolytic in these species and perhaps alterations in the secretion of gonadotrophins other than LH may be involved (Labhsetwar, 1973c; 1974).

6.2.1.3 Direct effect on the lutein cells

Behrman *et al.* (1971b) have postulated that rather than vascular or central effects, intracellular changes induced by a direct action of prostaglandins on the lutein cells may be involved in luteolysis. It is known that cholesterol in the lutein cells exist in two pools—esterified and free—the latter being utilised for the synthesis of progesterone. The relative size of the two pools is determined by cholesterol synthetase and esterase enzyme activity. Behrman *et al.* (1971a) found that in hypophysectomised immature rats treated with gonadotrophins to produce superovulation, cholesterol synthetase activity was stimulated by prolactin and this action was antagonised by $PGF_{2\alpha}$. However, cholesterol esterase activity was not affected to the same degree by the prostaglandin treatment. They postulated that $PGF_{2\alpha}$ antagonises the trophic influence of prolactin on cholesterol biosynthesis and results in the depletion of cholesterol stores, due to lack of precursors. This leads to a decline in progesterone secretion in the $PGF_{2\alpha}$-treated animals. The extent to which this theory is applicable to corpora lutea of pregnancy or pseudopregnancy of rats or to corpora of other species where prolactin may not be required for the luteal maintenance is not known. Additional changes occurring in the lutein cells as a result of $PGF_{2\alpha}$ administration involves loss of ability of luteal cells to bind to oestrogen in the rabbit (Jacobson *et al.*, 1972) and LH in the rat (Hichens *et al.*, 1974). These studies would indicate that luteolysis is not necessarily due to a withdrawal of the luteotrophic support but interference by $PGF_{2\alpha}$ with the action of that support as a result of loss of specific receptors.

6.2.2 Reversal of luteolytic effects by luteotrophic hormones

Although prostaglandins exert luteolytic effects, several investigators have shown that simultaneous administration of a luteotrophic hormone (or a combination of hormones which constitutes the luteotrophic hormone complex) can prevent the luteolytic effects of prostaglandins. Behrman *et al.* (1971b) found that a single injection of $PGF_{2\alpha}$ into pseudopregnant rats (hypophysectomised prior to prostaglandin treatment) on day 5 increased secretion of 20_α-dihydro-progesterone which is a characteristic feature of luteolysis in rats but simultaneous administration of LH prevented this rise. Chatterjee (1972a, b) reported that a decrease in the size of deciduoma in pseudopregnant rats given a single subcutaneous injection of PGE_2 or $PGF_{2\alpha}$ could be prevented by chronic treatment with ovine prolactin. However, antifertility effects of $PGF_{2\alpha}$ in rats could not be reversed by exogenous prolactin (Pharriss *et al.*, 1972 and unpublished observations), although exogenous progestin can maintain both decidual reaction and pregnancy in the prostaglandin-treated rats (Labhsetwar, 1972a, b). In the rabbit, where oestrogen is luteotrophic, exogenous oestrogen prevented luteolytic effect of $PGF_{2\alpha}$ (Pharriss *et al.*, 1972). In the hamster a minimum combination of prolactin and FSH is luteotrophic (Greenwald, 1967a). The same combination proved effective in overcoming the luteolytic effect of $PGF_{2\alpha}$. More recently it has been reported that luteolytic effects of $PGF_{2\alpha}$ infused directly into the ovarian artery of the monkey could be antagonised by treatment with HCG, a hormone believed to be luteotrophic in the human (Auletta *et al.*, 1973). This antagonism between the luteolytic effect of prostaglandins and the luteotrophic hormones may even be operative under physiological conditions. Inskeep (1973) reported that the uterus secreted increased amounts of PGF about two weeks after mating when the cyclic corpus luteum begins to regress. However, pregnancy is not interrupted, presumably because of protective effects of the luteotrophic hormone secreted by the early conceptus. The fact that the exogenous luteotrophic hormone counteracts the luteolytic effects of prostaglandins suggests that either prostaglandins alter the endogenous secretion of these trophic hormones or antagonise the action of these hormones at the ovarian level. Since data on the plasma levels of luteotrophic hormones in the prostaglandin-treated animals are not yet available, one cannot select between these alternatives at the present time.

6.2.3 Physiological implications of prostaglandin-induced luteolysis

The uterus exerts profound effects on the luteal function in many laboratory animals. Hysterectomy in pseudopregnant rats or hamsters and cyclic guinea-pigs leads to prolongation of luteal life span (Anderson *et al.*, 1969). Exactly how the uterus influences luteal function has been a mystery but ever since the knowledge of the luteolytic effects of prostaglandins, these lipids have been implicated in mediating the effects of the uterus on the corpus luteum. Thus the regression of the corpus luteum at the end of pseudopregnancy, pregnancy or luteal phase of the cycle may be brought about by prostaglandins secreted mostly by the uterus. Administration of indomethacin has been reported to prolong luteal function in the rabbit (O'Grady *et al.*, 1972a) and the guinea-pig (Poyser, 1972). Antiserum raised against $PGF_{2\alpha}$ also prolonged the length of the oestrous cycle in the treated guinea-pigs (Horton and Poyser, 1974). Ability of the guinea-pig uterus to synthesise prostaglandins is markedly increased at the end of the cycle when progesterone secretion is declining (Poyser, 1972; 1973). Thus the possibility that the uterus may regulate luteal function by secreting prostaglandins appears attractive. Exactly how the uterine prostaglandins are transported to the ovary is not known. It has been postulated that in the sheep prostaglandins in the uterine vein are transported to the ovarian artery by a counter-current exchange mechanism (McCracken *et al.*, 1973). Whether or not such a mechanism operates in the laboratory animals is not known (see also Chapter 7).

6.2.4 Prostaglandin and progesterone synthesis *in vitro*

In contrast to deleterious effects of prostaglandins on luteal function *in vivo*, results of studies *in vitro* have shown a dramatic stimulation of progesterone synthesis by the luteal tissue following addition of prostaglandins. In an attempt to demonstrate that $PGF_{2\alpha}$ does not exert a direct toxic effect on the corpus luteum, Pharriss *et al.* (1968) incubated pseudopregnant rat ovaries *in vitro* in the presence of prostaglandin and observed an increased incorporation of labelled acetate into progesterone. These results were confirmed using luteal slices from cows (Speroff and Ramwell, 1970) and rabbits (Sellner and Wickersham, 1970). Among several prostaglandins used, PGEs were found to be more potent than $PGF_{2\alpha}$ in promoting progesterone synthesis *in vitro* (Speroff and Ramwell, 1970). This contrasts with their relative luteolytic activity *in vivo* in rats and hamsters where $PGF_{2\alpha}$ was far more potent than PGE_2 (see page 256). Speroff and Ramwell (1970) further found that PGE_2 although most active in stimulating progesterone biosynthesis was only about 50% as potent as LH on a molar basis. At the present time it is not possible to reconcile contrasting effects of prostaglandins *in vivo* and *in vitro*. It may be that initially prostaglandins stimulate progesterone synthesis even *in vivo* but the effect is transitory so that it has not been so far observed. With the initial stimulation, precursors are probably depleted resulting in decreased progesterone secretion and eventual luteolysis. This unitary concept, however, lacks support and is inconsistent with the fact that potencies of $PGF_{2\alpha}$ and PGE_2 in inducing luteolysis in rats *in vivo* are reversed in stimulating progesterone biosynthesis in bovine luteal slices *in vitro*. Until more controlled studies are done, this concept must remain speculative.

So far two groups have reported luteotrophic effects of $PGF_{2\alpha}$ under *in vivo* conditions. Lukaszewska *et al.* (1972) reported that $PGF_{2\alpha}$ significantly increased progesterone content of corpora lutea of *both* ovaries when applied directly to *one* ovary of the hysterectomised hamster on day 7 of pseudopregnancy at a very low dose (2 ng). At a higher dose (>20 ng) the prostaglandin exerted a luteolytic effect. Similarly Auletta *et al.* (1973) reported that infusion of $PGF_{2\alpha}$ in very low doses (in ng range) into the ovarian artery stimulated progesterone output from the monkey ovary but the same prostaglandin exerted luteolytic effect when infused at a higher rate (50 μg min^{-1}). These data would suggest that the luteotrophic and luteolytic effects of $PGF_{2\alpha}$ may be dose-dependent.

6.2.5 Prostaglandin receptors

Each target organ seems to contain specific receptors which show a high degree of affinity and specificity for binding to a particular hormone. Such receptors have been demonstrated for many steroid and peptide hormones (Jensen and DeSombre, 1973). The same may be true for prostaglandins. Kuehl and Humes (1972) demonstrated a specific binding of PGEs to the isolated fat cells but such a binding could not be demonstrated for PGFs. Bito (1972) also noted binding of labelled prostaglandins to many tissues including uterine smooth muscle *in vitro*. Rao (1973) reported the presence of prostaglandin receptors in the cell membranes of the bovine corpus luteum. The receptors specifically bound to PGE_1 and E_2 but showed little binding to PGFs unless used in a very high concentration. Although both PGEs and HCG exert steroidogenic action on the bovine corpus luteum *in vitro* (Speroff and Ramwell, 1970) the receptors for PGEs appeared to be distinct from those for HCG (Rao, 1974). An inhibitor of prostaglandin biosynthesis (indomethacin), an antagonist of prostaglandin (7-oxa-13-prostynoic acid) and oestradiol-17β inhibited binding of PGE_1 to receptors but progesterone and HCG did not (Rao, 1974). This raises the possibility whether oestrogen may not exert its well-known luteolytic effect at least partly by inhibiting the binding of PGEs to receptors (see page 251).

In addition to the corpus luteum, the uterus (Wakeling et al., 1973) and the Fallopian tube (Wakeling and Spilman, 1973) also show binding to prosta-glandins. Wakeling and Wyngarden (1974) reported a high degree of uptake and binding of prostaglandins E_1 and $F_{2\alpha}$ to the human, monkey and hamster uterine tissues. The myometrium showed more binding than the endometrium in both the human and the monkey. In the hamster uterus the degree of binding of PGE_1 was greater on days 2 and 3 of the cycle than on day 1 (oestrus) or 4 (pro-oestrus) but such a difference could not be demonstrated for $PGF_{2\alpha}$ or $F_{1\alpha}$. Treatment of ovariectomised hamsters with oestrogen decreased and with progesterone increased the binding of prostaglandins E_1 and $F_{2\alpha}$. 15-keto-PGE_1 to which PGE_1 is metabolised showed a lower affinity for receptors than PGE_1 (Wakeling and Wyngarden, 1974). Thus there is little doubt about the existence of a protein in the reproductive tract which specifically binds to prostaglandins; but the nature of this interaction and its physiological signifi-cance remains to be elucidated.

6.2.6 Role of prostaglandins in mediating luteinising hormone action

LH causes a several-fold increase in the ovarian concentration of cAMP within minutes. Ovulatory as well as steroidogenic actions of LH are believed to be mediated through this cyclic nucleotide. However, it is also known that PGEs can dramatically stimulate cAMP production in the mouse or rat ovary incubated in vitro (Kuehl et al., 1970; Lamprecht et al., 1973). This observa-tion has given rise to the view that the action of LH on the ovary is mediated through PGEs (Kuehl et al., 1970; Kuehl, 1974). The role of PGFs in stimulating cAMP production is believed to be only minor as these prosta-glandins were more selective in stimulating cGMP synthesis (Kuehl, 1974). The concept that the action of LH is mediated through PGEs is primarily based on the fact that a prostaglandin antagonist (7-oxa-13-prostynoic acid) inhibited the action of LH in causing increased cAMP and progesterone production in the isolated mouse ovary (Kuehl et al., 1970). Others have failed to confirm this observation. Bedwani and Horton (1971) using bioassays observed no increase in the prostaglandin synthesis in the rabbit ovary under conditions where LH stimulated progesterone secretion. More recently Lamprecht et al. (1973) using the rat ovary incubated in vitro failed to suppress increased accumulation of cAMP in response to LH addition by 7-oxa-13-prostynoic acid and indomethacin. If the action of LH is mediated through PGEs, the ovary or the corpus luteum stimulated maximally by PGEs should not respond to a further stimulation by LH. However, this was not found to be the case (Speroff and Ramwell, 1970; Marsh, 1971; Lamprecht et al., 1973). This suggests that the actions of prostaglandins and LH are probably mediated via distinct pathways. A recent demonstration of different receptors for PGEs and HCG in the bovine luteal cell membranes may provide some support for this view (Rao, 1974). In contrast to the view of Kuehl (1974) that prostaglandin stimulates production of cAMP in the ovary and thus mediates the action of LH, Marsh et al. (1974) have proposed that cAMP stimulates the synthesis of both prostaglandin Fs and Es in the isolated rabbit ovarian follicle and thus mediates the action of LH. There seems to be little doubt about the existence of a functional relationship between LH and prostaglandins but the precise nature of this relationship is unclear. In mediating the action of LH on the ovary, it is not clear if prostaglandins stimulate cAMP production or cAMP enhances the synthesis of prostaglandins and/or whether both of these possibilities are true.

6.2.7 Effects on luteal morphology

When high doses of prostaglandins are administered, the decrease in progesterone secretion, i.e. luteolysis, is usually associated with morphological degeneration of old corpora lutea and subsequent appearance of fresh corpora lutea in the ovary. This is particularly true in the hamster (Labhsetwar, 1972a). Morphological degeneration of corpora lutea were also observed in the guinea-pig (Blatchley and Donovan, 1969) and rabbit (Koering and Kirton, 1973). An electron microscopic study of luteal tissue of rats receiving antifertility doses of $PGF_{2\alpha}$, has shown considerable accumulation of lipids in the cytoplasm, increased numbers of ribosomes and disappearance of the microvillous protrusions from the cell surface; the mitochondria, however, remained unaffected (Okamura et al., 1972b). Koering and Kirton (1973) reported appearance of autophagic vacuoles containing lipid droplets in lutein cells of pregnant rabbits treated with $PGF_{2\alpha}$. Other cytoplasmic components remained unaffected by the treatment. Furthermore, interstitial cells as well as follicles showed no morphological deviations from normal. Thus the effects of $PGF_{2\alpha}$ on the ovary are highly selective and only affect the luteal tissue to the virtual exclusion of other ovarian compartments.

6.3 ROLE OF PROSTAGLANDINS IN UTERINE PHYSIOLOGY

6.3.1 Uterine secretion of prostaglandins

Recent investigations have demonstrated the presence of prostaglandins in the uterine tissues of several laboratory animals such as the rat (Saksena and Harper, 1972b), mouse (Saksena and Lau, 1973), hamster (Shaikh and Saksena, 1972) and guinea-pig (Poyser, 1972, 1973). It is well-established that infusion of both PGEs and PGFs in humans and primates increases uterine motility in non-pregnant and pregnant subjects (see Chapters 1, 2 and 4). Such detailed in vivo studies have not been reported in the laboratory animals. Intravenous infusion of $PGF_{2\alpha}$ into pregnant rabbits caused increased uterine contractions (Smith et al., 1973). Similar results were obtained in rats (Buckle and Nathanielsz, 1973). Weeks (1973) infused prostaglandins through venous cannulae into unanaesthetised rats (retired breeders) and observed increased uterine motility in response to both prostaglandins $F_{2\alpha}$ and E_2, but after three hours the uterus became quiescent and no longer responded to another injection. It appears that such responses have not been reported for the human uterus. In any event the uterine response to prostaglandins depends upon the steroidal environment to which it is exposed. Isolated uterine segments of the guinea-pig (Sullivan, 1966) and rabbit (Porter and Behrman, 1971) uteri under the influence of progesterone showed decreased motility in response to prostaglandins.

Vane and Williams (1972) have suggested that prostaglandins may play a role in maintaining the uterine tonus and spontaneous motility. More recently uterine prostaglandins have been implicated in the oestrogen induced hyper-aemia (Ryan et al., 1974). These authors found that increased blood flow in the uterus of the spayed rat, induced by exogenous oestrogen, could be blocked by treatment with inhibitors of prostaglandin synthesis (indomethacin and meclophenamic acid). This block was associated with a parallel decrease in the uterine level of both prostaglandins Fs and Es. Thus it is quite probable that prostaglandins play a role in the uterine haemodynamics.

6.3.2 Hormonal control of prostaglandin synthesis

The synthesis of prostaglandins in the uterus is modulated by the ovarian steroids. The uterine concentration of PGF varied according to the stage of the oestrous cycle in the rat (Saksena and Harper, 1972b) and hamster (Shaikh and Saksena, 1972) although the pattern was different between the two species. Oestrogen appears to be a potent stimulant for prostaglandin synthesis in the uterus as the secretion of PGF into the utero-ovarian vein increased significantly following oestrogen treatment of guinea-pigs (Blatchley et al., 1971). Similarly oestrogen treatment of hamsters (Saksena and Harper, 1972a) and spayed mice (Saksena and Lau, 1973) also increased the uterine level of PGFs. However, a combined treatment of progesterone and oestrogen appears to be far more effective than the treatment with either hormone alone in stimulating uterine prostaglandin synthesis in the spayed guinea-pigs (Blatchley and Poyser, 1974) and mice (Saksena and Lau, 1973). The significance of these observations lies in the fact that during the terminal portion of the luteal phase of the guinea-pig oestrous cycle the uterus is exposed to both hormones thus resulting in an optimal secretion of prostaglandins for luteolysis. Indeed the ability of the uterus to synthesise prostaglandins increases significantly during the last few days of the oestrous cycle in the guinea-pig (Poyser, 1972; 1973) and sheep (Bland et al., 1971; Cox et al., 1973; McCracken, et al., 1973) when oestrogen secretion is known to be increasing (Joshi et al., 1973; McCracken et al., 1972a). An intra-arterial infusion of oestradiol-17β in sheep caused more than a 100-fold increase in the uterine secretion of PGF within 1–2 hours after the start of infusion (McCracken et al., 1973). These observations taken together suggest that oestrogen acting in concert with progesterone constitute a physiological trigger for increased prostaglandin synthesis in the uterus under in vivo conditions. It is probable that well-documented luteolytic effects of oestrogens in the hamster (Greenwald, 1965b) and sheep (Hawk and Bolt, 1970) may also be mediated through an increased uterine prostaglandin synthesis. In the sheep, the uterus is essential for the luteolytic effects of oestrogen (Bolt and Hawk, 1972).

6.3.3 Prostaglandins and IUD

The leucocytic infiltration of the endometrium and the uterine cavity is a constant feature of the uterus bearing an intrauterine device (IUD). This association was originally observed by Greenwald (1965a) in the rat. He reported that the inflammatory reaction was essential for the antifertility effects of the IUD since the absence of leucocytes was always correlated with the occurrence of implantation in the presence of the device. An increased leucocytic infiltration with an IUD has also been observed in the human (Sagiroglu and Sagiroglu, 1970) and baboon (Joshi, 1971; Breed et al., 1972). As is well known, leucocytes contain very high levels of lysomal enzymes including phospholipase A which is involved in prostaglandin synthesis. This fact coupled with the observation of Piper and Vane (1971) that an irritation of many tissues results in an increased prostaglandin synthesis suggest that increased prostaglandin levels may be associated with the presence of the device. This has been amply confirmed. Distension of the guinea-pig uterus with a plastic device, which leads to a unilateral luteal regression, induced a significant increase in $PGF_{2\alpha}$ release into the utero-ovarian vein (Poyser et al., 1971). Chaudhury (1973) found increased PGE_2-like material by bioassay in the flushings from the uterine horn of the rat bearing an IUD as compared to levels in the flushings from the control horn. The concentration of PGF in the uterine horn as well as in the uterine venous blood draining that horn were also increased (Saksena et al., 1974a). Similar increases in PGF levels were observed in the IUD-bearing horns of the rabbit (Saksena and Harper, 1974) and the hamster (Saksena et al., 1974a).

How increased prostaglandin levels brought about by IUDs contribute to a localised antifertility effect of the device in these species is not known. One possibility is that prostaglandins from the IUD-horn are transported to the adjacent ovary by a mechanism similar to that postulated for the sheep (McCracken et al., 1973) and the regression of the corpus luteum results in the termination of pregnancy on that side. The unilateral luteolytic effect of IUDs have already been reported in the guinea-pig (Ginther et al., 1966), rat (Prasad et al., 1973) and sheep (Ginther, 1974). Furthermore, administration of indomethacin reversed the antifertility effects of unilateral IUDs in the rabbit (Saksena and Harper, 1974) but not in the rat (Chaudhury, 1973). Another possibility is that increased prostaglandin synthesis evoked by IUD increases uterine motility and thereby causes expulsion of early embryos. A direct effect of prostaglandins on blastocysts leading to their degeneration should also be considered (see page 259).

Although there is no evidence to date to implicate prostaglandins in antifertility effects of IUDs in the human, a case can perhaps be made that these lipids might mediate the side-effects of IUDs such as bleeding, uterine cramps and expulsion of the device. It has been reported that IUDs containing CU^{++} or progesterone show reduced incidence of these side-effects (Mishell, 1974). It is known that CU^{--} suppresses PGE synthesis (which is a potent vasodilator and thus probably plays a role in bleeding) by directing it to PGF (Lands et al., 1971). As the latter prostaglandin is a potent vasoconstrictor agent it would be expected to reduce bleeding. Progesterone could suppress prostaglandin synthesis in the uterus by its well-known anti-oestrogenic property as oestrogen is known to be a potent stimulant for prostaglandin synthesis (see page 251). Thus the involvement of prostaglandins in the antifertility effects of the IUD and its side-effects is an intriguing possibility worthy of further exploration as it might offer means for making IUDs more effective and safe.

6.3.4 Prostaglandins and parturition

The precise role of prostaglandins in the process of parturition cannot be ascertained until changes in the uterine secretion of prostaglandins in relation to changes in other hormones are correlated with various stages of labour. Although the finding of increased prostaglandin-like material in the amniotic fluid of women approaching parturition first raised the possibility of involvement of prostaglandins in this process (Karim and Devlin, 1967) the experimental test of this hypothesis in subsequent studies for the most part has relied on the measurement of peripheral prostaglandin levels. Due to a widespread distribution of prostaglandins in the body and a probable modification of their synthesis due to a generalised stress accompanying parturition, the relation of peripheral prostaglandin levels to uterine prostaglandin levels must be regarded as tenuous (see Chapter 1). As far as the laboratory animals are concerned data obtained by using various approaches strongly implicate prostaglandins in the process of parturition. Two potentially complementary roles of prostaglandins must be considered—ability of prostaglandins to cause luteolysis could initiate or precipitate parturition simply by withdrawal of progesterone 'block' according to a pathway postulated by Csapo (1956). Secondly, such a withdrawal of progesterone could lead to a sensitisation of the uterine muscle to the contractile action of prostaglandins promoting uterine motility. The relative importance of these two factors cannot be evaluated at the present time.

Exogenous prostaglandins can induce premature parturition in mice (Horton and Marley, 1969), rats (Buckle and Nathanielsz, 1973), rabbits (Abel et al., 1973), hamster (Labhsetwar, 1972b) and guinea-pigs (unpublished observations). The relative potency of PGEs and PGFs is not known in all species. In the hamster PGEs are about 10 times more potent than PGFs (Labhsetwar, 1974) as in the human (Karim, 1972). This correlates well with their ability to cause smooth muscle contractions of gerbil colon in vitro (Labhsetwar, 1974). The $PGF_{2\alpha}$-induced parturition is associated with a rapid fall in the peripheral plasma progesterone levels in the rat (Buckle and Nathanielsz, 1973) and rabbit (Abel et al., 1973; Challis et al., 1974b). If endogenous $PGF_{2\alpha}$ causes similar changes in parturient rats, then the uterine secretion of prostaglandin should rise prior to a fall in the progesterone level. However, in the rat Labhsetwar and Watson (1974) observed increased PGF levels in the uterine vein plasma after a significant fall in progesterone and a significant rise in oestrogen. Even in the rabbit, PGF level in the peripheral plasma increased at the time of parturition but the rise did not precede the fall in progesterone in all animals (Challis et al., 1973). Thus the role of prostaglandins in causing progesterone withdrawal at the time of parturition in laboratory animals remains uncertain at this time.

Involvement of prostaglandins in parturition became further evident from the fact that several anti-inflammatory drugs which inhibit prostaglandin synthesis can delay parturition in rats (Aiken, 1972; Chester *et al.*, 1972; Csapo *et al.*, 1973). Aiken (1972) reported that delay of parturition in rats with indomethacin and aspirin was associated with a decrease in the ability of uterine strips to synthesise prostaglandins *in vitro*.

6.4 EFFECTS OF PROSTAGLANDINS IN PREGNANT ANIMALS

6.4.1 Egg transport

In establishing the role of prostaglandins in the egg or sperm transport, as in any other reproductive process, it is necessary to show that (1) prostaglandins are present in the fallopian tube and their concentration varies in relation to altered gamete transport; (2) exogenous prostaglandins can influence gamete transport and (3) inhibitors of prostaglandin synthesis can interfere with this process. Available information is only fragmentary and mostly confined to the rabbit as the fallopian tube of the rabbit is considerably larger than that of other laboratory species permitting easy manipulations. The conclusions reached, therefore, may not be applicable to other species.

Recent data suggest that the human fallopian tube contains prostaglandins. The human oviductal fluid contained more $PGF_{2\alpha}$ than the peripheral serum suggesting secretion or a selective concentration of prostaglandin by the fallopian tube (Ogra *et al.*, 1974). Using the indirect immunofluorescence technique, these authors further demonstrated that $PGF_{2\alpha}$ was localised in the mucosal surface before ovulation and in the oviductal lamina propria after ovulation. Wakeling and Spilman (1973) reported binding of $PGF_{2\alpha}$ and PGE_1 to the rabbit fallopian tube.

Effects of exogenous prostaglandins on tubal motility and/or egg transport have been studied by many workers. Horton *et al.* (1965) reported that $PGF_{2\alpha}$ increased and PGE_2 depressed motility of the rabbit fallopian tube *in vivo*. Similar effects were observed in the sheep (Horton and Thompson, 1964) and human (Coutinho and Maia, 1971). These contrasting effects of two types of prostaglandins in the rabbit have been recently confirmed (Spilman and Harper, 1973) and it has been suggested that prostaglandins may interact with adrenergic mechanisms in the tube to control the oviductal motility (Spilman and Harper, 1974). The fallopian tube is richly supplied with adrenergic nerve terminals. Whether or not changes brought about by prostaglandins in tubal motility also effect egg transport is not known. In the rabbit, Chang *et al.* (1973) reported that subcutaneous administration of $PGF_{2\alpha}$ and to some extent PGE_1 12 hours after ovulation severely disturbed egg transport; PGE_2 was found ineffective. At autopsy two days after ovulatory dose of HCG, either no eggs could be found in the entire reproductive tract or their passage was markedly accelerated so that many eggs were located in the uterus or vagina whereas in the control rabbits they were confined to the fallopian tubes. In the rat, administration of $PGF_{2\alpha}$ during the tubal sojourn of zygotes failed to either accelerate or delay the egg transport (Labhsetwar, 1972b), but PGE_2 or PGE_1 given during the same period caused tubal retention of zygotes (Labhsetwar, 1972a, 1973b). In the hamster, on the other hand, none of these prostaglandins significantly affected egg transport (Labhsetwar, 1972 a, b, 1973b). Whether the tubal retention of eggs in rats treated with PGEs is due to inhibition of tubal motility is not known because such inhibitory effects have not yet been demonstrated in this species.

Effects of inhibitors of prostaglandin synthesis on egg transport have not been reported.

As prostaglandins significantly affect the tubal motility and egg transport, these lipids could mediate the contraceptive effectiveness of the postcoitally administered oestrogen. The reason for suspecting such a link is the well-documented fact that oestrogen can stimulate prostaglandin synthesis in the uterus of several species (see page 251). The postcoital administration of oestrogen is known to interrupt pregnancy in several laboratory species such as the rat, mouse, hamster, guinea-pig and rabbit primarily by causing accelerated passage of eggs through the reproductive tract and their eventual expulsion through the vagina (Greenwald, 1967b). Thus the involvement of prostaglandins in the contraceptive effectiveness of the postcoitally administered oestrogens is an interesting speculation which needs to be experimentally tested.

6.4.2 Sperm transport

Unlike eggs, sperm must travel in the genital tract of the donor and the recipient before reaching their destination, i.e. the site of fertilisation in the fallopian tube. Prostaglandins could play a role in sperm transport in either sex. Prostaglandins are distributed throughout the reproductive tract of the male, the human semen being the richest vertebrate source containing at least 13 different prostaglandins (Horton, 1969). Distribution of prostaglandins in the seminal plasma of laboratory animals is not known. The semen of guinea-pigs and rabbits showed very little prostaglandins estimated by using bioassays (Horton and Thompson, 1964) although data using more sensitive radioimmunoassays are not available. Ability of various prostaglandins to influence motility of vas deferens, testicular capsules, seminal vesicles, etc. and to interact with adrenergic system in doing so (Horton, 1969) has led to the early suggestion that prostaglandins might contribute to the propulsion of sperm through the excretory ducts at the time of ejaculation (von Euler and Elliason, 1967). As the precise distribution of various prostaglandins in the male reproductive tract in relation to its various functional activities is not yet known, this suggestion has remained untested. Administration of exogenous prostaglandins to rabbits for a prolonged period hastened spermatogenesis by only two days (Hunt and Nicholson, 1972).

Effects of prostaglandins on sperm transport in the female reproductive tract has received only limited attention despite the early suggestion that one of the roles of high levels of prostaglandins in the seminal plasma of certain species may be to aid sperm transport in the female (von Euler and Ellison, 1967). Mandl (1972) observed significantly higher numbers of sperm in the uteri and tubes of rabbits inseminated with semen containing PGE_1. However, more recently Chang *et al.* (1973) failed to confirm the accelerating effect of PGE_1 on sperm transport in this species. Furthermore the physiological significance of the role of PGE_1 in aiding sperm transport remains unclear as the rabbit semen appears to contain very little prostaglandins (Horton and Thompson, 1964).

6.4.3 Antifertility effects

The luteolytic effect of prostaglandins implies that they can exert an antifertility effect by creating progesterone deficiency. Such an effect was first described in the rat (Gutknecht *et al.*, 1971a; Nutting and Cammarata, 1969) and then extended to other species.

6.4.3.1 Prostaglandins of the F series

Soon after demonstrating a luteolytic effect of $PGF_{2\alpha}$, Gutknecht *et al.* (1969) reported an antifertility effect of this prostaglandin in rats. They found that $PGF_{2\alpha}$ terminated pregnancy in 100% of the animals when given subcutaneously at the rate of 2 mg/day for any three consecutive days between days 4 and 13 of pregnancy. When administered earlier from days 1–4 or after day 13, the treatment proved much less effective (Gutknecht *et al.*, 1971a; Labhsetwar, 1972b). In subsequent experiments, it was found that even as little as 0.4 mg/day of $PGF_{2\alpha}$ was fully effective in terminating pregnancy in rats (Labhsetwar, 1972b). When given orally at 10 times the subcutaneously effective dose, $PGF_{2\alpha}$ proved inactive (Gutknecht *et al.*, 1971a). Similar effects were reported by Nutting and Cammarata (1969) and soon confirmed (Labhsetwar, 1970; 1972a). In addition to $PGF_{2\alpha}$, prostaglandins $F_{1\alpha}$ and $F_{3\alpha}$ (unpublished observations) have also been found to exert antifertility effects, although these compounds are somewhat less potent than $PGF_{2\alpha}$. Simultaneous administration of synthetic progestin—Provera (Gutknecht *et al.*, 1971a) or progesterone (Labhsetwar, 1970, 1972b) protected pregnancy implying that progesterone deficiency was the major cause of loss of pregnancy. $PGF_{2\alpha}$ has also been reported to exert an antifertility effect in hamsters (Labhsetwar, 1971b; 1972b; Gutknecht *et al.*, 1971b), rabbits (Gutknecht *et al.*, 1971a) and mice (Horton and Marley, 1969; Bartke *et al.*, 1972; Labhsetwar, 1972c). Only the hamster has been studied extensively partly because among the laboratory species studied it appears to be the most sensitive. Like the rat, the hamster also showed a relatively short circumscribed period from days 3–9 during which prostaglandins were most effective as antifertility agents. During the first three days of pregnancy or after day 9, relatively large doses were required as compared to those required between days 3 and 9 to achieve termination of pregnancy (Labhsetwar, 1972b).

$PGF_{2\alpha}$ is also active orally as an antifertility agent in the hamster (Labhsetwar, 1972b) and to date the hamster remains the only species other than humans (Karim, 1972) where oral activity of prostaglandins has been demonstrated. The doses required (0.1 to 1 mg/day for three days) were relatively high (50–80 times the subcutaneous dose) but no diarrhoea or loss in body weight was observed at these doses (Labhsetwar, 1972a). The oral activity means that $PGF_{2\alpha}$ is either not rapidly metabolised in the hamster or metabolites are biologically active. Since inactivation of prostaglandins by lungs was solely monitored by using smooth muscle bioassays (Piper and Vane, 1971), it is possible that metabolites emerging from lungs could still possess other biological activities including antifertility property. The reason for a marked difference in sensitivity between rats and hamsters to antifertility effects is not known but may be related to the rapidity with which prostaglandins are metabolised. It may be that the rat lungs contain a higher level of 15-hydroxy prostaglandin dehydrogenase compared to that of the hamster. When $PGF_{2\alpha}$ and PGE_2 were administered together to rats in doses which were virtually ineffective individually, the combination exerted synergistic effects in termination of pregnancy (Labhsetwar, 1972a). The basis for this potentiation of antifertility effects remains to be explored.

There appears to be no residual effect of $PGF_{2\alpha}$ on the subsequent fertility of hamsters. When $PGF_{2\alpha}$ is given to pregnant hamsters, the animals come into oestrus prematurely. When they are placed with males at this time, they mate and a new pregnancy is established which appears normal for all practical purposes (unpublished observations). Thus prostaglandins do not appear to interfere with the functional maintenance of corpora lutea during subsequent pregnancy.

The mechanism by which $PGF_{2\alpha}$ brings about the termination of pregnancy in rats and hamsters appears primarily to be due to the deficiency of progesterone stemming from its luteolytic action (see page 242). In view of the potent smooth muscle stimulating action of $PGF_{2\alpha}$, it is also possible to argue that antifertility effects result from the direct action of the prostaglandin on the uterus and the resulting loss of the luteotrophic influence of embryos causes luteolysis (Labhsetwar, 1972a, b; 1973b). In other words, luteolysis may be secondary to antifertility effects. The protective effect of exogenous progestins can be accounted for by the fact that the progesterone-dominated uterine muscle is less sensitive to prostaglandins (Porter and Behrman, 1971). However, this explanation can be discounted because $PGF_{2\alpha}$ suppresses plasma progesterone in pseudopregnant rats (Pharris and Wyngarden, 1969) and hamsters (Labhsetwar, 1972a, b) and reduces decidual growth in either species which could be maintained by exogenous progesterone (Labhsetwar, 1972a, b). This suggests that the antifertility effects stem from the action of the prostaglandin on the ovary rather than on the uterus. In fact $PGF_{2\alpha}$ can exert luteolytic effects in the absence of the uterus both in the guinea-pig (Blatchley and Donovan, 1969) and the hamster (Labhsetwar, 1971b).

6.4.3.2 Prostaglandins of the E series

Both PGE_2 and PGE_1 exert antifertility effects although in general they are much less potent than PGFs (Nutting and Cammarata, 1969; Labhsetwar, 1972b). PGE_2 was found to be some 10 times (Labhsetwar, 1972b) and PGE_1 (Labhsetwar, 1973b) some 25 times less potent than $PGF_{2\alpha}$ in terminating early pregnancy in hamsters. In rats PGE_2 was about 10 times less potent than $PGF_{2\alpha}$ (requiring twice daily injections and far higher doses than the hamster to achieve termination of pregnancy) (Labhsetwar, 1972b). In fact, PGE_1 even when administered in sublethal doses (7.5 mg kg^{-1}) for three days proved inactive in pregnant rats (Labhsetwar, 1973b). The most sensitive period for antifertility effects in hamsters was the same as that for $PGF_{2\alpha}$, i.e. between days 3 and 9 (Labhsetwar, 1972b; 1973b). When administered outside this period prostaglandins proved inactive unless given in very high doses. Both PGE_2 and PGE_1 also exerted oral and antifertility effects in hamsters, although this has not been demonstrated in rats. The doses required were rather high (over 25 mg/kg/day) and at this dose level profuse diarrhoea and loss in body weight were observed (Labhsetwar, 1972a; 1973b). In hamsters, doses required to terminate pregnancy by the subcutaneous route, i.e. 150 μg/animal/day of PGE_2 and 300 μg/animal/day of PGE_1, did not induce diarrhoea. In rats, on the other hand, all doses used (0.5 mg or more/injection twice daily for three days) caused diarrhoea whether they exerted antifertility effects or not (Labhsetwar, 1972a; 1973b). It is not known whether these two effects, i.e. one on the gastrointestinal tract and the other on the reproductive tract, are interrelated. Occurrence of diarrhoea in rats at doses which exerted no antifertility effects (Labhsetwar, 1973b) suggests that the smooth muscle of the gastrointestinal tract is more sensitive than that of the uterus. Alternatively an increased uterine motility alone does not lead to detectable antifertility effects. The fact that antifertility doses of PGE_2 by subcutaneous route induced diarrhoea in rats but not in hamsters should not be construed as species difference because the doses required in hamsters were much lower than those in rats. When oral doses are increased in hamsters, diarrhoea occurs even in this species.

The mechanism by which PGEs exert antifertility effects in rats and hamsters is not known. As stated earlier both PGE_1 and PGE_2 exert luteolytic effects in hamsters as peripheral progesterone levels drop, development of deciduomata is inhibited, corpora lutea atrophy and administration of exogenous progesterone can maintain pregnancy (Labhsetwar 1972a; 1973b). However, deficiency of progesterone alone may not be the sole mode of action as the drop in plasma progesterone following treatment with PGE_2 is not as marked in hysterectomised hamsters as in intact pregnant hamsters (Labhsetwar, 1972a). Thus a contributory action at the uterine level cannot be totally excluded at this time although the predominant factor appears to be luteolysis.

6.4.3.3 Other prostaglandins

Prostaglandins of A series (A_1 and A_2) when administered at 40 times the minimum effective dose of $PGF_{2\alpha}$ to hamsters failed to terminate pregnancy (unpublished observations). Administration of very high doses of arachidonic acid (2 mg/day), a precursor of prostaglandins, also did not exert antifertility effects. This suggests that despite the widespread distribution of prostaglandin synthetase enzyme in the body enough of the precursor is not converted to PGFs or PGEs to obtain termination of pregnancy. So far no data on the effects of PGBs or PGC on pregnancy have been reported.

6.4.4 Prostaglandins and implantation

It is now well-recognised that implantation of blastocyst is a complex process involving coordinated interplay of several endocrine factors. The antifertility effect of prostaglandins described above could be due in part to inhibition of implantation. The most likely step susceptible to prostaglandins (because of their potent vasoactive properties) is an early blastocyst–endometrial inter-action which involves vasodilatation and increased vascular permeability to macromolecules. These changes can be visualised in the normal rats, hamsters, mice and perhaps other species by injecting a dye such as Pontamine blue and observing blue spots in the uterus which represent sites of blastocyst implan-tation (Finn and Mclaren, 1967).

The effects on implantation have been tested in rats and hamsters treated with antifertility doses of prostaglandins $F_{2\alpha}$, E_2 and E_1 (Labhsetwar, 1971a; 1972a, b; 1973b). A marked difference was observed between PGFs and PGEs: the latter inhibited the implantation of blastocysts while the former had no significant effects. Of the prostaglandins so far tested, PGE_1 was the most potent in inhibiting implantation. Twice daily administration of 1.0 mg/day from days 1–5 inclusive of pregnancy inhibited implantation in virtually all rats (Labhsetwar, 1973b). PGE_2 was somewhat less potent. Flushing of uteri on the morning of day 6 when blastocysts in the control rats have already implanted showed unimplanted blastocysts, many of which appeared normal under the microscope. It is apparent that PGE_1 and PGE_2 cause delayed implantation of blastocysts in rats. Such effects were not observed in hamsters. It is unlikely that the delayed implantation stems from the luteolytic effects of prostaglandins as PGE_1 did not terminate pregnancy when given from days 4–6 of pregnancy even when administered in sublethal doses. Simultaneous administration of progesterone did not overcome the implantation delaying action of PGE_1 in rats (Labhsetwar, 1973b). Perhaps prostaglandins may have inhibited or attenuated the oestrogen surge on day 4 of pregnancy which is essential for implantation in rats. Whether this was a direct action of PGE_1 on the blastocyst and uterus or an indirect one through the pituitary–hypothalamic complex is not known. Thus PGEs seem to exert anti-implantation effects in rats but for some unknown reason $PGF_{2\alpha}$ does not share this property. In unpublished studies we have found that $PGF_{1\alpha}$ also did not exert anti-implantation effects in rats under conditions where antifertility effects were observed. Thus, implantation represents one of the few physiologic processes which is differentially affected by PGEs and PGFs and highlights the importance of studying effects of both types of prostaglandins on various reproductive processes.

6.5 ROLE OF PROSTAGLANDINS IN GONADOTROPHIN SECRETION AND OVULATION

6.5.1 Stimulation of gonadotrophin secretion

The stimulatory effects of prostaglandins on gonadotrophin secretion was first postulated by Labhsetwar (1970). Administration of antifertility doses of

$PGF_{2\alpha}$ to pregnant rats raised the pituitary LH stores several-fold over those normally found at a comparable stage of pregnancy or pseudopregnancy and even over those found on the day of pro-oestrus and two weeks after bilateral ovariectomy. Since $PGF_{2\alpha}$ did not inhibit ovulation in cyclic rats (Labhsetwar, 1970) but induced it in pregnant rats (Labhsetwar, 1972b) and hamsters (Labhsetwar, 1971b), it was postulated that $PGF_{2\alpha}$ stimulates LH secretion. Although blood levels of LH were not directly measured in this study, increased pituitary LH stores correlated with the target organ stimulation clearly supported such a conclusion. In a later study using hamsters significantly higher levels of LH in blood of pregnant hamsters treated with antifertility doses of $PGF_{2\alpha}$ were observed (Labhsetwar, 1972b). The stimulatory effects of prostaglandins on gonadotrophin secretion have been amply confirmed in subsequent studies. Thus ovulation in the cyclic rat blocked by barbiturates could be reversed by subcutaneous (Tsafriri et al., 1972a) or intraventricular injections of PGEs (Spies and Norman, 1973). In the latter study PGFs were found to be much less effective. In the bilaterally ovariectomised rats, PGE_2 but not PGE_1 or $PGF_{2\alpha}$ injected into the third ventricle stimulated both LH and FSH secretion (Harms et al., 1973). Parenteral injections of PGEs in castrated rats primed with oestrogen alone (Batta et al., 1974) or a combination of oestrogen and progesterone (Sato et al., 1974a) also induced release of gonadotrophins, again in these studies PGFs were less potent. In sheep, intracarotid infusion of $PGF_{2\alpha}$ during the luteal phase of the cycle caused a sharp increase in LH secretion (Carlson et al., 1973).

These results taken together leave little doubt about the stimulatory effects of prostaglandins on gonadotrophin secretion. However, there is considerable uncertainty about the kind of prostaglandin involved in this response under physiological conditions. Thus Spies and Norman (1973) reported stimulatory effects of PGE_1 on LH secretion in *cyclic* rats blocked with barbiturates and failed to find the same with PGE_2. Using castrated rats Harms et al. (1973) found stimulation of gonadotrophin secretion only with PGE_2 (PGE_1 being inactive). It is quite clear that the endocrine status of the experimental animal can crucially affect the response to prostaglandin administration.

In addition to stimulating release of LH and FSH, prostaglandins also stimulate secretion of prolactin. Vermouth and Deis (1972) observed a significant increase in prolactin secretion following intravenous injection of $PGF_{2\alpha}$ in pregnant rats. More recently intraventricular injection of different doses of PGE_1 induced a dose-related increase in plasma prolactin 15 min after the injection in spayed rats; other prostaglandins (E_2, $F_{2\alpha}$ or $F_{1\alpha}$) were ineffective (Ojeda et al., 1974).

The mechanism by which prostaglandins exert stimulatory effect on gonadotrophin secretion and whether or not they subserve this function under physiological conditions is not known. However, they could bring about increased gonadotrophin secretion and ovulation by acting at various levels in the hypothalamicopituitary–ovarian axis. Evidence for this is reviewed below.

6.5.2 Action at hypothalamic level

Brains of many species are known to contain prostaglandins. The hypo-thalamus of the dog was found to contain both PGEs (E_1 and E_2) and PGFs ($F_{2\alpha}$ and $F_{1\alpha}$) (Horton, 1969). Cerebrospinal fluid from the third and lateral ventricles of the cat contains prostaglandin-like material (Feldberg and Myers, 1966) and electrical stimulation of the cat brain evoked release of prosta-glandins (Ramwell and Shaw, 1966). Prostaglandins are also present in the brains of the mouse, rat, and rabbit (see Horton, 1969). Detailed information about the type of prostaglandins (Es $v.$ Fs) and the changes, if any, in relation to the oestrous cycle is not available. The hypothalamic prostaglandins probably play a role in the gonadotrophin secretion as intrahypothalamic injection of aspirin interferes with ovulation (Labhsetwar and Zolovick, 1973). Precisely how they function in this role is speculative. One possibility is that they could function as neurotransmitters to evoke LRF secretion but evidence is against such a possibility (Baldessarini and Karobath, 1973). Another possibility is that they could interact with catecholamines (CA) which are present in very high concentrations in the hypothalamus (Cuello et $al.$, 1973) and thus either inhibit (Hedqvist, 1973) or potentiate (Brody and Kadowitz, 1974) adrenergic transmission which is normally required for gonadotrophin secretion (McCann et $al.$, 1973). The potentiation of adrenergic transmission for gonadotrophin secretion by $PGF_{2\alpha}$ was postulated by Labhsetwar and Zolovick (1973) when they found that the inhibitory effects of the intra-hypothalamically administered aspirin could be overcome by the simultaneous injection of excess dopamine. Although the inhibitory effect of PGEs on adrenergic transmission with respect to gonadotrophin secretion has not been reported, so far, such an effect has been documented for the peripheral nervous system (Hedqvist, 1973). Available evidence, however, is too meagre to permit a definitive conclusion that PGFs potentiate and PGEs inhibit adrenergic transmission for gonadotrophin secretion in the hypothalamus or brain. Several studies already cited have shown stimulatory effect of PGEs and lesser effectiveness of PGFs on the gonadotrophin secretion. It is not yet known if the positive results with PGEs are due to in $vivo$ transformation of PGEs to PGFs, although enzymes for such a transformation are present in many tissues including the brain (Levine, 1973) and such a conversion is known to occur under certain conditions (Hamberg and Israelsson, 1970).

6.5.3 Action at pituitary level

The anterior pituitary like many other tissues probably contains prostaglandins, although the type of prostaglandin (Es or Fs) and variation in its concentra-tion in relation to the functional state of the gland is not known. Nevertheless attempts have been made to demonstrate an intermediary role of prosta-glandins in the action of LRF on the pituitary cells in $vitro$. Addition of antagonists of prostaglandins to pituitary cell cultures or fragments inhibited, in a dose-related manner, stimulation of LH secretion in response to the addition of LRF (Vale et $al.$, 1971; Dowd et $al.$, 1973). Furthermore, the presence of PGE_1 in the medium also caused a significant increase in LH release from the pituitary fragments incubated without LRF and this stimulation was associated with a parallel increase in the accumulation of cAMP in the gland (Ratner *et al.*, 1974). Thus the relationship between prostaglandins and secretion of LH may be similar to the one already discussed in connection with the action of LH on the ovary.

6.5.4 Action at ovarian level

Role of prostaglandins in causing ovulation by action at the ovarian level has become apparent from several recent studies. It has long been known that the ovary contains prostaglandins (Pickles, 1967) but their precise distribution with respect to various ovarian compartments (corpus luteum, follicle and interstitium), different stages of the reproductive cycle and the type (PGEs *v.* PGFs) remain to be elucidated. The ovarian follicle of rabbits in oestrus contains detectable levels of both PGFs and PGEs and the amount increases following an injection of an ovulatory dose of HCG (LeMaire *et al.*, 1973). These authors reported that the PGF level in the whole follicle increased more than 60-fold and PGE level more than 15-fold when examined nine hours after the injection of HCG. The rise precedes the time of actual rupture of the follicle by about one hour (Harper, 1961). Similar increases in prostaglandin content were observed after mating or LH injection and these increases could be completely suppressed by a single intravenous injection of indomethacin (20 mg kg^{-1}) 30 min prior to the gonadotrophin treatment or mating (Yang *et al.*, 1973). Isolated follicles incubated *in vitro* also synthesised both types of prostaglandins and the rate of synthesis could be markedly enhanced by the addition of LH or cAMP (Marsh *et al.*, 1974). The granulosa cells of the follicle are most probably the source of prostaglandins as incubation of these cells from the preovulatory follicle also synthesise PGF and the synthesis could be completely suppressed by the addition of indomethacin to the medium (Challis *et al.*, 1974a). However, unlike the response of the whole follicles (Marsh *et al.*, 1974) the response of the isolated granulosa cells to LH or cAMP was different; LH failed to augment the prostaglandin synthesis and dibutyryl cAMP in fact caused a 50% reduction in the prostaglandin synthesis (Challis *et al.*, 1974a). The reason for this discrepancy is not known but emphasises the difficulty of extrapolating *in vitro* results to *in vivo* situations and is reminiscent of differences in *in vivo* and *in vitro* effects of prostaglandins on the corpus luteum (see page 247).

One is tempted to speculate that these changes in prostaglandin levels at the time of ovulation are somehow involved in the actual rupture of the follicle. Some support for this speculation is derived from several studies which show that indomethacin can block ovulation. This has been demonstrated in the rabbit (Armstrong and Grinwich, 1972; O'Grady *et al.*, 1972a), rat (Behrman *et al.*, 1972; Orczyk and Behrman, 1972; Tsafiri *et al.*, 1972b) and mouse (Saksena *et al.*, 1974b). In each species indomethacin blocked ovulation even when administered after the LH surge. In the rabbit, in fact, indomethacin blocks ovulation after intrafollicular injection while the control follicles injected with vehicle ovulate normally (Armstrong *et al.*, 1973). LH surge occurs normally after the ovulation blockade with indomethacin in the mouse

(Sato *et al.*, 1974b). These results collectively suggest that indomethacin interferes with ovulation by directly acting on the ovary and thus implicate prostaglandins in the rupture of the follicle.

The question as to how prostaglandins participate in the actual rupture of the follicle remains to be resolved. Numerous biochemical and physiological events occur in the follicular wall prior to its rupture (Rondell, 1974). Prostaglandins could trigger ovulation by affecting vascular permeability, vasodilation or by altering contractile activity of the ovary. The smooth muscle fibres are present in the ovarian stroma as well as in the follicular wall (Okamura *et al.*, 1972a). These authors found that administration of $PGF_{2\alpha}$ to rabbits increased and PGE_2 decreased the frequency and amplitude of ovarian contractions and the ovary was more responsive to prostaglandins just prior to than after ovulation. Stimulation of ovarian contractions were also observed following administration of $PGF_{2\alpha}$ to non-pregnant women (Coutinho and Maia, 1970). In this study PGE_2 showed very little activity. The fact that the rabbit ovarian follicle shows greater increase in PGF than PGE levels prior to ovulation (LeMaire *et al.*, 1973) and that this rise appears to coincide with an increased ovarian sensitivity to prostaglandins (Virutamasen *et al.*, 1972) lends credence to the idea that PGFs may play a role in the follicular rupture and ovulation.

Acknowledgements

Unpublished observations in the author's laboratory were supported by a grant from the Ford Foundation and a contract from the Agency for International Development. The author is grateful to Annette Murray and Doris Marx for typing the manuscript.

References

Abel, M., Taurog, J. and Nathanielsz, P. W. (1973). A comparison of the luteolytic effect of $PGF_{2\alpha}$ and cortisol in the pregnant rabbit. *Prostaglandins*, 4, 431–440

Aiken, J. W. (1972). Aspirin and indomethacin prolong parturition in rats: Evidence that prostaglandins contribute to expulsion of foetus. *Nature (London)*, 240, 21–25

Aldridge, R. R., Barrett, B., Brown, J. B., Funder, J., Goding, J. R., Kaltenback, C. C. and Mole, B. C. (1970). The effect of prostaglandins on ovarian steroidogenesis *in vivo*. *J. Reprod. Fert.*, 21, 369–370

Anderson, L., Bland, K. and Melampy, R. M. (1969). Comparative aspects of uterine luteal relationships. *Recent Progr. Hormone Res.*, 25, 57

Armstrong, D. T. and Grinwich, D. L. (1972). Blockade of spontaneous and LH induced ovulation in rabbits by indomethacin—an inhibitor of prostaglandin biosynthesis. *Prostaglandins*, 1, 21–28

Armstrong, D. T., Moon, Y. S. and Grinwich, D. L. (1973). Possible role of prostaglandins in ovulation. *Adv. Biosciences*, 9, 709–715

Auletta, F. J., Caldwell, B. V., van Wagenen, G. and Morris, J. M. (1972). Effects of postovulatory estrogen on progesterone and prostaglandin F levels in the monkey. *Contraception*, 6, 411–421

Auletta, F. J., Speroff, L. and Caldwell, B. V. (1973). Prostaglandin $F_{2\alpha}$ induced steroidogenesis and luteolysis in the primate corpus luteum. *J. Clin. Endocrinol. Metab.*, 36, 405–407

Baldessarini, R. J. and Karobath, M. (1973). Biochemical physiology of central synapses. *Ann. Rev. Physiol.*, 35, 273–304

Bartke, A., Merrill, A. and Baker, C. (1972). Effects of prostaglandin $F_{2\alpha}$ on pseudopregnancy and pregnancy in mice. *Fertility and Sterility*, 23, 543–547

Batta, S., Zanisi, M. and Martini, L. (1974). Prostaglandins and gonadotropin secretion. *Neuroendocrinology*, 14, 224–232

Bedwani, J. R. and Horton, E. W. (1971). Interaction between prostaglandins and gonadotrophins in the rabbit ovary. *Brit. J. Pharmacol.*, 43, 794–803

Behrman, H. R., MacDonald, G. and Greep, R. O. (1971a). Regulation of ovarian cholesterol esters: Evidence for the enzymatic sites of prostaglandin-induced loss of corpus luteum function. *Lipids*, 6, 791–796

Behrman, H. R., Orczyk, G. P. and Greep, R. O. (1972). Effects of synthetic Gn-Rh on ovulation blockade by aspirin and indomethacin. *Prostaglandins*, 1, 245–258

Behrman, H. R., Yoshinaga, K. and Greep, R. O. (1971b). Extraluteal effects of prostaglandins. *Ann. N.Y. Acad. Sci.*, 180, 426–433

Bergstrom, S., Carlson, L. and Weeks, J. C. (1968). The prostaglandins: A family of biologically active lipids. *Pharmacol. Rev.*, 20, 1–48

Bito, L. Z. (1972). Accumulation and apparent active transport of prostaglandins by some rabbit tissues *in vitro*. *J. Physiol.*, 221, 371–387

Bland, K. P. and Donovan, B. T. (1966). Uterine distension and the function of the corpora lutea in the guinea pig. *J. Physiol.* 186, 503–515

Bland, K. P. and Donovan, B. T. (1969). Control of luteal function during early pregnancy in the guinea pig. *J. Reprod. Fert.*, 20, 491–501

Bland, K. P., Horton, E. and Poyser, N. (1971). Levels of prostaglandin $F_{2\alpha}$ in the uterine venous blood of sheep during the oestrous cycle. *Life Sci.*, 10 (Part 1), 509–517

Blatchley, F. R. and Donovan, B. T. (1969). Luteolytic effect of prostaglandin in the guinea-pig. *Nature (London)*, 221, 1065–1066

Blatchley, F. R. and Donovan, B. T. (1972). The effect of prostaglandin $F_{2\alpha}$ and prostaglandin E_2 upon luteal function and ovulation in the guinea-pig. *J. Endocrinol.*, 53, 493–501

Blatchley, F. R., Donovan, B., Poyser, N. L., Horton, E., Thompson, C. and Los, M. (1971). Identification of prostaglandin $F_{2\alpha}$ in the utero-ovarian blood of guinea-pig after treatment with oestrogen. *Nature (London)*, 230, 243–244

Blatchley, F. R. and Poyser, N. L. (1974). The effect of oestrogen and progesterone on the release of prostaglandins from the uterus of the ovariectomized guinea pig. *J. Reprod. Fert.*, 40, 205–209

Bolt, D. J. and Hawk, H. (1972). Failure of exogenous estrogens to induce CL regression in hysterectomized ewes. *J. Anim. Sci.*, 35, 237 (Abst.)

Breed, W. G., Fraser, A., Eckstein, P. and Peplow, P. V. (1972). Phagocytic cells in smears from intrauterine devices in the baboon. *J. Reprod. Fert.*, 30, 143–146

Brody, M. J. and Kadowitz, P. J. (1974). Prostaglandins as modulators of the autonomic nervous system. *Fed. Proc.*, 33, 48–60

Buckle, J. W. and Nathanielsz, P. W. (1973). The effect of low doses of prostaglandin $F_{2\alpha}$ infused into the aorta of unrestrained pregnant rats: Observations on induction of parturition and effect on plasma progesterone concentration. *Prostaglandins*, 4, 443–457

Carlson, J., Barcikowski, B. and McCracken, J. (1973). Prostaglandin $F_{2\alpha}$ and the release of LH in sheep. *J. Reprod. Fert.*, 34, 359–363

Challis, J., Davies, I. J. and Ryan, K. J. (1973). The relationship between progesterone and prostaglandin F concentrations in the plasma of pregnant rabbits. *Prostaglandins*, 4, 509–516

Challis, J., Erickson, G. F. and Ryan, K. J. (1974a). Prostaglandin F production *in vitro* by granulosa cells from rabbit pre-ovulatory follicles. *Prostaglandins*, 7, 183–193

Challis, J., Porter, D. G. and Ryan, K. J. (1974b). The effects of prostaglandin $F_{2\alpha}$ and ovariectomy on the peripheral plasma steroid concentrations and the evolution of myometrial activity in the pregnant rabbit. *Endocrinology*, 95, 783–792

Chamley, W. A. and Christie, M. (1973). Failure of prostaglandin to affect LH secretion in the ovariectomized ewe. *Prostaglandins*, 3, 405–412

Chang, M. C., Hunt, D. and Polge, C. (1973). Effects of prostaglandins (PGs) on sperm and egg transport in the rabbit. *Adv. Biosciences*, 9, 805–810

Chatterjee, A. (1972a). The possible mode of action of prostaglandins. I. Interruption of decidual reaction by $PGF_{2\alpha}$ and its prevention by using prolactin or progesterone. *Acta Endocrinol. (Kbh)*, 70, 781–785

Chatterjee, A. (1972b). The possible mode of action of prostaglandins. IV. Reversal of the detrimental effects of prostaglandin E$_2$ in the termination of decidual growth in pseudo-pregnant rats by using prolactin or progesterone. *Prostaglandins*, 2, 417–425

Chaudhury, G. (1973). Release of prostaglandins by the I.U.C.D. *Prostaglandins*, 3, 773–784

Chester, R., Dukes, M., Slater, S. R. and Walpole, A. (1972). Delay of parturition in the rat by anti-inflammatory agents which inhibit biosynthesis of prostaglandins. *Nature (London)*, 240, 37–38

Coutinho, E. M. and Maia, H. S. (1971). The contractile response of the human uterus, fallopian tubes and ovary to prostaglandins *in vivo*. *Fertility and Sterility*, 22, 539–543

Cox, R., Thorburn, G., Currie, W., Restall, B. and Schneider, W. (1973). Prostaglandin F group (PGF), progesterone and estrogen concentrations in the utero-ovarian venous plasma of the conscious ewe during the estrous cycle. *Adv. Biosciences*, 9, 625–630

Csapo, A. I. (1956). Progesterone 'block'. *Amer. J. Anat.*, 98, 273–291

Csapo, A. I., Csapo, E., Fay, E., Henzl, M. and Salau, G. (1973). The delay of spontaneous labor by naproxen in the rat model. *Prostaglandins*, 3, 827–837

Cuello, A., Horn, A., Mackay, A. and Iversen, L. (1973). Catecholamines in the median eminence: New evidence for a major noradrenergic input. *Nature (London)*, 243, 465–467

Dowd, A. J., Hoffman, D. C. and Speroff, L. (1973). Direct effect of prostaglandins and prostaglandin inhibitors on pituitary LH release demonstrated by *in vitro* perfusion. *Proc. Endocrine Soc. 55th Meeting, Chicago*, p. 135

DuCharme, D. W., Weeks, J. and Montgomery, R. (1968). Studies on the mechanism of the hypertensive effect of prostaglandin F$_{2\alpha}$. *J. Pharmacol. Exp. Ther.*, 160, 1–10

Duncan, G. W. and Pharriss, B. (1970). Effect of nonsteroidal compounds on fertility. *Fed. Proc.*, 29, 1232–1239

Feldberg, W. and Myers, R. D. (1966). Appearance of 5-hydroxytryptamine and an unidentified pharmacologically active lipid acid in effluent from perfused cerebral ventricles. *J. Physiol. (London)*, 184, 837–855

Finn, C. and McLaren, A. (1967). A study of the early stages of implantation in mice. *J. Reprod. Fert.*, 13, 259–267

Gibori, G. and Kraicer, P. F. (1972). Histological and functional analysis of the auto-transplanted corpus luteum of pregnancy in the rat. *J. Reprod. Fert.*, 31, 179

Ginther, O. J. (1974). Internal regulation of physiological processes through local venoarterial pathways: A review. *J. Anim. Sci.*, 39, 550–564

Ginther, O. J., Mahajan, S. and Casida, L. (1966). Local ovarian effects of an intrauterine device in intact and unilaterally ovariectomized guinea pigs. *Proc. Soc. Exp. Biol. Med.*, 123, 775–778

Greenwald, G. S. (1965a). Interruption of pregnancy in the rat by a uterine suture. *J. Reprod. Fert.*, 9, 9–17

Greenwald, G. S. (1965b). Luteolytic effect of estrogen on the corpora lutea of pregnancy of the hamster. *Endocrinology*, 76, 1213–1219

Greenwald, G. S. (1967a). Luteotropic complex of the hamster. *Endocrinology*, 80, 118–130

Greenwald, G. S. (1967b). Species differences in egg transport in response to exogenous estrogen. *Anat. Rec.*, 157, 163–172

Gutknecht, G. D., Cornette, J. and Pharriss, B. B. (1969). Antifertility properties of PGF$_{2\alpha}$. *Biol. Reprod.*, 1, 367–371

Gutknecht, G. D., Cornette, J. and Pharriss, B. B. (1971a). The effect of prostaglandin F$_{2\alpha}$ on ovarian and plasma progesterone levels in the pregnant hamster. *Proc. Soc. Exp. Biol. Med.*, 136, 1151–1157

Gutknecht, G. D., Duncan, G. and Wyngarden, L. (1970). Effect of prostaglandin F$_{2\alpha}$ on ovarian blood flow in the rabbit as measured by hydrogen desaturation. *Physiologist*, 13, 214 (Abst.)

Gutknecht, G. D., Wyngarden, L. J. and Pharriss, B. (1971b). The effect of prostaglandin F$_{2\alpha}$ on the ovarian and plasma progesterone levels in the pregnant hamster. *Proc. Soc. Exp. Biol. Med.*, 136, 1151–1157

Hamberg, M. and Israelsson, U. (1970). Metabolism of prostaglandin E$_2$ in guinea pig liver. I. Identification of seven metabolites. *J. Biol. Chem.*, 245, 5107–5114

Harms, P. G., Ojeda, S. R. and McCann, S. (1973). PG involvement in hypothalamic control of gonadotropin and prolactin release. *Science*, 181, 760–761

Harper, M. J. K. (1961). The time of ovulation in the rabbit following the injection of lutenizing hormone. *J. Endocrinol.*, 22, 147–152

Harper, M. J. K. (1968). Pharmacological control of reproduction in women. *Prof. Drug Res.*, 12, 47–131

Hawk, H. W. and Bolt, D. (1970). Luteolytic effect of estradiol-17β when administered after midcycle in the ewe. *Biol. Reprod.*, 2, 275–278

Hedqvist, P. (1973). Prostaglandin mediated control of sympathetic neuroreflector transmission. *Adv. Biosciences*, 9, 461–473

Hichens, M., Grinwich, D. L. and Behrman, H. R. (1974). PGF$_{2\alpha}$-induced loss of corpus luteum gonadotrophin receptors. *Prostaglandins*, 7, 449–458

Horton, E. W. (1969). Hypotheses on physiological roles of prostaglandins. *Physiol. Rev.*, 49, 122–161

Horton, E. W., Main, I. and Thompson, C. (1965). Effects of prostaglandins on the oviduct, studied in rabbits and ewes. *J. Physiol.*, 180, 514–528

Horton, E. W. and Marley, P. B. (1969). An investigation of the possible effects of prostaglandins E$_1$, F$_2$$_\alpha$ and F$_{2\alpha}$ on pregnancy in mice and rabbits. *Brit. J. Pharmacol.*, 36, 188P

Horton, E. W..and Poyser, N. L. (1974). Elongation of oestrous cycle in the guinea-pig following active immunization against prostaglandin F$_{2\alpha}$. *Prostaglandins*, 5, 349–354

Horton, E. W. and Thompson, C. J. (1964). Thin layer chromatography and bioassay of prostaglandins in extracts of semen and tissues of the male reproductive tract. *J. Pharmacol.*, 22, 183–188

Hunt, W. L. and Nicholson, N. (1972). Studies on semen from rabbits injected with ^{3}H-thymidine and treated with prostaglandins E$_2$ and F$_{2\alpha}$. *Fertility and Sterility*, 23, 763–768

Inskeep, E. K. (1973). Potential uses of prostaglandins in control of reproductive cycles of domestic animals. *J. Anim. Sci.*, 36, 1149–1157

Jacobson, H., Bullock, D. and Keyes, P. L. (1972). Effect of prostaglandin F$_{2\alpha}$ on oestrogen receptor in corpus luteum and uterus. *Fourth Int. Congr. Endocrinol., Washington, D.C.* (Abst.) 472

Jensen, E. V. and DeSombre, E. R. (1973). Estrogen–receptor interaction. *Science*, 182, 126–134

Joshi, S. G. (1971). Accumulation of macrophages in the uterine cavity of baboons bearing an intrauterine foreign body (IUFB). *Contraception*, 4, 45–49

Joshi, H. S. and Labhsetwar, A. (1972). The pattern of ovarian secretion of oestradiol and oestrone during pregnancy and the post-partum period in the hamster. *J. Reprod. Fert.*, 31, 299–302

Joshi, H. S., Watson, D. J. and Labhsetwar, A. P. (1973). Ovarian secretion of oestradiol, oestrone, progesterone and 20-dihydroprogesterone during the oestrous cycle of the guinea pig. *J. Reprod. Fert.*, 35, 177–181

Karim, S. M. M. (1972). *The Prostaglandins: Progress in Research* (S. M. M. Karim, editor) (Lancaster: M.T.P.)

Karim, S. M. M. and Devlin, J. (1967). Prostaglandin content of amniotic fluid during pregnancy and labour. *J. Obstet. Gynaecol. Brit. Cwlth.*, 74, 230–234

Keyes, P. L. and Bullock, D. W. (1974). Effects of prostaglandin F$_{2\alpha}$ on ectopic and ovarian corpora lutea of the rabbit. *Biol. Reprod.*, 10, 519–525

Kirton, K. T., Gutknecht, G., Bergstrom, K., Wyngarden, L. and Forbes, A. (1972). Prostaglandins and reproduction. *J. Reprod. Med.*, 9, 266–269

Koering, M. J. and Kirton, K. T. (1973). The effects of prostaglandin F$_{2\alpha}$ on the structure and function of the rabbit ovary. *Biol. Reprod.*, 9, 226–245

Kuehl, F. A., Jr (1974). Prostaglandins, cyclic nucleotides and cell function. *Prostaglandins*, 5, 325–340

Kuehl, F. A., Jr. and Humes, J. (1972). Direct evidence for a prostaglandin receptor and its application to prostaglandin measurements. *Proc. Nat. Acad. Sci.*, 69, 480–484

Kuehl, F. A., Jr., Humes, J., Tarnoff, J., Cirillo, V. and Hamm, E. A. (1970). Prostaglandin receptor site: Evidence for an essential role in the action of luteinizing hormone. *Science*, 169, 883–886

Labhsetwar, A. P. (1970). Effects of prostaglandin F$_{2\alpha}$ on pituitary luteinising hormone content of pregnant rats: A possible explanation for the luteolytic effect. *J. Reprod. Fert.*, 23, 155–159

Labhsetwar, A. P. (1971a). Prostaglandin F$_{2\alpha}$ and the implantation process in the rat. *J. Endocrinol.*, 50, 353–354

Labhsetwar, A. P. (1971b). Luteolysis and ovulation induced by prostaglandin F$_{2\alpha}$ in the hamster. *Nature (London)*, 230, 528–354

Labhsetwar, A. P. (1972a). Prostaglandin E₂: Analysis of effects on pregnancy and corpus luteum in hamsters and rats. *Acta Endocrinol. (Kbh)*, suppl. 170, **71**, 1–35

Labhsetwar, A. P. (1972b). Effects of prostaglandin F$_{2\alpha}$ on some reproductive processes of hamsters and rats. *J. Endocrinol.*, **53**, 201–213

Labhsetwar, A. P. (1972c). Luteolytic and ovulation inducing properties of prostaglandin F$_{2\alpha}$ in pregnant mice. *J. Reprod. Fert.*, **28**, 451–452

Labhsetwar, A. P. (1972d). A new antifertility agent—an orally active prostaglandin—ICI 74205. *Nature (London)*, **238**, 400–401

Labhsetwar, A. P. (1973a). Neuroendocrine basis of ovulation in hamsters treated with prostaglandin F$_{2\alpha}$. *Endocrinology*, **92**, 606–610

Labhsetwar, A. P. (1973b). Prostaglandin E₁: Studies on antifertility and luteolytic effects in hamsters and rats. *Biol. Reprod.*, **8**, 103–111

Labhsetwar, A. P. (1973c). Do prostaglandins stimulate LH release and thereby cause luteolysis? *Prostaglandins*, **3**, 729–732

Labhsetwar, A. P. (1974). Prostaglandins and the reproductive cycle. *Fed. Proc.*, **33**, 61–77

Labhsetwar, A. P. and Watson, D. (1974). Temporal relationship between secretory patterns of gonadotropins, estrogens, progestins and prostaglandin F in periparturient rats. *Biol. Reprod.*, **10**, 103–110

Labhsetwar, A. P. and Zolovick, A. (1973). Evidence for the hypothalamic interaction between prostaglandins and catecholamines in promoting gonadotrophin secretion for ovulation. *Nature, New Biol.*, **249**, 55–56

LeMaire, W., Yang, N., Behrman, H. R. and Marsh, J. (1973). Preovulatory changes in the concentration of prostaglandins in rabbit Graafian follicles. *Prostaglandins*, **3**, 367–376

Lamprecht, S. A., Zor, U., Tsafriri, A. and Lindner, H. R. (1973). Action of prostaglandin E₂ and of luteinising hormone on ovarian adenylate cyclase, protein kinase and ornithine decarboxylase activity during postnatal development and maturity in the rat. *J. Endocrinol.*, **57**, 217–233

Lands, W., Lee, R. and Smith, W. (1971). Factors regulating the biosynthesis of various prostaglandins. *Ann. N.Y. Acad. Sci.*, **180**, 107–122

Levine, L. (1973). Antibodies to pharmacologically active molecules: Specificities and some applications of anti-prostaglandins. *Pharmacol. Rev.*, **25**, 293–307

Lukaszewaska, J., Wilson, J., Jr and Hansel, W. (1972). Luteotropic and luteolytic effects of prostaglandins in the hamster. *Proc. Soc. Exp. Biol. Med.*, **140**, 1302–1307

Mandl, J. P. (1972). The effect of prostaglandin E₁ on rabbit sperm transport *in vivo. J. Reprod. Fert.*, **31**, 263–269

Marley, P. B. (1972). Effects of prostaglandins F$_{2\alpha}$, E₂ and E₁ on fertility in mice. *Nature, New Biol.*, 235–214

Marley, P. B. (1973). Indomethacin lengthens the oestrous cycle of the guinea-pig when given orally with oestrogen or when implanted within the uterine lumen. *Prostaglandins*, **4**, 251–261

Marsh, J. (1971). The effect of prostaglandins on the adenyl cyclase of the bovine corpus luteum. *Ann. N.Y. Acad. Sci.*, **180**, 416–425

Marsh, J., Yang, S. and LeMaire, W. (1974). Prostaglandin synthesis in rabbit Graafian follicles *in vitro*: Effect of luteinising hormone and cyclic AMP. *Prostaglandins*, **7**, 269–283

McCann, S., Krulich, L., Cooper, J., Kalra, P., Kalra, S., Libertun, C., Negro-Vilar, A., Orias, R., Ronnekleiv, O. and Fawcett, C. (1973). Hypothalamic control of gonadotrophin and prolactin secretion; implications for fertility control. *J. Reprod. Fert.*, **Suppl. 20**, 43–59

McCracken, J. A., Baird, D. and Goding, J. R. (1972a). Factors affecting the secretion of steroids from the transplanted ovary in the sheep. *Rec. Prog. Hormone Res.*, **27**, 537–582

McCracken, J. A., Carlson, J., Glew, M., Goding, J. R., Baird, D., Green, K. and Samuelson, B. (1972b). Prostaglandin F$_{2\alpha}$ identified as a luteolytic hormone in sheep. *Nature New Biol.*, **238**, 129–134

McCracken, J. A., Barcikowski, B., Carlson, J., Gréen, K. and Samuelson, B. (1973). The physiological role of prostaglandin F$_{2\alpha}$ in corpus luteum regression. *Adv. Biosciences*, **9**, 599–624

Mishell, D. R., Jr (1974). Current status of contraceptive steroids and the intrauterine device. *Clin. Obstet. Gynecol.*, **17**, 35–51

Nutting, E. F. and Cammarata, P. (1969). Effects of prostaglandins on fertility in female rats. *Nature (London)*, **222**, 287–288

Ogra, S. S., Kirton, K. T., Tomasi, T. and Lippes, J. (1974). Prostaglandins in the human Fallopian tube. *Fertility and Sterility*, **25**, 250–255

O'Grady, J. P., Caldwell, B. V., Auletta, F. J. and Speroff, L. (1972a). The effects of an inhibitor of prostaglandin synthesis (indomethacin) on ovulation, pregnancy and pseudopregnancy in the rabbit. *Prostaglandins*, 1, 97–106

O'Grady, J. P., Kohorn, E., Glass, R. H., Caldwell, B. V., Brock, W. and Speroff, L. (1972b). Inhibition of progesterone synthesis *in vitro* by prostaglandin $F_{2\alpha}$. *J. Reprod. Fert.*, 30, 153–156

Ojeda, S., Harms, P. G. and McCann, S. (1974). Central effect of prostaglandin E_1 (PGE_1) on prolactin release. *Endocrinology*, 95, 613–618

Okamura, H., Virutamasen, P., Wright, K. and Wallach, E. (1972a). Ovarian smooth muscle in the human being, rabbit and cat. *Amer. J. Obstet. Gynecol.*, 112, 183–191

Okamura, H., Yang, S., Wright, K. and Wallach, E. (1972b). The effect of prostaglandin $F_{2\alpha}$ on the corpus luteum of the pregnant rat—an ultra-structural study. *Fertility and Sterility*, 23, 475–483

Orczyk, G. P. and Behrman, H. R. (1972). Ovulation blockade by aspirin or indomethacin —*in vivo* evidence for a role of prostaglandin in gonadotrophin secretion. *Prostaglandins*, 1, 3–20

Pharriss, B. B. (1970). The possible vascular regulation of luteal function. *Perspect. Biol. Med.*, 13, 434–444

Pharriss, B. B., Cornette, J. and Gutknecht, G. D. (1970). Vascular control of luteal steroidogenesis. *J. Reprod. Fert.*, Suppl, 10, 97–103

Pharriss, B. B., Tillson, S. and Erickson, R. (1972). Prostaglandins in luteal function. *Rec. Prog. Hormone Res.*, 28, 51–89

Pharriss, B. B. and Wyngarden, L. J. (1969). The effect of prostaglandin $F_{2\alpha}$ on the progestogen content of ovaries from pseudopregnant rats.*Proc. Soc. Exp. Biol. Med.*, 130, 92–94

Pharriss, B. B., Wyngarden, L. J. and Gutknecht, G. D. (1968). Biological interactions between prostaglandins and luteotrophins in the rat. In: *Gonadotrophins*, 121–129 (E. Rosenberg, editor) (Palo Alto, California: Geron-X, Inc.)

Pickles, V. R. (1967). Prostaglandins. *Biol. Rev.*, 42, 614–652

Piper, P. and Vane, J. (1971). The release of prostaglandins from lung and other tissues. *Ann. N.Y. Acad. Sci.*, 180, 363–383

Porter, D. G. and Behrman, H. R. (1971). Prostaglandin-induced myometrial activity inhibited by progesterone. *Nature (London)*, 232, 627–628

Poyser, N. L. (1972). Production of prostaglandins by the guinea-pig uterus. *J. Endocrinol.*, 54, 147–159

Poyser, N. L. (1973). The formation of prostaglandins by the guinea-pig uterus and the effect of indomethacin. *Adv. Biosciences*, 9, 631–634

Poyser, N. L., Horton, E. W., Thompson, C. L. and Los, M. (1971). Identification of $PGF_{2\alpha}$ released by distension of guinea-pig uterus *in vitro*. *Nature (London)*, 230, 526–529

Prasad, D. S. M., Joshi, H. and Labhsetwar, A. (1973). Effects of an intrauterine device (IUD) on ovarian secretion of progestogens and oestrogens in pregnant rats: evidence for local effects. *J. Reprod. Fert.*, 33, 519–522

Ramwell, P. W. and Shaw, J. E. (1966). Spontaneous and evoked release of prostaglandins from cerebral cortex of anesthetized cats. *Amer. J. Physiol.*, 211, 125–133

Rao, C. V. (1973). Receptors for prostaglandins and gonadtrophins in the cell membranes of bovine corpus luteum. *Prostaglandins*, 4, 567–576

Rao, C. V. (1974). Differential properties of prostaglandin and gonadotrophin receptors in the bovine corpus luteal cell membranes. *Prostaglandins*, 6, 313–328

Ratner, A., Wilson, M. C., Srivastava, L. and Peake, G. T. (1974). Stimulatory effects of prostaglandin E_1 on rat anterior pituitary cyclic AMP and luteinising hormone release. *Prostaglandins*, 5, 165–171

Rondell, P. (1974). Role of steroid synthesis in the process of ovulation. *Biol. Reprod.*, 10, 199–215

Rothchild, I. (1965). The corpus luteum—hypophysis relationship: The luteolytic effect of LH in the rat. *Acta Endocrinol. (Kbh)*, 49, 107–117

Ryan, M. J., Clark, K., Van Orden, D., Farley, D., Edvisson, L., Sjoberg, N. O., Van Orden, L., III and Brody, M. J. (1974). Role of prostaglandins in estrogen-induced uterine hyperemia. *Prostaglandins*, 5, 257–268

Sagiroglu, N. and Sagiroglu, E. (1970). Biologic mode of action of the Lippes loop in intrauterine contraception. *Amer. J. Obstet. Gynecol.*, 106, 506–515

Saksena, S. K. and Harper, M. J. K. (1972a). Levels of F-prostaglandin (PGF) in uterine tissue during the oestrous cycle of hamster: Effects of estradiol and progesterone. *Prostaglandins*, 2, 405–411

Saksena, S. K. and Harper, M. J. K. (1972b). Level of F prostaglandin (PGF) in peripheral plasma and uterine tissue of cyclic rats. *Prostaglandins*, 2, 511–517

Saksena, S. K. and Harper, M. J. K. (1974). Prostaglandin-mediated action of intrauterine devices: F-prostaglandins in the uterine horns of pregnant rabbits with unilateral intrauterine devices. *Fertility and Sterility*, 25, 121–126

Saksena, S. K. and Lau, I. F. (1973). Effect of exogenous estradiol and progesterone on the uterine tissue levels of PGF (PGF$_{2\alpha}$) in ovariectomized mice. *Prostaglandins*, 3, 317–322

Saksena, S. K., Lau, I. F. and Castracane, V. (1974a). Prostaglandin-mediated action of IUDs. (II). F-prostaglandins (PGF) in the uterine horn of pregnant rats and hamsters with intra-uterine devices. *Prostaglandins*, 5, 97–106

Saksena, S. K., Lau, I. F. and Shaikh, A. A. (1974b). Cyclic changes in the uterine tissue content of F-prostaglandins and the role of prostaglandins in ovulation in mice. *Fertility and Sterility*, 25, 636–643

Sato, T., Taya, K., Jyujo, T., Hirono, M. and Igarashi, M. (1974a). The stimulatory effect of prostaglandins on luteinizing hormone release. *Amer. J. Obstet. Gynecol.*, 118, 875–876

Sato, T., Taya, K., Jyujo, T. and Igarashi, M. (1974b). Ovulation block by indomethacin, an inhibitor of prostaglandin synthesis: A study of its action in rats. *J. Reprod. Fert.*, 39, 33–40

Sellner, R. G. and Wickersham, E. (1970). Effects of prostaglandins on steroidogenesis. *J. Anim. Sci.*, 31, 230 (Abst.)

Shaikh, A. A. and Saksena, S. K. (1972). Cyclic changes in uterine venous and peripheral plasma levels of F prostaglandins correlated with peripheral progesterone levels in the golden hamster. *Adv. Biosciences*, 9, 635–639

Smith, G. W., Abel, M. and Nathanielsz, P. (1973). Uterine sensitivity to prostaglandins in the pregnant rabbit: a method for testing the effect of previous administration of small doses of PGF$_{2\alpha}$ for short periods. *Prostaglandins*, 3, 525–530

Speroff, L. and Ramwell, P. W. (1970). Prostaglandin stimulation of *in vitro* progesterone synthesis. *J. Clin. Endocrinol. Metab.*, 30, 345–350

Spies, H. and Norman, R. (1973). LH release and ovulation induced by the intraventricular infusion of PGE into pentobarbital-blocked rats. *Prostaglandins*, 4, 131–142

Spilman, C. H. and Harper, M. (1973). Effect of prostaglandins on oviduct motility in estrous rabbits. *Biol. Reprod.*, 9, 36–45

Spilman, C. H. and Harper, M. (1974). Comparison of the effects of adrenergic drugs and prostaglandins on rabbit oviduct motility. *Biol. Reprod.*, 10, 549–554

Stormshak, F. and Casida, L. (1965). Effects of LH and ovarian hormones on corpora lutea of pseudopregnant and pregnant rabbits. *Endocrinology*, 77, 337–342

Sullivan, T. (1966). Response of the mammalian uterus to prostaglandins under differing hormonal conditions. *Brit. J. Pharmacol. Chemother.*, 26, 678–685

Tsafriri, A., Lindner, H. R., Zor, U. and Lamprecht, S. A. (1972a). Physiological role of prostaglandins on the induction of ovulation. *Prostaglandins*, 2, 1–10

Tsafriri, A., Lindner, H. R., Zor, U. and Lamprecht, S. A. (1972b). *In vitro* introduction of meiotic division in follicle-enclosed rat oocytes by LH, cyclic AMP and prostaglandin E$_2$. *J. Reprod. Fert.*, 31, 39–50

Vale, W., Rivier, C. and Guillemin, R. (1971). A prostaglandin receptor in the mechanisms involved in the secretion of anterior pituitary hormones. *Fed. Proc.*, 30, 363 (Abst.)

Vane, J. R. (1971). Inhibition of prostaglandin synthesis as a mechanisms of action of aspirin-like drugs. *Nature New Biol.*, 231, 232–235

Vane, J. R. and Williams, K. (1972). Prostaglandin production contributes to the contractions of the rat isolated uterus. *Brit. J. Pharmacol.*, 45, 146P

Vermouth, N. T. and Deis, R. P. (1972). Prolactin release induced by prostaglandin F$_{2\alpha}$ in the pregnant rats. *Nature New Biol.*, 238–248

Virutamasen, P., Wright, K. and Wallach, E. (1972). Effects of prostaglandins E$_2$ and F$_{2\alpha}$ on ovarian contractility in rabbit. *Fertility and Sterility*, 23, 675–682

Von Euler, U. S. and Elliason, R. (1967). *Prostaglandins*. Medicinal Chemistry Series of Monographs, Academic Press, N.Y., Vol. 8

Wakeling, A. E. and Spilman, C. H. (1973). Prostaglandin specific binding in the rabbit oviduct. *Prostaglandins*, 4, 405–414

Wakeling, A. E., Kirton, K. T. and Wyngarden, L. J. (1973). Prostaglandin receptors in the hamster uterus during the estrous cycle. *Prostaglandins*, 4, 1–8

Wakeling, A. E. and Wyngarden, L. J. (1974). Prostaglandin receptors in the human, monkey and hamster uterus. *Endocrinology*, 95, 55–64

Weeks, J. R. (1972). Prostaglandins. *Ann. Rev. Pharmacol.*, 12, 317–336

Weeks, J. R. (1973). Tachyphylactic response of the rat uterus to prostaglandins E_2 and $F_{2\alpha}$. *Adv. Biosciences*, 9, 773–777

Yang, N., Marsh, J. M. and LeMaire, W. J. (1973). Prostaglandin changes induced by ovulatory stimuli in rabbit Graafian follicles. The effect of indomethacin. *Prostaglandins*, 3, 395–404

Zor, U., Lamprecht, S., Kaneko, T., Schneider, H. P., McCann, S. M., Field, J., Tsafriri, A. and H. R. Lindner, H. (1972). Functional relations between cyclic AMP, prostaglandins and luteinising hormone in rat pituitary and ovary. *Adv. Cyclic Nucleotide Res.*, 1, 503–520

7
Prostaglandins and Reproductive Processes in Female Sheep and Goat

A. P. F. FLINT and K. HILLIER

7.1 INTRODUCTION

Certain characteristics of the sheep have made it an extensively investigated animal in reproductive physiology, particularly in the study of luteal function. It is large enough to permit major operative techniques, such as chronic vascular catheterisation, both in the adult and in the fetus *in utero*, allowing repetitive blood sampling. The ease with which fetal catheters can be maintained for long periods of time allows the study of endocrine changes in relation to pregnancy and parturition.

Before the total synthesis of prostaglandins had been accomplished, sheep vesicular glands served as a major source of these compounds and enzymes for their biosynthesis. The animal has provided important information on the role of prostaglandins in reproduction and has been important in the overall genesis of knowledge of prostaglandin physiology.

Much less experimental data is available in the goat. This animal, however, is of interest because in contrast to the sheep the maintenance of pregnancy throughout gestation is totally dependent upon a functional corpus luteum.

7.2 THE ROLE OF PROSTAGLANDINS IN OVULATION AND LUTEINISATION

An essential role for prostaglandins in ovulation has been demonstrated in the rabbit (Grinwich *et al.*, 1972; Armstrong *et al.*, 1973; Lemaire *et al.*, 1973;

Armstrong et al., 1974) and rat (Armstrong and Grinwich, 1972; Orczyk and Behrman, 1972) by a variety of techniques, including direct measurement of follicular prostaglandins and intrafollicular administration of prostaglandins, indomethacin (prostaglandin synthesis inhibitor) and prostaglandin antiserum. There appear to be no published reports of elevated prostaglandin levels in the ovulatory follicle in the sheep. However, as in the rabbit (Virutamasen et al., 1972), $PGF_{2\alpha}$ causes increased contractility of strips of ovine follicular tissue in vitro, with concentrations as low as 30 ng ml^{-1} (O'Shea and Phillips, 1974).

Little is known of the involvement of prostaglandins in luteinisation in the sheep. Studies in the rabbit indicate that 'normal' luteinisation of follicles occurs after ovulation blockade with indomethacin (Grinwich et al., 1972) suggesting that prostaglandins are not involved in the process of luteinisation of the follicle. Luteinisation in sheep is not prevented by administration of luteolytic doses of $PGF_{2\alpha}$ on days 1 and 2 of the cycle (Hearnshaw et al., 1973).

7.3 UTERINE $PGF_{2\alpha}$ AND THE CONTROL OF LUTEAL FUNCTION DURING THE OESTROUS CYCLE

7.3.1. Evidence that there is a uterine luteolysin in sheep

Two forms of evidence suggest that the ovine uterus produces a luteolysin: that based on hysterectomy, or other surgical intervention; and that obtained by administration of extracts of uterus or uterine venous blood in test systems.

Extension of the luteal phase of the cycle by hysterectomy was first demonstrated in sheep by Wiltbank and Casida (1956), who observed prolonged luteal phases (up to 107 days) in 9 out of 10 ewes hysterectomised on days 3–8 of the oestrous cycle. Denamur and Mauleon (1963) and Moor and Rowson (1964) subsequently corroborated this observation, and numerous similar experiments have since confirmed and extended the basic finding. The uterine luteolytic effect has been shown to be local, in that hemihysterectomy results only in maintenance of an ipsilateral corpus luteum (Inskeep and Butcher 1966; Moor and Rowson, 1966a; Caldwell et al., 1969). This local action has been confirmed in a ewe with congenital absence of one uterine horn (McCracken and Caldwell, 1969). Furthermore it has been shown that a quantitative relationship exists between the amount of uterus removed and the degree to which the luteal phase is lengthened (Rowson and Moor, 1964).

Further evidence for a locally acting ovine uterine luteolytic factor is derived from experiments with animals bearing autotransplanted ovaries, uteri, or both. Where both ovary and uterus are transplanted to the neck, either subcutaneously (Harrison et al., 1968) or in a jugulo-carotid loop (McCracken et al., 1970a), cycle length (as indicated by duration of progesterone secretion) is generally normal. However, when the ovary alone is transplanted to the neck with the uterus remaining in situ (Goding et al., 1967a, 1967b) corpora lutea are maintained for up to 22 days and there are no normal cycles. Extended luteal function has likewise been observed in one animal where the uterus was transplanted to the neck and the ovaries left in situ (Goding et al., 1969, 1967b) (Figure 7.1).

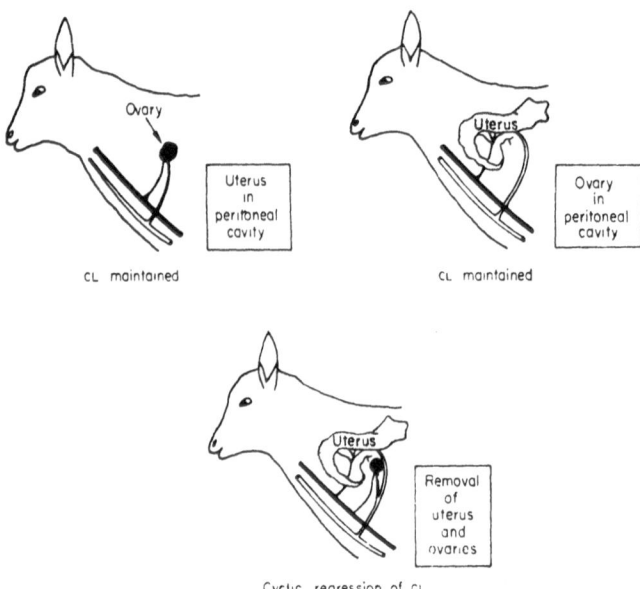

Figure 7.1 Luteal function after autotransplantation of uterus, ovary or both. (From Caldwell *et al.*, 1969, by courtesy of *J. Reprod. Fert.*)

Ginther *et al.* (1973) have recently provided further evidence for a local effect of the uterine luteolysin. In unilaterally hysterectomised ewes, luteolysis occurred normally when the uterine vein on the intact side was anastomosed to that on the hysterectomised side (and where at autopsy the anastomosis was found to be patent). Likewise, luteolysis was observed in animals where the ovarian artery on the intact side ('donor') was anastomosed to that on the hysterectomised ('recipient') side.

Experiments in which utero–ovarian venous blood or plasma has been administered to cycling animals in the luteal phase provide a second line of evidence for the existence of an ovine uterine luteolysin. This type of evidence is important, since it does not depend on surgical intervention in the genital tract. Freeze-dried extracts of uterine venous plasma obtained on day 14 were luteolytic on infusion into the ovarian artery of an intact sheep on day 8 (Caldwell and Moor, 1971). Uterine venous plasma extracts obtained on day 8, or freeze-dried jugular venous plasma obtained on day 14, were not active. When luteolysis occurred, ovarian venous progesterone levels were reduced by approximately 50% during a 6–8 hour infusion and the sheep returned to oestrus prematurely.

Similar results have been obtained by Caldwell *et al.* (1968) in pseudo-pregnant hamsters after administration of ovine endometrial extracts or insertion of endometrial transplants. Material obtained on days 14 and 15 was luteolytic, whereas that obtained between days 3 and 9 had no effect on the recipient hamster's pseudopregnancy.

Cross-circulation experiments provide similar data. McCracken *et al.* (1972) tested utero–ovarian venous blood from sheep with organs transplanted to the neck for luteolytic activity by infusing it into the ovarian arteries of haemocompatible recipients with autotransplanted luteal ovaries in the neck. Blood from the donor was luteolytic on day 15 of the cycle, but not on days 2, 6, 10 or 13, when there was minimal ($<20\%$) depression of progesterone output. Peripheral arterial blood from the day 15 donor was only mildly luteolytic. These experiments have subsequently been confirmed and extended by Baird *et al.* (1973).

Mono-layer cultures of ovarian granulosa cells have also been used to assess the timing of the appearance of the uterine luteolysin in the ovine uterus. Caldwell *et al.* (1969) showed that sterile endometrial extracts were luteolytic when added to cultured granulosa cells; the activity being highest in the day 14 and 15 extracts. In two cases 'lytic' endometrial extracts were also lytic to fibroblast mono-layer cultures, whereas one 'non-lytic' extract had no deleterious effect on fibroblasts. The extracts therefore lacked tissue specificity and were in one out of four cases lytic at the 'wrong' time.

Taken together this evidence strongly indicates that the ovine uterus secretes a luteolytic substance at the end of the normal oestrous cycle. The luteolysin is not active systemically, but has a local action on the ovary. This latter point is significant in considering the identity of the luteolytic factor. Since $PGF_{2\alpha}$, the only substance so far considered in depth for the role, is almost quantitatively removed from the circulation during one passage through the lungs, it would be unlikely to exert a physiological action systemically.

7.3.2 Attempts to purify the uterine luteolytic factor

So far, attempts to extract, purify and identify the uterine luteolysin(s) have not been successful. This approach is the only one likely to lead to the absolute and positive identification of the compound.

Caldwell *et al.* (1969), using luteolytic ovine endometrial extracts, have shown the active component to be non-dialysable and heat labile at 50 °C for 30 min. On gel filtration using Sephadex G-25, the molecular weight was below 1500. In these experiments, the compound was assayed by its effect on cultured ovine ovarian granulosa cells. Mazer and Wright (1968) and Lukaszewska and Hansel (1970), using preparations of hamster and bovine uteri respectively, have found that in these species also, the luteolytic factor in crude extracts is heat labile and non-dialysable. This would suggest that the active component is a protein or other macromolecule. However, more recent work has indicated that the active factor in crude preparations of bovine endometrium can be separated from the protein by lipid extraction, and that it subsequently behaves (on TLC, GLC and mass spectrometry) as arachidonic acid (Hansel *et al.*, 1975). On injection into the ovarian bursae of hysterectomised pseudopregnant hamsters (the luteolytic 'assay' system used by Hansel and his co-workers), arachidonic acid was luteolytic in amounts consistent with its concentration in endometrial extracts. However, it was active systemically and not in the unilateral fashion of the uterine luteolysin and therefore does not possess all of the characteristics of the sought-after luteolytic compound.

7.3.3 Evidence that PGF$_{2\alpha}$ is luteolytic in sheep

Following the demonstration that PGF$_{2\alpha}$ is a venoconstrictor in dogs (DuCharme and Weeks, 1968) and the initial finding that the human uterus and menstrual fluid contain high concentrations of PGF$_{2\alpha}$ (Pickles *et al.*, 1965), Pharris and Wyngarden (1969) hypothesised that PGF$_{2\alpha}$ may be the uterine luteolytic factor, acting by reducing luteal blood flow. In pseudo-pregnant rats Pharris and Wyngarden (1969) found that 1 mg kg^{-1}/day subcutaneously would cause luteolysis. Although an effect via a reduction in luteal blood flow is now disputed, this is of historical interest, being the first demonstration of the luteolytic effect of PGF$_{2\alpha}$. It has since been shown that PGF$_{2\alpha}$, PGF$_{1\alpha}$ and PGE$_2$ are all luteolytic in a variety of laboratory and domestic animals.

Two lines of evidence suggest that PGF$_{2\alpha}$ is luteolytic in the sheep. Firstly it is luteolytic on administration; and secondly, cycle length can be extended by immunising against PGF$_{2\alpha}$.

PGF$_{2\alpha}$ is luteolytic in the cycling ewe when infused into the ovarian artery, both in animals with ovaries *in situ* (Thorburn and Nicol, 1971) and where the ovaries have been autotransplanted to the neck (McCracken *et al.*, 1970b; Barrett *et al.*, 1971; Chamley *et al.*, 1972). In animals with intact ovaries, the minimum intra-arterial dose required is in the region of 10 μg/hour for three hours. Treatment is followed by a return to oestrus in about 60 hours and a normal ovulation. In these experiments, PGF$_{2\alpha}$ was infused via a side-branch of the ovarian artery through an indwelling catheter. Similarly, intra-arterial doses are luteolytic in the autotransplanted ovary in a dose-dependent fashion (2 μg/hour for 9.5–18 hours; 10 μg/hour for 7 hours; or 40 μg/hour for 4 hours are all effective luteolytic doses). Treatment is followed by decreased progesterone secretion, increased levels of oestrogens and luteinising hormone and oestrus.

Prostaglandin F$_{2\alpha}$ is also luteolytic when infused via the uterine vein. This point is of paramount importance in consideration of the possibility that it is the physiological luteolysin. In one animal with ovaries *in situ*, Thorburn and Nicol (1971) observed luteolysis after infusion of 40 μg/hour for six hours into the uterine vein; infusion of this dose for three hours was not luteolytic. The animals returned to oestrus 60 hours later. Using animals with utero–ovarian autotransplants, Barrett *et al.* (1971) obtained luteolysis in two out of three sheep following administration of 20 μg/hour for nine hours. In the third animal the progesterone level dropped transiently, but increased after stopping treatment. These authors suggest a minimum effective dose of 20 μg/hour for seven hours for luteolysis. They found 200 μg/hour for three hours infused via the jugular vein had no luteolytic effect; nor did infusion of saline via the uterine vein. Assuming an ovarian arterial blood flow of 10–15 ml min^{-1} minimum effective doses of PGF$_{2\alpha}$ administered through the ovarian artery result in levels of 2–4 ng ml^{-1} in ovarian arterial blood. Given a blood flow of about 20 ml min^{-1} in the uterine vein, minimum effective doses result in concentrations of about 15 ng ml^{-1} in the uterine vein. It seems likely that 5–10% of the PGF$_{2\alpha}$ administered via the uterine vein finds its way into the ovarian artery in the autotransplanted utero–ovarian system (Barrett *et al.*, 1971).

It has subsequently been shown that $PGF_{2\alpha}$ administered via one uterine vein has a unilaterally luteolytic effect reminiscent of unilateral hysterectomy; that is, only the ipsilateral corpus luteum lyses (Goding et al., 1972a).

The luteolytic effect of $PGF_{2\alpha}$ is confirmed by the fact that actively immunising cycling ewes against $PGF_{2\alpha}$ results in cessation of the normal luteolytic mechanism (Scaramuzzi et al., 1973). Prolonged cycles were observed in four out of six animals within one month of the first inoculation with $PGF_{2\alpha}$-protein conjugate. The circulating level of antibody was not determined, nor whether the effect was specific for $F_{2\alpha}$ antibodies. Surgical removal of corpora lutea in these animals was followed by oestrus and mating of all ewes within three days, but none of the animals came into oestrus during the subsequent 42 days. At laparotomy, all were shown to have normal corpora lutea and none was pregnant.

7.3.4 Concentration of $PGF_{2\alpha}$ in utero–ovarian venous blood and in uterine tissue of cycling ewes

Data on uterine blood $PGF_{2\alpha}$ levels are generally consistent with a role for $PGF_{2\alpha}$ as a uterine luteolytic agent in the sheep.

Bland et al. (1971) using GLC-mass spectrometry found concentrations of up to 8.8 ng ml^{-1} $PGF_{2\alpha}$ in uterine venous blood on days 14–16 of the cycle whereas levels up to day 13 were <2–3 ng ml^{-1}. McCracken et al. (1972), also using GLC-mass spectrometry, observed utero–ovarian venous plasma levels of 20–40 ng ml^{-1} during the two days preceding oestrus. Thorburn et al. (1973) found PGF levels of up to 22.3 ng ml^{-1} by radioimmunoassay, in cycling animals bearing indwelling utero–ovarian venous catheters. Elevated PGF concentrations were found only on days 13–17 and preceded the fall in progesterone concentrations (Figure 7.2).

The physiological levels of $PGF_{2\alpha}$ detected in uterine venous blood are of the same order as those required for a luteolytic effect. Correcting plasma levels for packed cell volume and assuming a utero–ovarian venous blood flow of about 2 litres/hour (estimated by summing the previously quoted flows, for ovarian artery and uterine vein, Barrett et al., 1971) levels in plasma of 20 ng ml^{-1} are equivalent to a secretion rate of about 20 μg/hour. This may just be sufficient to cause luteolysis if infused into the uterine vein. Thorburn and Nicol (1971) showed that it was necessary to administer 40 μg/hour for nine hours to get a return to oestrus in intact animals. Barrett et al. (1971) quote a minimum effective dose of 20 μg/hour for seven hours, in animals with autotransplanted ovaries. These calculations are complicated by the fact that PGF secretion apparently occurs in surges or peaks of relatively short duration of less than six hours (Thorburn et al., 1973; see Figures 7.2a and 7.2b). It is therefore possible that the individual concentrations measured in the uterine vein were not maximal, since peaks might have been missed. Alternatively continuous doses effective when given for nine hours are lower than physiologically effective doses, as the surges do not last that long. It remains to be seen therefore whether this quantitative approach confirms the hypothesis that $PGF_{2\alpha}$ is the uterine luteolysin.

Elevated $PGF_{2\alpha}$ concentrations have also been found in peripheral blood

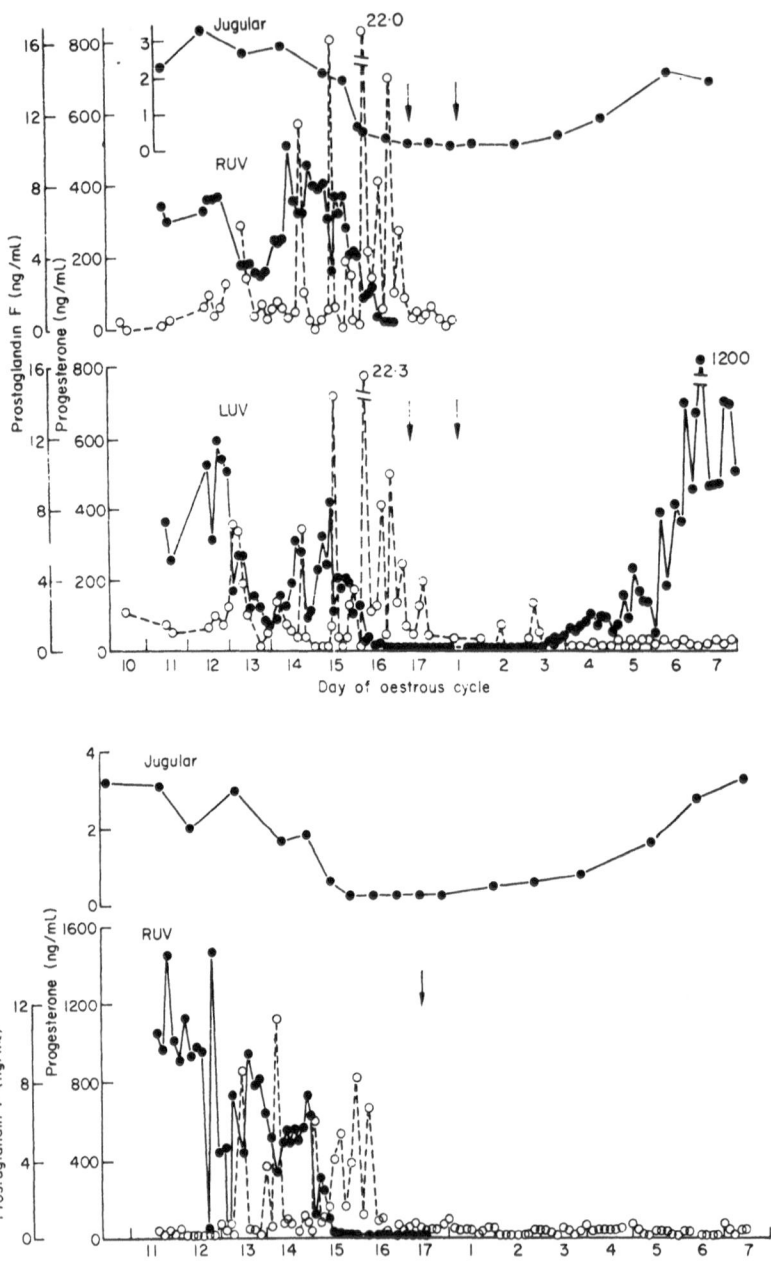

Figure 7.2 Plasma concentrations of progesterone (•) and PGF (○) in two ewes during the oestrous cycle.

(a) Levels in right and left utero–ovarian veins and in jugular vein; during the first cycle a corpus luteum was present in each ovary, after oestrus a corpus luteum was present on the left ovary only. Arrows signify days of oestrus.

(b) Levels in utero–ovarian and jugular veins; a corpus luteum was present in the right ovary. (From Thorburn *et al.*, 1973, by courtesy of *J. Reprod. Fert.*)

(Caldwell *et al.*, 1972; Coudert *et al.*, 1972), in uterine lumen fluid (Harrison *et al.*, 1972) and endometrium (Wilson *et al.*, 1972a), at times coincident with luteal regression.

7.4 ROUTES BY WHICH UTERINE PGF$_{2\alpha}$ MAY REACH THE OVARY

Following the suggestion that there may be a uterine luteolysin, speculation arose as to how it might be transported to the ovary in a manner consistent with its local mode of action. Five possible routes have been suggested:

7.4.1 Via the oviduct

This does not seem likely. Ligation of the oviduct in the rat (Butcher *et al.*, 1969), or removal of part of the oviduct in the guinea-pig (Bland and Donovan, 1969) does not result in prolongation of pseudopregnancy. In the sheep, the luteolytic influence of an intrauterine plastic coil is not reduced by previous complete salpingectomy (Stormshak *et al.*, 1967). Furthermore, experiments in sheep with intact oviducts indicate that luteal maintenance can be achieved by ligating the uterine veins. Oviductal transport of luteolysin therefore does not seem likely in the sheep.

7.4.2 Via the lymphatics

Work of Morris and Sass (1966) and Morris and McIntosh (1971) on the lymphatic drainage of the ovine uterus and ovary indicates that lymph ducts arising in the uterus do not anastomose with those of the ovary until well down in the mesometrium. This would seem to rule out possible involvement of the lymphatics.

7.4.3 Vascular shunts

Arterio–venous anastomoses have been identified between the ovarian artery and the utero–ovarian vein. These are unlikely to be of importance in the transfer of the uterine luteolysin because flow through them is likely to be in the direction of the vein as a result of the blood pressure difference. Collection of ovarian arterial blood after infusion of radio-labelled serum albumin into the uterine vein has shown that no blood crosses in this direction (Coudert *et al.*, 1974a, b).

7.4.4 The counter-current transfer mechanism

Counter-current transfer is the name given to the partitioning of a solute between two liquid phases travelling in opposite directions past one another.

The transfer of compounds between vascular currents has been named by analogy to the method used in chemistry. Counter-current transfer mechanisms have been said to be important in the placenta (Ramsey, 1960; Assali, 1968), the kidney (Wirz *et al.*, 1951) and the testis (Waites and Moule, 1961). The possible involvement of such a mechanism in the transfer of the uterine luteolytic factor between the utero–ovarian vein and the ovarian artery has attracted considerable attention.

Initial investigations of the role of the uterus in luteolysis included experiments in which the utero–ovarian vein was ligated. Kiracofe *et al.* (1966) showed that luteal maintenance resulted from ligation of the uterine vein and the uterine artery, but not from ligation of the uterine artery alone. Inskeep and Butcher (1966) obtained similar results. These experiments were repeated more recently by Baird and Land (1973), who ligated the uterine vein proximal to its junction with the ovarian artery, in order to prevent $PGF_{2\alpha}$ from getting to that part of the uterine vein apposing the ovarian artery (Figure 7.3). Control animals had all connections (except the uterine vein) severed between the uterus and the ovarian pedicle. All ten control animals had normal cycles. In the experimental group, however, ligation of the uterine vein alone resulted in luteal maintenance in only four out of ten animals. Baird and Land (1973)

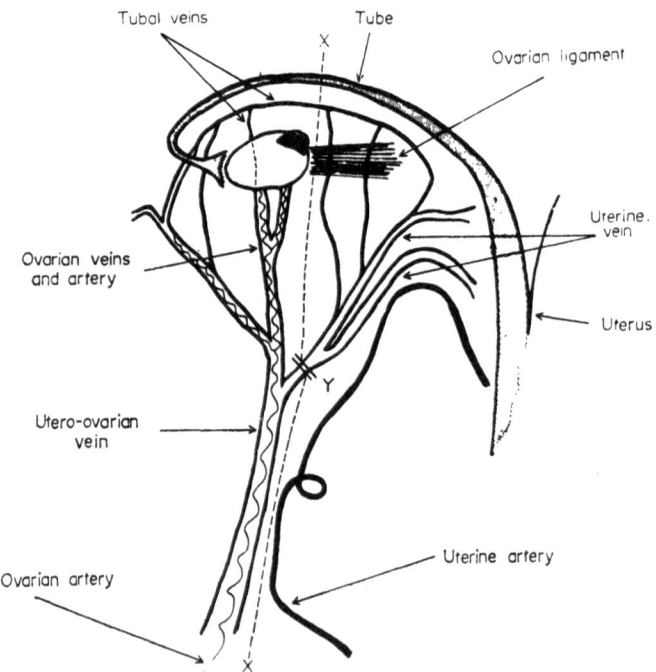

Figure 7.3 Diagrammatic representations of the vascular supply to the uterus, ovary and fallopian tube in the ewe. In the control group all connections along the line X (-----) were cut, leaving the uterine vein intact. (All animals had normal cycles.) In the experimental group the uterine vein was divided and ligated at Y (four of ten animals had maintained corpora lutea.) (From Baird and Land, 1973, by courtesy of *J. Reprod. Fert.*)

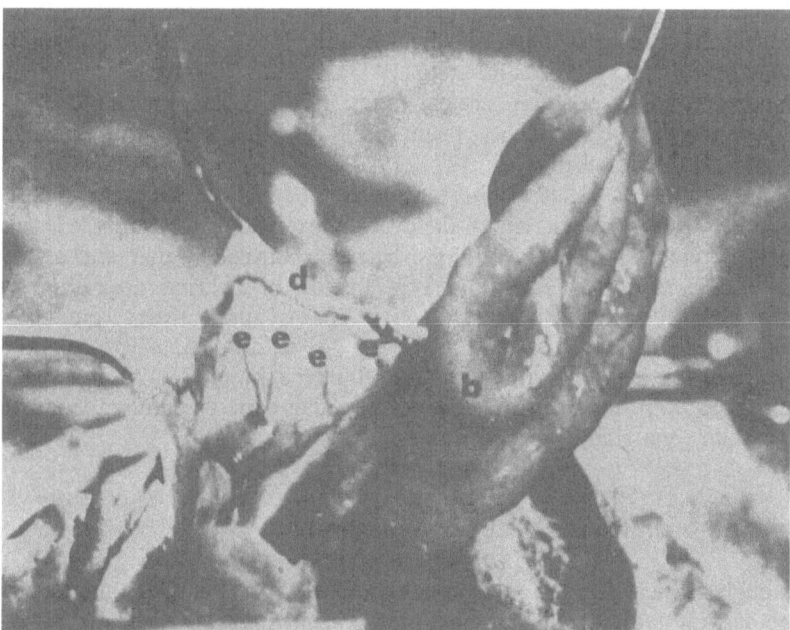

Figure 7.4 Photograph of the vascular supply to the uterus, fallopian tube and ovary in the ewe. a—distended middle uterine vein; b—uterine horns; c—ovary; d—fallopian tube; e— tubal veins; f—twin ovarian veins. The middle uterine vein has been ligated near its origin with the ovarian vein. The arcade of tubal veins can be seen clearly anastomosing with the uterine and ovarian veins. (From Baird and Land, 1973, by courtesy of *J. Reprod. Fert.*)

suggest that this low level of luteal maintenance may have been due to the opening of uterine venous drainage along the oviduct, the resulting venous arcade forming an anastomotic pathway from the uterine venous system to the ovarian veins (Figure 7.4) and allowing the luteolysin access to the utero—ovarian vein. Interruption of this channel resulted in luteal maintenance in six out of seven of the original experimental group that had returned to heat (see Section 7.4.1).

These experiments suggest that normal luteolysis depends on an intact uterine venous drainage, but they do not prove the counter-current transfer hypothesis. Attempts to prove it have taken two forms. Initially, the possibility was investigated by separating the ovarian artery from the utero—ovarian vein without interfering with blood flow in either vessel. When Barrett *et al.* (1971) carried out this operation in four ewes on days 2–3 of the cycle, corpora lutea were maintained in three animals up to day 25. Three sham operated animals cycled normally. (Subsequent investigation of the one experimental failure showed that the vessels were incompletely separated.) In these animals the vessels were separated by inserting a fold of broad ligament between them. Similar results have been reported by Restall *et al.* (1973), who showed that separation of the vessels resulted in prolonged luteal function in both of two ewes. However, in two other identically prepared animals $PGF_{2\alpha}$ 80 μg/hour for six hours infused into the uterine vein, resulted in luteolysis. Since this dose of $PGF_{2\alpha}$ was shown to be inactive systemically, it is important to find an explanation for this result which does not support the counter-current theory. Goding (1974) suggests that it may be due to the type of oviductal anastomotic pathway observed by Baird and Land (1973).

Further evidence of a non-surgical nature for the counter-current theory has been supplied by experiments where ^{3}H-PGF$_{2\alpha}$ has been infused into the uterine vein (McCracken et al., 1971, 1972). [9-^{3}H]-PGF$_{2\alpha}$ was infused at 0.1 μCi min^{-1} into the uterine vein of four sheep on day 14 of the cycle and blood was collected from the cut end of the ovarian artery and also from the left iliac artery. After extraction, partitioning between petroleum ether and aqueous alcohol and extensive TLC, the PGF region of ovarian arterial plasma contained up to 30 times more radioactivity than similar extracts from the iliac artery. This indicated a transfer of about 7% of intravenously administered PGF$_{2\alpha}$ and is consistent with the data of Barrett et al. (1971). An unexplained finding was that there was a 20–30 min time lag between ending the infusion and reaching maximum radioactivity in the ovarian artery.

7.4.5 Autonomic innervation of the ovary

Although surgical separation of artery and vein supports the counter-current hypothesis, it does not rule out other mechanisms that might depend on a close relationship between the utero–ovarian vein and the ovarian artery, for example neural mechanisms. Restall et al. (1973) have presented preliminary evidence to suggest that the antiluteolytic effect of separating the utero–ovarian vein from the ovarian artery might be due to disruption of the local autonomic nervous system. Prostaglandin F$_{2\alpha}$-induced luteolysis (which occurred on administration into the utero–ovarian vein) was prevented in three out of four sheep by guanethidine sulphate (8 mg/hour). In a control group of four animals given PGF$_{2\alpha}$ alone in the same regime, three returned to oestrus. The effect of PGF$_{2\alpha}$ was not blocked by lignocaine. This postulated mechanism is difficult to reconcile with the observed luteolytic effect of PGF$_{2\alpha}$ in the autotransplanted ovary.

7.5 EVIDENCE THAT PGF$_{2\alpha}$ IS NOT THE UTERINE LUTEOLYSIN IN THE SHEEP

Niswender et al. (1970) reported that autotransplantation of the whole uterus to a peritoneal site in the abdomen did not affect cyclic behaviour in five out of 13 animals. Uterine secretions were accessible to the ovary in these preparations, since the cut, unligated end of the uterus was left within the abdomen to allow drainage of lumen fluid. This may, therefore, account for maintained cyclicity in some animals. In the ewes with uterine autotransplants that did not show oestrus, Niswender et al. (1970) found that at subsequent laparotomy either the endometrium had degenerated, or the entire uterus was being resorbed. This, rather than inaccessibility of uterine secretions to the ovary, may therefore account for the failure of the other animals to cycle.

Wilson et al. (1972b) found higher concentrations of PGF in the uterine venous blood of pregnant ewes than of non-pregnant ewes on day 13 of the cycle. The concentrations were, however, considerably higher than those obtained by others, possibly because they were measured by bioassay. (See objections to bioassays in the measurement of utero–ovarian venous $PGF_{2\alpha}$ raised by Goding, 1974.) Elevation of utero–ovarian venous PGF levels in early pregnancy is disputed by Thorburn et al. (1973).

A third objection has been raised by Coudert et al. (1972), who after assaying PGF in posterior vena caval serum by radioimmunoassay, have suggested that levels of PGF peak on day 12, considerably before the start of luteolysis. Several criticisms have been made of this work (Goding, 1974). Most significant among them are that serum was obtained only once daily, which in the light of Thorburn et al.'s (1973) findings may be too infrequent to allow detection of PGF surges. Also the cyclic behaviour was induced early in the breeding season in these animals by administration of progesterone + PMSG. Such treatment can lead to irregular cycles, which in turn could interfere with dating the stages of the cycle. Furthermore the use of serum rather than plasma can lead to variable PGF levels.

Lastly, normal regression of corpora lutea in the left ovaries of two ewes with congenital absence of the left uterine horn has been cited as evidence against the unilateral effect of the uterine luteolysin (Hunter, 1970). The recent description by O'Shea et al. (1974) of the presence of normal left ovarian/ uterine vasculature in five congenitally unicornuate ewes (all with absence of the left horn but with left uterine veins carrying uterine venous effluent) has not only satisfactorily explained these findings, but also suggests that the ipsilateral uterine horn itself is unnecessary for luteolysis.

7.5.1 Objections to the counter-current transfer hypothesis

Coudert et al. (1974b) have been unable to confirm the results of McCracken et al. (1971, 1972) obtained by infusing ^{3}H-$PGF_{2\alpha}$ into the uterine vein and collecting from the ovarian and iliac arteries. Coudert et al. (1974b) suggest that less than 0.7% of the ^{3}H-$PGF_{2\alpha}$ in the utero–ovarian vein crossed to the artery, this being the lower limit of detection of their method. This percentage is very much lower than that suggested by Barrett et al. (1971) and is also less than that required to cause luteolysis as judged from infusion experiments. At present these differences are unresolved.

The concept that counter-current transfer is the only means by which uterine PGF may reach the ovary has been questioned recently by Lamond and Drost (1973), on the basis of their finding that ligating the ovarian artery in four ewes had no effect on luteal demise. This criticism has been refuted by McCracken (1973) on the grounds that too few experiments were done, that laparotomy to check for luteal regression was not done early enough after operation and that ligating the ovarian artery might be expected to lead to non-specific effects due to anoxia.

Although no conclusive evidence has been forthcoming *against* $PGF_{2\alpha}$ being the uterine luteolytic factor, the positive evidence although weighty, is essentially circumstantial. This situation is likely to endure until the uterine luteolysin is extracted, purified and identified. Evidence for a counter-current transfer mechanism is likewise inconclusive. The only direct evidence for it is that of McCracken *et al.* (1971, 1972), which shows that the same $PGF_{2\alpha}$ that is infused into the vein reaches the artery, although in similar experiments Coudert *et al.* (1974b) could not confirm these findings. An additional unexplained factor is the time lag between administration of $PGF_{2\alpha}$ into the vein and identification in the artery.

7.6 FACTORS INFLUENCING UTERINE $PGF_{2\alpha}$ PRODUCTION IN NON-PREGNANT SHEEP

7.6.1 Control by ovarian steroids

Oestradiol-17β administered to the ewe on days 9–11 of the cycle causes premature luteolysis. This effect is blocked by hysterectomy (Stormshak *et al.*, 1969; Hawk and Bolt, 1970; Akbar *et al.*, 1971; Kann and Denamur, 1973) but not by hypophysectomy or pituitary stalk section (Denamur and Kann, 1973). This suggests that the uterine luteolytic effect may be stimulated by oestrogens and this conclusion is confirmed by the finding that removal of Graafian follicles (the source of ovarian oestrogens) by X-irradiation or cautery results in some degree of luteal maintenance (Karsch *et al.*, 1970; Ginther, 1971).

Caldwell *et al.* (1972) provided direct evidence by measuring PGF (by radioimmunoassay) in peripheral plasma of cycling animals and of ovariectomised animals treated with progesterone and oestrogen. Progesterone alone had no effect on peripheral PGF levels, but progesterone administered every other day for 11 days, followed on the thirteenth day by a single dose (50 μg) of oestradiol-17β, resulted in peripheral PGF levels comparable to those in normal animals at day 14 of the cycle. This effect was blocked by hysterectomy or by immunisation against oestradiol; in either case PGF was not detectable in peripheral plasma.

The stimulatory effect of oestrogens has been confirmed in animals bearing uteri autotransplanted to the neck. McCracken *et al.* (1973) demonstrated elevated PGF levels in uterine venous effluent two hours after infusing a physiological dose (1 ng min^{-1}) of oestradiol-17β into the uterine artery; the uterine production rate of PGF reached 100 μg/hour, from a basal rate of about 5 μg/hour. Barcikowski *et al.* (1973) have confirmed this effect and have in addition shown that in order to elicit it, the uterus must be previously exposed to progesterone. Also using the ovariectomised, autotransplanted uterus model, Scaramuzzi *et al.* (1974) reported elevated PGF production after oestrogen treatment only when the animals were pretreated with progesterone; oestrogen alone had no effect and progesterone alone stimulated a relatively small increase. Harrison and Heap (1975) have similar results (Figure 7.5).

Whereas the stimulatory effects of oestrogen on PGF production are well documented, those of progesterone are less well known. Dutt and Casida (1948) first observed a luteolytic action of progesterone in intact animals, when given early in the cycle; Woody *et al.* (1967) confirmed this effect and Ginther (1968) showed it could be blocked by hysterectomy. Ginther (1968) also showed progesterone was luteolytic unilaterally, in unilaterally hysterectomised animals where the remaining horn was adjacent to the corpus

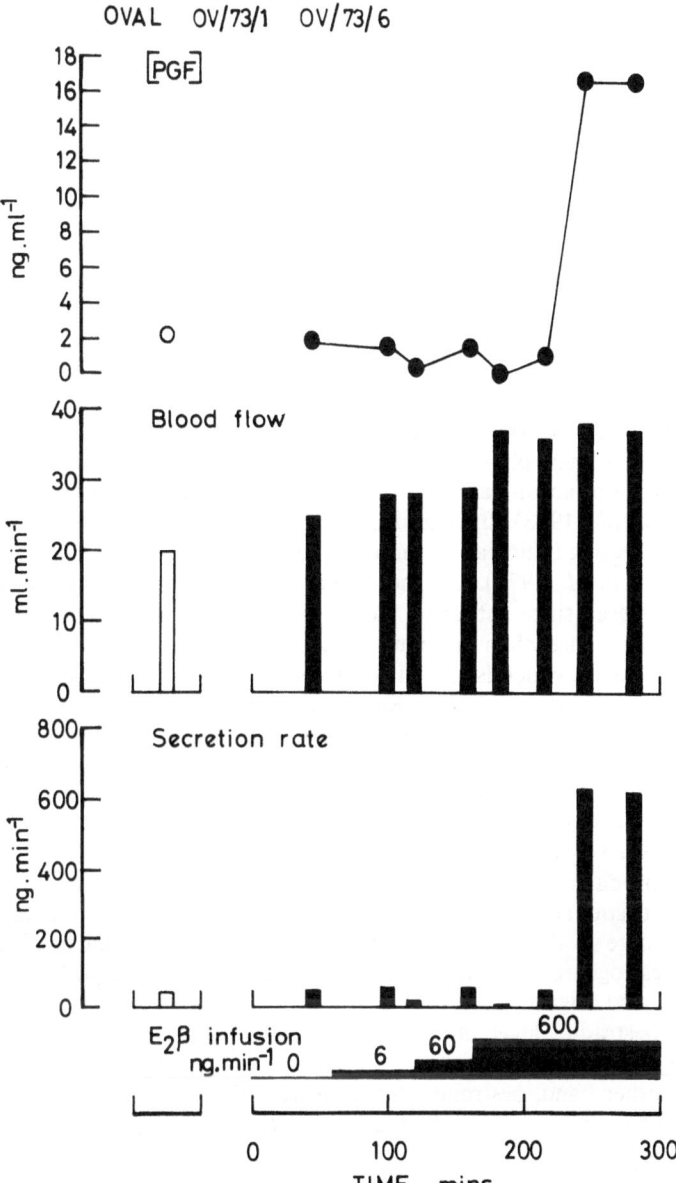

Figure 7.5 The effect of a close-arterial infusion of oestradiol-17β ($E_{2\beta}$) on the concentration of prostaglandin F (PGF) compounds in uterine-jugular blood, on uterine blood flow and on the uterine secretion of PGF. The left uterine horn was transplanted to the neck and the uterine artery was anastomosed to the left carotid artery and the uterine vein to the left jugular vein. Both ovaries were removed and the sheep was treated with progesterone (20 mg/day) for 84 days. Note the marked increase in uterine secretion of PGF during the infusion of oestradiol-17β at 600 ng min^{-1}, a rate approximately equivalent to the production rate at parturition. (From Harrison and Heap, 1975, by courtesy of *J. Endocrinol.*)

luteum. The effect of progesterone on the uterine PGF level is consistent with its luteolytic action. Wilson et al. (1971) showed elevated endometrial levels of PGF after progesterone treatment. A similar action of progesterone has been demonstrated by Harrison et al. (1972), who observed the accumulation of high levels of PGF in the uterine lumen fluid (up to 4 μg ml^{-1}) in animals with autotransplanted ovaries and persistent corpora lutea. Amoroso et al. (1973) have noted the same effect in unilaterally pregnant animals with one horn isolated with a septum inserted surgically. Thus although both oestrogen after progesterone pretreatment and progesterone alone can cause release of PGF, it appears that the main effect of progesterone may be to cause PGF to accumulate in the uterus, that of oestrogen being to allow release into the uterine vein.

Control of uterine PGF production during the normal cycle has been considered mainly in terms of oestrogen and progesterone. Oestrogens are secreted during the luteal phase in sheep, as well as on days 15 and 16, at the pre-ovulatory surge (Moore et al., 1969; Cox et al., 1971; Mattner and Braden, 1972). The first luteal phase elevation occurs on day 3 of the cycle (Cox et al., 1971); this is not accompanied by elevated utero–ovarian venous PGF levels (Thorburn et al., 1973). Increased oestrogen levels next occur on days 6–9, probably reflecting follicular maturation (Scaramuzzi et al., 1970; Obst et al., 1971; Barrett et al., 1971). The increase at this time apparently does not lead to PGF release (since luteolysis does not occur). Thorburn et al. (1973) observed no increase when sampling infrequently at day 10. The pre-ovulatory surge of oestrogen, which is responsible for stimulating the ovulatory LH surge (Goding et al., 1969, 1970; Radford, Wheatley and Wallace, 1969; Scaramuzzi et al., 1971) generally occurs on days 15 and 16, by which time progesterone levels are already low, luteolysis having occurred. Cox et al. (1972), the only workers to assay oestrogens and PGF simultaneously to date, also showed (in two animals) a rise in peripheral oestradiol-17β on days 11–12, followed by low levels until the ovulatory surge on day 15. The peak of oestradiol on days 11 and 12 preceded PGF release by about 48 hours. It is therefore questionable whether this peak is responsible for stimulating the luteolytic surge in PGF. McCracken et al. (1973) showed that physiological doses of oestrogen could raise uterine venous PGF to very high levels in 2–4 hours; see also Figure 7.5. None of the three luteal and one pre-ovulatory surges in oestradiol level therefore seems responsible for stimulating PGF production.

On the other hand, oestrone, also measured by Cox et al. (1972) between day 10 and ovulation, instead of dropping on days 12–15 like oestradiol, remained high (100–500 pg ml^{-1} in utero–ovarian venous plasma). Furthermore Bjersing et al. (1973) observed an increase in total oestrogen (oestradiol + oestrone), before the fall in progesterone on day 13. It may therefore be that oestrone, rather than oestradiol, stimulates PGF release on days 13–16.

7.6.2 The influence of oxytocin

Relatively large doses of oxytocin (400–10 000 mU) administered as bolus intravenous injections will elicit elevated posterior vena caval PGF levels in oestrogen-primed anoestrous sheep (Sharma and Fitzpatrick, 1974). These doses of oxytocin have no effect on untreated anoestrous animals. It is not clear to what extent this stimulatory effect is due to the uterine contractions caused by oxytocin, perhaps in a way analogous to PGF release following manipulation of the uterus (Roberts *et al.*, 1974), or whether a metabolic action of oxytocin is involved.

7.6.3 The influence of an intrauterine device

It has been known for some time that an intrauterine device (usually an IUCD-type plastic coil) causes shortening of the cycle. Ginther *et al.* (1966) showed that in seven sheep, insertion of an IUD on the side of the luteal ovary on day 3 of the cycle resulted in a return to oestrus on days 8–13 (oestrus = day 0). These results were confirmed by Stormshak *et al.* (1967). The effect is local, applying to the corpus luteum in the ipsilateral ovary (Ginther *et al.*, 1966; Stormshak *et al.*, 1967; Ginther and Bisgard, 1972).

Levels of PGF in the uteri of animals bearing IUDs are consistent with a role for PGF as the uterine luteolysin. Wilson *et al.* (1972a) found that an IUD caused a premature rise in PGF level; after insertion on day 2, PGF levels typical of day 14 in a normal cycle were found in the uterus on day 5. Spilman and Duby (1972) have recently confirmed this and have in addition shown that the luteolytic effect of an IUD inserted on days 2–4 can be blocked by concurrent administration of indomethacin, a prostaglandin synthetase inhibitor. They have also shown that PGF is raised preferentially in the endometrium immediately adjacent to the IUD (control horn: 34.4 ng g^{-1}; in the IUD-containing horn, away from the IUD: 48.7 ng g^{-1}; under the IUD: 216.6 ng g^{-1}), as well as being elevated in the utero–ovarian vein. PGF levels in the utero–ovarian vein are also elevated unilaterally (Pexton *et al.*, 1973). This local action is consistent with the unilaterally luteolytic effect of the IUD. As might be expected from its inhibitory effect on the luteolytic action of an IUD, indomethacin prevented the rise in PGF levels.

Increased PGF concentrations in IUD-bearing uterine horns may also explain the increased uterine activity noted in them by Spilman *et al.* (1972) and the interference by an IUD with sperm transport and fertilisation (Hawk, 1967).

7.6.4 Effects of intrauterine infections

Introduction of *E. coli* to the uterus on day 2 of the cycle results in consistently smaller corpora lutea by day 8, than in animals treated with intrauterine saline, or in which *E. coli* were injected into the broad ligament at the base of the mesovarium (Brinsfield and Hawk, 1968). This suggests that intrauterine infections mimic an IUD. However, in contrast are the findings of Coudert and Short (1966), who showed luteal maintenance in six out of 11 ewes inoculated with *C. pyrogenes* or *Vibrio fetus* into the uterine lumen on day 10 of the cycle. This apparent disagreement may reflect the stage of the cycle at which the infection was introduced, rather than the use of different organisms.

As prostaglandin synthesis is elevated in inflammation, a shortened cycle might be expected and the results of Coudert and Short (1966) are therefore at present inexplicable.

7.6.5 The luteotrophic effect of oestrogen

Daily administration of oestradiol (1 mg/day) starting early in the cycle results in further ovulations and subsequently in luteal maintenance for several weeks (Denamur and Mauleon, 1963; Piper and Foote, 1965, 1968; Ginther, 1970). Both natural and oestrogen-induced corpora are maintained and are functional (Denamur et al., 1970; Piper and Foote, 1970). It seems unlikely that (as in the rabbit) this effect is brought about through a direct stimulation of the corpus luteum, since oestrogen is not luteotrophic in hypophysectomised sheep (Denamur and Mauleon, 1963; Kaltenbach et al., 1968; Denamur et al., 1970). On the other hand it does not appear to be due to stimulation of LH or prolactin secretion (Kann and Denamur, 1973). Although the effect occurs in intact animals in association with raised levels of LH and prolactin, it is also seen, in pituitary stalk-sectioned sheep, without any concomitant elevation in LH and under circumstances where the stimulatory effect of oestrogen on prolactin release is very much reduced (Kann and Denamur, 1973). Since prolactin alone is not luteotrophic in intact sheep (Denamur and Mauleon, 1963; Denamur, 1968; Kaltenbach et al., 1968) these experiments suggest that the pituitary is not involved in the luteotrophic effect of oestrogen. It has been concluded, therefore, that its effect may be due to direct inhibition of the luteolytic activity of the uterus (Kann and Denamur, 1973). It is difficult to reconcile the apparent paradox of an inhibitory effect of oestrogen early in the cycle with a stimulatory one later. It is possible though that oestrogen without progesterone pretreatment inhibits, whereas oestrogen following progesterone stimulates production of luteolysin. It would be instructive to measure uterine PGF after oestrogen treatment early in the cycle.

7.6.6 The luteotrophic effect of gonadotrophins

Continuous infusion of LH causes luteal maintenance in intact animals (Kaltenbach et al., 1968). This finding confirms the observation that hypophysectomy late in the cycle causes immediate luteolysis (by removing luteotrophin) and is consistent with the later finding that corpora lutea regress after treatment with anti-LH (Nalbandov and Cook, 1968; Fuller and Hansel, 1970). The luteotrophic properties of hormones with LH activity has also been demonstrated by the observation that HCG prevents the luteolytic effect of oestradiol on days 8–11 (Ginther, 1970) and prevents the luteolytic effect of an IUD (Stormshak et al., 1967). This ability of LH to suppress the luteolytic influence of the uterus is consistent with the suggestion that the corpus luteum is under luteotrophic control by the pituitary, as well as luteolytic control by the uterus and that luteal function may be determined by the interplay between these influences (Short, 1964).

It has been suggested that the trophic effect of LH may be due to stimulation of oestrogen synthesis (Denamur, 1968). This hypothesis is attractive, since if true it would mean that in the three situations where luteal maintenance is obtained in intact animals (pregnancy, continuous LH and early administration of oestrogen) the antiluteolytic effect may result from oestrogenic inhibition of luteolysin synthesis.

7.6.7 The mechanism of the luteolytic action of $PGF_{2\alpha}$

An antiluteotrophic effect of $PGF_{2\alpha}$ on the hypothalamic–pituitary axis can be ruled out. Intracarotid infusion of $PGF_{2\alpha}$ has no inhibiting effect on LH secretion in ovariectomised ewes (Chamley and Christie, 1973). Also LH and prolactin levels do not change at the time of PGF production in intact sheep (Goding et al., 1973). Furthermore, separation of the uterus and ovary is associated with prolongation of the cycle (see Section 7.3.1) thus precluding a systemic effect.

$PGF_{2\alpha}$ does not cause luteolysis by reducing overall ovarian blood flow. Although high doses of $PGF_{2\alpha}$ administered via the ovarian artery will reduce blood flow in the autotransplanted ovary (McCracken et al., 1971), lower doses will cause luteolysis in the absence of any change in blood flow (McCracken et al., 1971; Chamley et al., 1972). Furthermore PGE_1 reduces progesterone secretion but increases blood flow (Aldridge et al., 1970). An effect on the intraovarian distribution of blood flow (i.e. an effect on the corpus luteum alone) has been suggested on the basis of labelled microsphere trapping (Thorburn and Hales, 1972). This has not been confirmed by studies on $PGF_{2\alpha}$ induced luteolysis in the rabbit (Bruce and Hillier, 1974), where a transient increase in blood flow in the interstitium was noted after $PGF_{2\alpha}$ treatment and no decrease in luteal blood flow occurred until after the progesterone level had dropped. Functional luteolysis in the absence of blood flow changes in rabbit corpora lutea is corroborated by the occurrence of luteolysis on administration of $PGF_{2\alpha}$ to rabbit corpora in organ culture (O'Grady et al., 1972), and in ectopic corpora lutea (Keyes and Bullock, 1974). The role of luteal blood flow in luteolysis in the ewe is therefore open to question.

Behrman et al. (1971), investigating cholesterol metabolism during $PGF_{2\alpha}$-induced luteolysis in the rat ovary, have demonstrated an antagonistic effect of $PGF_{2\alpha}$ on the maintenance of cholesterol ester synthetase activity by prolactin. The suggestion has therefore been made that $PGF_{2\alpha}$ causes luteolysis by preventing storage of cholesterol ester. There is, however, no indication that cholesterol ester storage is a necessary step in the conversion of cholesterol to progesterone: unesterified cholesterol, not cholesterol ester, is the substrate for cholesterol side-chain cleavage. It appears likely in fact that in most species, including the sheep (Bjersing et al., 1973) cholesterol ester accumulates during luteolysis, probably after the steroid content of the gland decreases (Flint et al., 1973, 1974b). No data are available on the effects of $PGF_{2\alpha}$ on the metabolism of the ovine corpus luteum, although it has been noted that an increase in lysosomal fragility occurs during luteolysis (Dingle et al., 1968), in which prostaglandins may be involved (Weiner and Kaley, 1972).

Little is known about the hormonal requirements for the luteolytic action of $PGF_{2\alpha}$. Studies of progesterone and oestrogen concentrations in cows during

$PGF_{2\alpha}$-induced luteolysis have shown that oestrogen levels are raised (Hixon *et al.*, 1973). This may also occur in sheep (Barrett *et al.*, 1971). A mandatory requirement for oestrogen in luteolysis in these species is suggested as its removal by X-irradiation results in luteal phase prolongation (see Section 7.6.1). The corpora lutea of sheep and cows contain a specific cytoplasmic oestrogen receptor protein (Cook and Taylor, 1973; Kimball and Hansel, 1974).

Experiments to test this more directly in sheep have also demonstrated a requirement for oestrogen in the luteolytic response to $PGF_{2\alpha}$ (Hixon *et al.*, 1974; J. E. Hixon, personal communication). X-irradiation of the ovaries of five ewes, on day 7 of the cycle and thus removal of oestrogen, followed by administration of $PGF_{2\alpha}$ (7 mg, intramuscular), resulted in decreased jugular venous progesterone during the subsequent 96 hours in only one case. (This animal was found to have a luteinised cystic follicle at autopsy.) Adminis-tration of this dose of $PGF_{2\alpha}$ to five sham-irradiated animals resulted in luteolysis after 36 hours and a return to oestrus by 96 hours. Plasma oestrogen levels were raised by $PGF_{2\alpha}$ in the intact group but no increase was observed in the X-irradiated animals. Treatment with oestrogen caused luteolysis in both X-irradiated and intact groups, with progesterone levels falling after 54–60 hours. However, treatment of both groups with $PGF_{2\alpha}$ plus oestrogen resulted in decreased progesterone levels after 1–12 hours, thus demonstrating an interaction between $PGF_{2\alpha}$ and oestrogen in the luteolytic response. The results are presented in Table 7.1. This experiment indicates an absolute requirement for oestrogen in $PGF_{2\alpha}$-induced luteolysis. It does not rule out a separate stimulatory effect on uterine PGF production. The mechanism by which oestrogen has this effect is not known; it is presumably a direct action on the corpus luteum.

Table 7.1 Time taken for treatment to significantly decrease jugular venous pro-gesterone levels (From Hixon *et al.*, 1974. *Proc. 7th Meeting of the Soc. for the Study of Reproduction, Ottawa*)

Treatment	Time taken for treatment to cause a significant fall in progesterone (hours)	
	Sham irradiated	X-irradiated
None	96 (5)	96 (5)
$PGF_{2\alpha}$	36 (5)	96 (4)*
Oestradiol	54–60 (5)	54–60 (5)
PGF_2 + oestradiol	1 (5)	12 (5)

( ) = number of ewes/group
* One animal, in which luteolysis occurred, had a luteinised cystic follicle at autopsy and therefore should be excluded

7.6.8 Control of PGF release during the oestrous cycle

A satisfactory explanation of the factors controlling the surge of PGF observed on days 13–16 has not yet been presented. Progesterone alone is probably not the only factor involved. Although it may be capable of stimulating the release of luteolytic quantities of PGF, it is present throughout the luteal phase and not only at the time of the observed prostaglandin surge. Good evidence for an oestradiol surge at the right time has not been presented to date; the importance of oestrone (which is present in high concentration from days 11–15) needs clarification.

The ability of oxytocin to elicit PGF release suggests that it may be involved during the cycle; oxytocin is luteolytic in the cow (Armstrong and Hansel, 1959) and the intermittent pattern of PGF release is reminiscent of the way in which oxytocin is secreted during suckling (Folley and Knaggs, 1966; Cleverley and Folley, 1970; Thorburn et al., 1973). However, there is no direct evidence that oxytocin release is involved in the normal luteolytic mechanism. Increased oxytocin release has not been demonstrated at the end of the cycle in many species and in fact oxytocin release may be inhibited by progesterone (Roberts and Share, 1969).

7.7 UTERINE $PGF_{2\alpha}$ PRODUCTION IN THE FERTILE CYCLE

The corpus luteum is required for the maintenace of pregnancy in the ewe up to day 50 (Denamur and Martinet, 1955). The embryo must be in the uterus before days 12–13 if the corpus luteum of the non-pregnant cycle is to be maintained during early pregnancy (Moor and Rowson, 1966a, b, c, d). Although it seems clear that the conceptus has an antiluteolytic effect, there is also evidence to suggest it is luteotrophic. For instance, pituitary stalk section on day 10 of the cycle in a hysterectomised sheep (i.e. an animal deprived of the uterine luteolytic effect) results in luteal maintenance for 15 days (Denamur et al., 1966). The same operation carried out on days 10, 20 or 30 of gestation results in continuation of pregnancy for a much longer period (Denamur, 1968). This therefore suggests a luteotrophic effect of the pregnant uterus. Any such effect must initially be weak, however, since hypophysectomy up to day 50 of gestation results in luteal involution and abortion. Additionally $PGF_{2\alpha}$ (67 μg/hour for nine hours, infused via the uterine vein) is still luteolytic on days 13–16 after mating in 10 out of 12 pregnant sheep (Hearnshaw et al., 1973).

Better evidence is available for the antiluteolytic effect of the conceptus. The embryo has a local effect, maintaining the corpus luteum ipsilateral to the pregnant horn (Moor and Rowson, 1966a, b; Moor et al., 1969). The simplest explanation for this is that the conceptus overcomes the local luteolytic effect of the uterus (Caldwell et al., 1969). Furthermore, for luteal maintenance the conceptus must be implanted by day 12 or 13, which is when utero–ovarian venous PGF levels begin to rise. The antiluteolytic effect has been confirmed in three ewes by Thorburn et al. (1973), who showed that in early pregnancy, surges in utero–ovarian venous PGF levels were either absent on days 12–16, or were very much reduced relative to the levels observed at a similar time in the non-pregnant cycle (Figures 7.6 and 7.7).

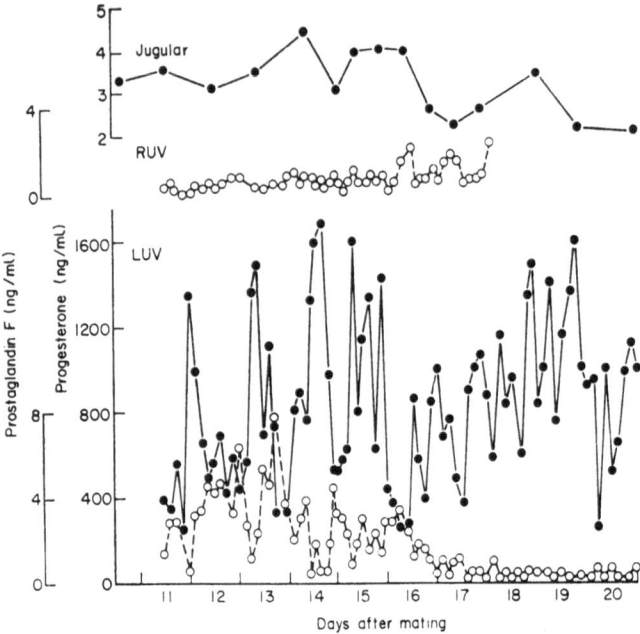

Figure 7.6 Plasma concentration of PGF (O) in the right and left utero–ovarian veins and of progesterone (●) in the jugular and left ovarian veins of a ewe during early pregnancy. Embryos were present in both uterine horns on day 25 and two corpora lutea were present in the left ovary. (From Thorburn *et al.*, 1973, by courtesy of *J. Reprod. Fert.*)

7.8 UTERINE PROSTAGLANDIN PRODUCTION AT PARTURITION

The only prostaglandin identified in utero–ovarian venous plasma at term, by GLC or GLC-mass spectrometry is $PGF_{2\alpha}$ (Liggins and Grieves, 1971; Challis *et al.*, 1972). Since most of the measurements were made by radio-immunoassays, which frequently do not distinguish between $PGF_{2\alpha}$ and other F series prostaglandins, we refer below mostly to $PGF_{2\alpha}$ equivalents (PGF).

7.8.1 Changes in utero–ovarian venous PGF levels at term

Levels of PGF in utero–ovarian venous plasma (Liggins and Grieves, 1971; Liggins *et al.*, 1972; Thorburn *et al.*, 1972) and in uterine tissues (Liggins *et al.*, 1972, 1973) rise before parturition. Utero–ovarian venous plasma levels may exceed 200 ng ml^{-1} at delivery (Mitchell *et al.*, 1974), which is ten times the concentration measured at the end of the oestrous cycle. When one considers that utero–ovarian venous blood flow at term is at least 700 ml min^{-1} (Ladner *et al.*, 1970; Bedford *et al.*, 1972) it is evident that relatively high production rates are possible (in the region of 0.1–0.2 mg min^{-1}). After delivery, utero–ovarian venous plasma levels decrease gradually. In non-suckling animals it reaches basal, prelabour levels some 2–4 days later; the effect of suckling (which, in view of the possible control of PGF production by oxytocin, could be significant) has not been investigated.

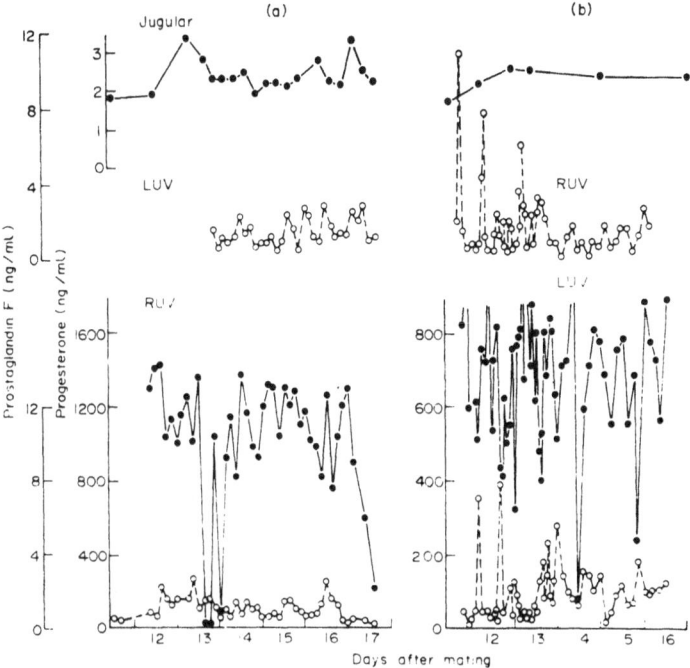

Figure 7.7 (a) Plasma concentration of progesterone (•) in the jugular and right utero–ovarian veins and PGF (○) in both utero–ovarian veins of a ewe with a persistent corpus luteum following mating with an entire ram. A corpus luteum was present in right ovary.
(b) Plasma concentrations of progesterone (•) in the jugular and left utero-ovarian veins and PGF (○) in both utero–ovarian veins of a ewe with a persistent corpus luteum following mating to an entire ram. A corpus luteum was present in left ovary. These results are a continuation of data in Figure 7.2 a. (From Thorburn *et al.*, 1973, by courtesy of *J. Reprod. Fert.*)

7.8.2 Control of uterine PGF production at parturition

In addition to changes in utero–ovarian venous levels of PGF at term, the maternal peripheral concentration of progesterone drops (Bassett *et al.*, 1969; Fylling, 1970) and unconjugated oestrogen (mostly oestrone) increases (Challis, 1971; Obst and Seamark, 1972). The studies of Liggins and others indicate that in sheep these changes are precipitated by trophic stimulation of the fetal adrenal cortex, which results in rising fetal cortisol levels during the last 5–10 days of pregnancy (Bassett and Thorburn, 1969; Comline *et al.*, 1970; Liggins *et al.*, 1973).

The time course of these hormonal changes is as follows (Figure 7.8). Fetal cortisol levels rise, and maternal progesterone levels fall 4–8 days before delivery. These changes appear to be simultaneous, though concurrent measurements have apparently not been made in the same animals. Subsequently, unconjugated oestrogen and PGF levels rise approximately 24–48 hours before delivery; again these changes are apparently simultaneous. Finally, uterine contractions start from 1–12 hours before delivery. At the onset of the second stage of labour (which in the sheep as in man is

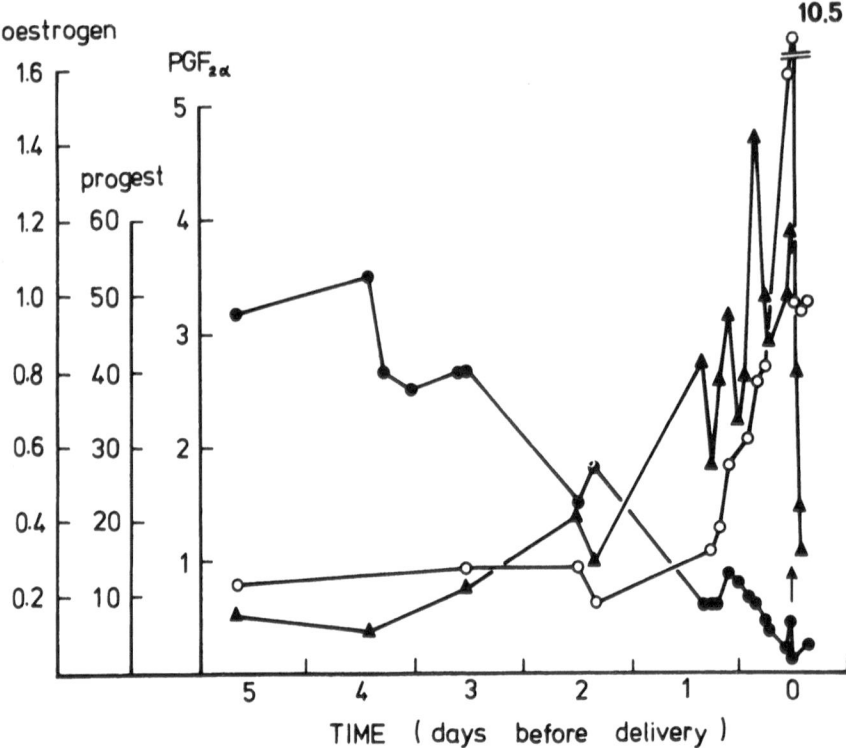

Figure 7.8 Changes in posterior vena caval plasma concentrations of progesterone (•), ng ml⁻¹, total unconjugated oestrogen (▲), ng ml⁻¹ and PGF (○), ng ml⁻¹ at parturition following the natural onset of labour. A single lamb was born on day=0 (arrow indicates time of delivery), 148 days *post coitus*. (From Flint *et al.*, 1973, by courtesy of *J. Endocrinol.*)

characterised by contractions of the abdominal musculature—'bearing down'—in addition to uterine contractions), PGF levels surge rapidly to peak as oxytocin secretion occurs. These temporal inter-relationships have been described by a number of authors (Fitzpatrick and Walmsley, 1965; Liggins *et al.*, 1972; Currie *et al.*, 1973; Liggins, 1973; Flint *et al.*, 1974a). Because of the way in which levels of fetal cortisol, maternal progesterone, oestrogens and oxytocin change before parturition, it is possible that all of these hormones play a part in controlling PGF production.

7.8.3 Fetal cortisol

Intrafetal administration of glucocorticoid (usually cortisol or dexamethasone) leads to all the endocrine changes associated with spontaneous labour, including increased levels of PGF in utero–ovarian venous plasma, maternal placenta and myometrium and to labour itself (Liggins, 1968; Liggins *et al.*, 1972). It is possible therefore that glucocorticoids act via their effects on progesterone and oestrogen.

Because of the regularity with which apparently normal parturition can be induced by fetal administration of glucocorticoids after about day 120 *post coitus*, widespread use has been made of glucocorticoids (usually dexamethasone) in experimental studies to cause delivery in a predictable way. This facilitates frequent sampling of plasma in the period immediately preceding delivery, because the experimenter knows with increased accuracy when parturition will occur.

7.8.4 Progesterone

In the sheep towards the end of pregnancy, the rise in PGF levels follows a decrease in maternal peripheral progesterone whereas during the oestrous cycle the reverse is the case (Currie *et al.*, 1973). It is not clear, however, that *ovarian* progesterone production drops before the PGF surge at term. Bedford *et al.* (1973) have estimated that about one-third of the progesterone produced in late pregnancy is of ovarian origin. Ovarian progesterone secretion drops before or at the same time as placental and peripheral progesterone levels reach those found at delivery some 24–48 hours prepartum.

In the sheep, as in other species, labour can be halted, or its onset postponed, by the systemic administration of progesterone in large doses (Bengtsson and Schofield, 1963; Liggins *et al.*, 1972; Bedford *et al.*, 1973). This treatment prevents the rise in utero–ovarian venous PGF in glucocorticoid-stimulated labour (Liggins, 1973), but in contrast does not block the increase in maternal placental or myometrial PGF levels (Liggins, 1973). This effect in pregnancy is reminiscent of the stimulatory effect of progesterone on PGF levels in the uterus, which occurs in the absence of marked increases in utero–ovarian venous plasma levels (see Section 7.6.1).

7.8.5 Oestrogens

As already stated, maternal peripheral total unconjugated oestrogen levels (i.e. oestradiol-17α + oestradiol-17β + oestrone) rise before delivery, from below 20 ng ml^{-1} to 1–2 ng ml^{-1} at delivery (Challis, 1971; Obst and Seamark, 1972; Thorburn *et al.*, 1972). In maternal peripheral plasma oestrone, oestradiol-17*b* and oestradiol-17α are present in a ratio of about 2 : 1 : 1 (Thorburn *et al.*, 1972); the ratio of sulphoconjugated to unconjugated oestrogens at least 2 : 1. Levels of oestrogen sulphates in fetal plasma are much higher (5.4 ng oestrone sulphate and 0.4 ng oestradiol sulphate/ml fetal plasma 48 hours before delivery rising to 22.8 ng and 48.4 ng ml^{-1} respectively six hours before delivery). Similar levels have been found by Findlay and Seamark (1973). The source of these oestrogens is probably the fetal placenta (Ainsworth and Ryan, 1966; Steele *et al.*, 1974). The tissue source of the androgens aromatised is, however, unknown (Liggins, 1973).

Labour can be induced by administration of oestrogens to the ewe. Hindson *et al.* (1967) observed apparently normal labour about 24 hours after administration of 20 mg of stilboestrol to the ewe during mid- or late pregnancy and this has been confirmed by Liggins *et al.* (1972). However, although oestrogen-induced *labour* may appear normal, *delivery* is frequently delayed under these circumstances due to failure of the cervix to dilate (Hindson *et al.*, 1967; Liggins *et al.*, 1972). This cervical distocia may be associated with the fact that progesterone levels do not drop after oestrogen administration (Liggins, 1973). Administration of progesterone at term in doses not sufficient to block labour (150 mg/day), can also cause cervical distocia (Liggins *et al.*, 1972).

Concentrations of PGF in utero–ovarian venous plasma, maternal placenta and in myometrium increase during oestrogen-induced labour in a manner similar to that seen after intrafetal administration of glucocorticoid (Liggins *et al.*, 1973). As in dexamethasone-induced labour, treatment of the ewe with progestin, in doses sufficient to block labour, prevents the oestrogen-induced rise in PGF in utero–ovarian venous plasma, but not the rise in maternal placenta and myometrium. Neither oestrogen nor dexamethasone raise PGF in the fetal cotyledons (Liggins *et al.*, 1973).

The parallel influences of dexamethasone and oestrogens on PGF levels again suggest that the effects of the former may be mediated via the latter. Furthermore, it seems that the effects of oestrogens and progesterone on uterine activity may be explained in terms of their effects on uterine PGF production as measured in utero–ovarian venous plasma. The significance of the reduction in utero–ovarian PGF levels by progesterone (while placental and myometrial concentrations remain unaltered), is unclear, although the release mechanism may be affected.

The significance of the decrease in circulating progesterone levels near term is not clear. Since the drop in progesterone is not seen in labour stimulated by oestrogens, it seems this fall is not a necessary prelude to labour. On the other hand labour of spontaneous onset, or labour induced by dexamethasone, can be blocked by large doses of progesterone. The fall in progesterone levels may be of importance in the clearance of the cervical mucus plug, or in cervical softening and dilatation.

7.8.6 Oxytocin

Maternal oxytocin secretion does not occur before the onset of second stage labour in the sheep (Fitzpatrick and Walmsley, 1965). Fetal oxytocin levels increase as long as 40 hours before term and reach 16–18 μU ml^{-1} before delivery (Forsling *et al.*, 1974). Oxytocin in the fetal circulation may exert a uterine stimulatory effect, since infusion of oxytocin to the fetus has been shown to cause uterine contractions (Nathanielsz *et al.*, 1973).

Observations that utero–ovarian venous PGF levels were elevated after vaginal distension in sheep during labour (Flint *et al.*, 1974a) led to the suggestion that oxytocin may influence utero–ovarian venous PGF levels at delivery (Figure 7.9). Oxytocin has been shown to be secreted in response to vaginal distension in the ewe (Debackere *et al.*, 1961; Roberts and Share, 1968; Flint *et al.*, 1975) and physiological doses of oxytocin raise utero–ovarian venous PGF levels (Mitchell *et al.*, 1975) (Figure 7.10). Control of PGF levels by oxytocin as well as by oestrogens and progesterone is consistent with earlier suggestions that release occurs in two phases, one before first stage

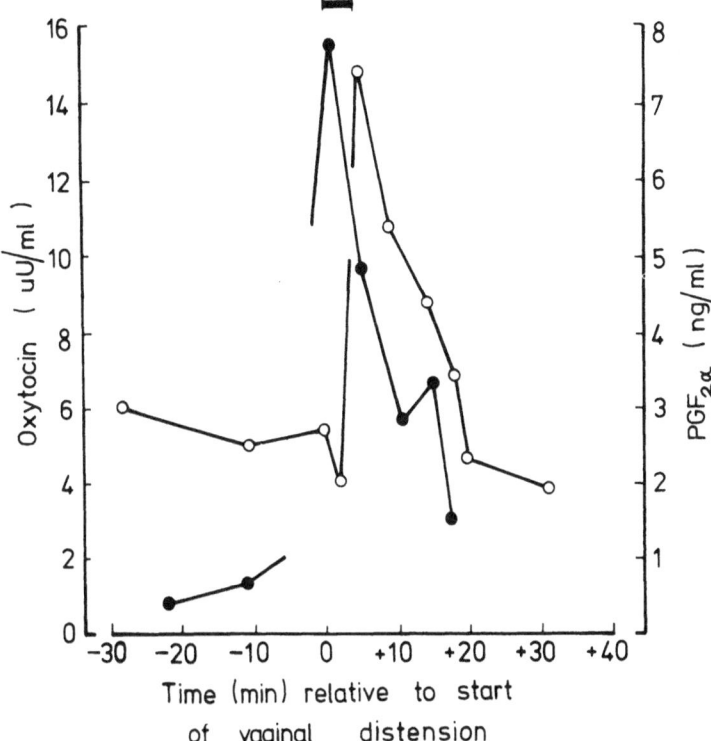

Figure 7.9 Effect of vaginal distension on maternal jugular venous oxytocin (●) and utero–ovarian venous PGF (○) levels. The vagina was distended manually, for 4 min, starting at time zero (indicated by the bar); the experiment was carried out on day 142 *post coitus*; live twins were delivered on day 147. (From Flint *et al.*, 1975, by courtesy of *J. Reprod. Fert.*)

labour and the other at the onset of second stage labour, when the fetal snout and fore-limbs enter the upper vagina (Currie *et al.*, 1973; Flint *et al.*, 1974a). It is now envisaged that the earlier increase is controlled by steroid hormones and the second by oxytocin, although a role for vasopressin in the latter cannot at present be ruled out.

7.8.7 Effects of maternal administration of PGF$_{2\alpha}$

Unlike the pregnant human uterus, that of the sheep is rather insensitive to acute stimulation by PGF$_{2\alpha}$. Infusion of large (by human standards) doses of PGF$_{2\alpha}$ (up to 22 μg min^{-1} for up to 30 hours) via the fetal posterior vena cava or the maternal uterine artery does not induce labour between 118 and 140 days of pregnancy (Keirse *et al.*, 1973; Oakes *et al.*, 1973). However, Liggins *et al.* (1973) have recently reported that intra-aortic infusions of 5–10 μg PGF$_{2\alpha}$ min^{-1} for 24–48 hours does lead to labour 'indistinguishable from normal labour'. The effect of infusion of large amounts of PGF$_{2\alpha}$ in this way has not been tested in animals in which the preterm drop in circulating progesterone level has occurred and it may be that nearer to term the uterus becomes more sensitive to prostaglandins.

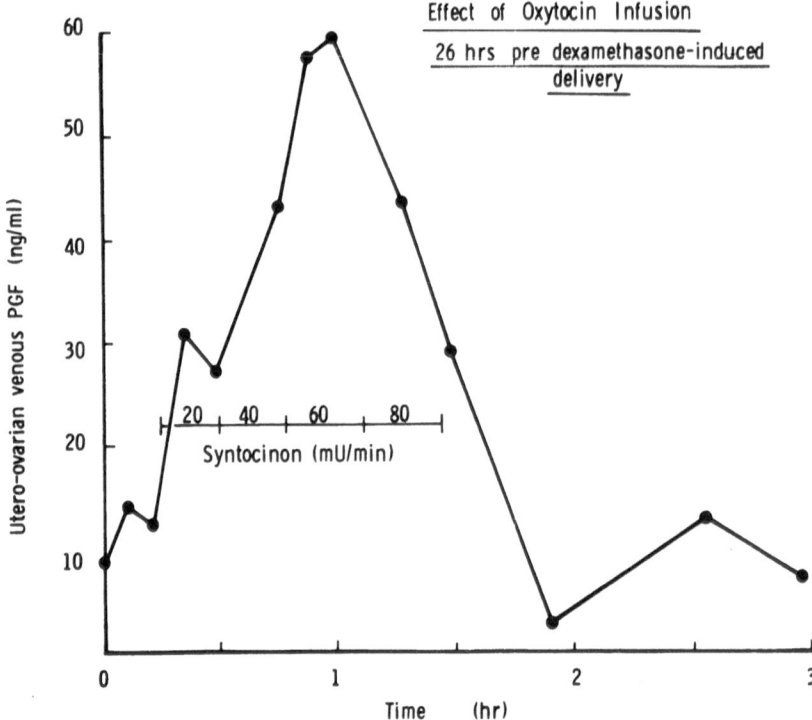

Figure 7.10 Effect of oxytocin on utero–ovarian venous PGF levels in one ewe 26 hours before delivery induced by administration of dexamethasone to the fetus. (From Mitchell *et al.* 1975, by courtesy of *Prostaglandins*)

A more acute effect of $PGF_{2\alpha}$ administered in late pregnancy is that on the oxytocic threshold. Liggins *et al.* (1972) have described a tenfold reduction in the dose of oxytocin required to make the uterus contract (from 100–300 mU to 5–50 mU) after intra-aortic administration of $PGF_{2\alpha}$ (5 μg min^{-1} for 24 hours). This effect may be of importance in reducing the oxytocic threshold when the octapeptide is secreted late in labour. The decrease in threshold cannot be prevented by the simultaneous administration of progesterone in doses (200 mg/day) sufficient to prevent the onset of labour (Liggins *et al.*, 1972). Also the reduction in threshold, or the induction of labour caused by chronic $PGF_{2\alpha}$ infusion, occurs in the absence of any changes in progesterone or oestrogen levels (Liggins *et al.*, 1973). The effect of $PGF_{2\alpha}$ on the oxytocic threshold is mimicked by administration of oestrogen to the ewe (Liggins *et al.*, 1973), as might be expected from the effect of oestrogen on myometrial PGF levels. The lack of effect of progesterone, on the reduction in oxytocic threshold by $PGF_{2\alpha}$, is consistent with the observed elevation of myometrial PGF levels by oestrogen in the presence of progesterone (Liggins *et al.*, 1973). The effects of oestrogen and progesterone on the myometrial oxytocic threshold are consistent therefore with the effects of these steroids on myometrial, rather than utero–ovarian venous, PGF levels. This is in contrast to their effects on uterine contractility.

It is unlikely that the intra-aortic infusion of large doses of $PGF_{2\alpha}$ in late pregnancy causes luteolysis, since Liggins *et al.* (1973) noted no change in peripheral progesterone level. This may be because the ovary (blood flow 10–15 ml min^{-1}) probably received less than 1% of aortic blood flow, i.e. less than 1% of the $PGF_{2\alpha}$ administered. In the experiments of Liggins *et al.* (1973) where 5 μg min^{-1}, i.e. 300 μg/hour was infused, the ovarian dose would amount to 3 μg/hour, which is only slightly higher than the luteolytic dose when administered for 9.5–18 hours in the autotransplanted ovary (Barrett *et al.*, 1971). However, the corpus luteum of pregnancy may be maintained under these circumstances by the luteotrophic effect of the conceptus (see Section 7.7).

7.8.8 Interaction between oxytocin and $PGF_{2\alpha}$ at the cellular level

Work of Goldberg *et al.* (1973) and of Carsten (1969, 1972, 1973, 1974) has drawn attention to the possible mediation of the effects of oxytocin and $PGF_{2\alpha}$ through levels of 3', 5'-(cyclic)-guanosine monophosphate (cyclic-GMP) and Ca^{2+}. Both oxytocin and $PGF_{2\alpha}$ raise cyclic-GMP levels in myometrium and decrease ATP-dependent binding of Ca^{2+} by isolated sarcoplasmic reticulum *in vitro*. These observations may lead to the recognition of common intracellular pathways for the effects of these two oxytocic agents. This work has not, however, been carried out on ovine tissue.

7.8.9 Transfer of $PGF_{2\alpha}$ from site of synthesis to site of action

It is assumed that $PGF_{2\alpha}$ produced at term has its effect directly on the myometrium, although PGF receptors have not been identified in ovine myometrium. It is not known in what tissue these prostaglandins are produced; one possibility appears to be the maternal placenta, since levels rise in this tissue before they rise in myometrium, following administration of glucocorticoid (Liggins *et al.*, 1972). Since oxytocin will cause PGF levels to rise for some time postpartum (Mitchell *et al.*, 1975) and in the oestrogen-treated anoestrous ewe (Sharma and Fitzpatrick, 1974), other uterine tissues should be considered.

In an attempt to account for the time lapse between the appearance of PGF in maternal placenta and myometrium, Liggins *et al.* (1973) conducted an experiment to test possible counter-current distribution of PGF from uterine veins to uterine arteries. The uterine arteries in the pregnant ewe are closely applied to the veins and such a transfer may be possible. However, Liggins *et al.* (1973) were unable to demonstrate a transfer, following infusion of ^{3}H-$PGF_{2\alpha}$ to the uterine vein, and concluded that PGF was either synthesised in the myometrium, or reached it by diffusion from the maternal cotyledons.

7.8.10 Metabolism of $PGF_{2\alpha}$ by uterine tissues

In man, the organs within the pregnant uterus contain enzymes capable of converting prostaglandins to less active metabolites (Keirse and Turnbull, 1975; Sykes *et al.*, 1975). This is also true of the sheep, though to a lesser degree. The activity of prostaglandin 15-hydroxy dehydrogenase in ovine maternal placenta is at most one-tenth that in human placental villi (M. J. N. C. Keirse, personal communication; see Table 7.2).

Table 7.2   Rate of disappearance of ^{3}H-PGF$_{2\alpha}$. This was determined during incubations containing 0.9 μg PGF$_{2\alpha}$ per gram of tissue homogenate in 0.1 M potassium phosphate, pH 7.4 containing 20 mM EDTA and 2mM NAD$^+$. Incubations were for 60 min at 37 °C (From M. Keirse, unpublished data)

Tissue	Percentage of ^{3}H-PGF$_{2\alpha}$ remaining after incubation	
	Human	Sheep
Fetal placenta	<2	92
Decidua or maternal cotyledons	91	<2
Myometrium	79	11
Membranes	<1	98

7.9 PROSTAGLANDINS IN REPRODUCTIVE PROCESSES IN THE GOAT

7.9.1 In the oestrous cycle

It is not known whether PGF$_{2\alpha}$ is luteolytic in the cycling goat; as far as we are aware PGF levels have not been measured.

7.9.2 At parturition

In contrast to the sheep, pregnancy in the goat is corpus luteum-dependent and can be terminated at any time by hypophysectomy or ovariectomy (Meites *et al.*, 1951; Cowie *et al.*, 1963). Arterio-venous differences across the uterus, and the drastic effect of ovariectomy on progesterone levels suggest that the corpus luteum is the major site of progesterone synthesis in the pregnant goat (Linzell and Heap, 1968; Thorburn and Schneider, 1972). The goat is therefore a useful model for the study of utero–ovarian interactions at parturition. Like the sheep, chronic indwelling catheters can be maintained in the goat to allow sampling of fetal and maternal utero–ovarian blood, and gestational length (150 days) allows experimentation with the kid *in utero* for some time before delivery.

Luteolysis occurs and circulating progesterone levels drop 2–4 days before delivery in the doe (Irving *et al.*, 1972; Thorburn and Schneider, 1972). Luteolysis can be induced prematurely by administration of PGF$_{2\alpha}$ (1.9–15 μg min^{-1} for 5–6 hours) to the uterine vein (Currie and Thorburn, 1973); the kid is delivered 30–35 hours after starting the treatment. Measurements of PGF in utero–ovarian venous blood indicate that the level rises markedly after luteolysis has occurred (Thorburn *et al.*, 1972), but some transient increases also occur at the time of luteolysis (Currie *et al.*, 1973). These findings therefore suggest that the preterm decrease in progesterone levels may be mediated via uterine PGF production.

What stimulates PGF production at this time is open to speculation. Unconjugated oestrogen levels are higher in the goat than in the sheep during late gestation. However, levels do increase before parturition, but the increase is not so marked as in the sheep. In parturition of spontaneous onset, the oestrogen rise does not precede the fall in progesterone (Thorburn *et al.*, 1972), suggesting that PGF output is not stimulated by oestrogens. Other factors have not been investigated in labour of natural onset. Labour can be induced in the doe, as in the ewe, by infusing ACTH to the fetus. Under these conditions, oestrogen levels do rise before the progesterone falls (at the same time as the fetal corticosteroids increase) and PGF production may be stimulated by oestrogens (Thorburn *et al.*, 1972).

7.10 PRACTICAL APPLICATIONS OF PROSTAGLANDINS IN ANIMAL HUSBANDRY

Prostaglandins are likely to be of limited use in induction of labour in sheep; the myometrium is relatively insensitive to prostaglandins and maternally administered dexamethasone would provide a superior alternative method. On the other hand prostaglandins may become of practical importance in synchronisation of oestrus, particularly as a means of improving the efficiency of artificial insemination (Goding *et al.*, 1972b; Inskeep, 1973). The subject is discussed in detail in Chapter 8.

References

Ainsworth, L. and Ryan, K. J. (1966). Steroid hormone transformations by endocrine organs from pregnant mammals. I. Estrogen biosynthesis by mammalian placental preparation *in vitro*. *Endocrinology*, 79, 875–883

Akbar, A. M., Rowe, K. E. and Stormshak, F. (1971). Estradiol induced luteal regression in unilaterally hysterectomized and luteinizing hormone treated ewes. *J. Anim. Sci.*, 33, 426–429

Aldridge, R. R., Barrett, S., Brown, J. B., Funder, J. W., Goding, J. R., Kaltenbach, C. C. and Mole, B. J. (1970). The effect of prostaglandins on ovarian steroidogenesis *in vivo*. *J. Reprod. Fert.*, 21, 369–370

Amoroso, E. C., Harrison, F. A., Heap, R. B. and Poyser, N. L. (1973). The production of prostaglandin $F_{2\alpha}$ by the uterus of the sheep. *J. Endocrinol.*, 57, lix

Armstrong, D. T. and Grinwich, D. L. (1972). Blockade of spontaneous or LH induced ovulation in rats by indomethacin, an inhibitor of prostaglandin biosynthesis. *Prostaglandins*, 1, 21–28

Armstrong, D. T., Grinwich, D. L., Moon, Y. S. and Zamecnik, J. (1974). Inhibition of ovulation in rabbits by intrafollicular injection of indomethacin and PGF antiserum. *Life Sci.*, 14, Part 1, 129–140

Armstrong, D. T. and Hansel, W. (1959). Alteration of the bovine oestrous cycle with oxytocin. *J. Dairy Sci.*, 42, 533–542

Armstrong, D. T., Moon, Y. S. and Grinwich, D. L. (1973). Possible role of prostaglandins in ovulation. *Adv. Biosciences*, 9, 709–715

Assali, N. S. (1968). Placental transfer—transport systems and transfer of specific substances. In: *Biology of Gestation*, Vol. 1, 250–273 (N. S. Assali, editor) (N.Y.: Academic Press)

Baird, D. T., Collett, R. A., Fraser, J. S., Kelly, R. W., Land, R. B. and Wheeler, A. G. (1973). Progesterone secretion from the ovary in the ewe following infusion of uterine venous plasma. *J. Reprod. Fert.*, 35, 13–22

Baird, D. T. and Land, R. B. (1973). Division of the uterine vein and the function of the adjacent ovary in the ewe. *J. Reprod. Fert.*, 33, 393–397

Barcikowski, B., Carlson, J. C., Wilson, L. and McCracken, J. A. (1973). Effect of endogenous and exogenous estradiol-17β on the release of prostaglandin $F_{2\alpha}$ from the ovine uterus. *Biol. Reprod.*, 9, 70

Barrett, S., Blockley, M. A. de B., Brown, J. M., Cumming, I. A., Goding, J. R., Mole, B. J. and Obst, J. M. (1971). Initiation of the oestrous cycle in the ewe by infusions of $PGF_{2\alpha}$ to the autotransplanted ovary. *J. Reprod. Fert.*, 24, 136–137

Bassett, J. M., Oxborrow, T. J., Smith, I. D. and Thorburn, G. D. (1969). The concentration of progesterone in the peripheral plasma of the pregnant ewe. *J. Endocrinol*, 45, 449–457

Bassett, J. M. and Thorburn, G. D. (1969). Foetal plasma corticosteroids and the initiation of parturition in sheep. *J. Endocrinol.*, 44, 285–286

Bedford, C. A., Challis, J. R. G., Harrison, F. A. and Heap, R. B. (1972). The role of oestrogens and progesterone in the onset of parturition in various species. *J. Reprod. Fert.*, **Suppl. 16**, 1–23

Bedford, C. A., Harrison, F. A. and Heap, R. B. (1973). The kinetics of progesterone metabolism in the pregnant sheep. In: *The Endocrinology of Pregnancy and Parturition: Experimental studies in the Sheep*, 83–93 (C. G. Pierrepoint, editor) (Cardiff: Alpha-Omega-Alpha Press)

Behrman, H. R., McDonald, G. J. and Greep, R. O. (1971). Regulation of ovarian cholesterol esters. Evidence for the enzymatic sites of prostaglandins induced loss of corpus luteum function. *Lipids*, 6, 791–796

Bengtsson, L. P. and Schofield, B. M. (1963). Progesterone and the accomplishment of parturition in the sheep. *J. Reprod. Fert.*, 5, 423–431

Bjersing, L., Hay, M. F., Kann, G., Moor, R. M., Naftolin, F., Scaramuzzi, R. J., Short, R. V. and Younglai, E. V. (1973). Changes in gonadotrophins, ovarian steroids and follicular morphology in sheep at oestrus. *J. Endocrinol.*, 52, 465–479

Bland, K. P. and Donovan, B. T. (1969). Observations on the time of action and the pathway of the uterine luteolytic effect in the guinea-pig. *J. Endocrinol.*, 43, 259–264

Bland, K. P., Horton, E. W. and Poyser, N. L. (1971). Levels of prostaglandin $F_{2\alpha}$ in the uterine venous blood of sheep during the oestrous cycle. *Life Sci.*, 10, Part 1, 509–517

Brinsfield, T. H. and Hawk, H. W. (1968). Luteolytic effect of induced uterine infection in the ewe. *J. Anim. Sci.*, 27, 150–152

Bruce, N. W. and Hillier, K. (1974). Effect of prostaglandin $F_{2\alpha}$ on ovarian blood flow and corpus luteum regression in the rabbit. *Nature (London)*, 249, 176–177

Butcher, R. L., Barley, D. A. and Inskeep, E. K. (1969). Local relationship between the ovary and uterus of rats and guinea pigs. *Endocrinology*, 84, 476–487

Caldwell, B. V. and Moor, R. M. (1971). Further studies on the role of the uterus in the regulation of corpus luteum function in sheep. *J. Reprod. Fert.*, 26, 133–135

Caldwell, B. V., Moor, R. M. and Lawson, R. A. S. (1968). Effects of endometrial grafts and extracts on the length of pseudopregnancy in the hysterectomised hamster. *J. Reprod. Fert.*, 17, 567–569

Caldwell, B. V., Rowson, L. E. A., Moor, R. M. and Hay, M. F. (1969). The utero–ovarian relationship and its possible role in fertility. *J. Reprod. Fert.*, **Suppl. 8**, 59–76

Caldwell, B. V., Tillson, S. A., Brock, W. A. and Speroff, L. (1972). The effects of exogenous progesterone and estradiol on prostaglandin F levels in ovariectomised ewes. *Prostaglandins*, 1, 217–228

Carsten, M. E. (1969). Role of calcium binding by sarcoplasmic reticulum in the contraction and relaxation of uterine smooth muscle. *J. Gen. Physiol.*, 53, 414–426

Carsten, M. E. (1972). Prostaglandin's part in regulating uterine contraction by transport of calcium. *J. Reprod. Med.*, 9, 277–281

Carsten, M. E. (1973). Prostaglandins and cellular calcium transport in the pregnant human uterus. *Amer. J. Obstet. Gynecol.*, 117, 824–832

Carsten, M. E. (1974). Prostaglandins and oxytocin. Their effects on uterine smooth muscle. *Prostaglandins*, 5, 33–40

Challis, J. R. G. (1971). Sharp increase in free circulating oestrogens immediately before parturition in sheep. *Nature (London)*, 229, 208

Challis, J. R. G., Harrison, F. A., Heap, R. B., Horton, E. W. and Poyser, N. L. (1972). A possible role of oestrogens in the stimulation of prostaglandin $F_{2\alpha}$ output at the time of parturition in a sheep. *J. Reprod. Fert.*, 30, 485–488

Chamley, W. A., Buckmaster, J. M., Cain, M. D., Cerini, J. C., Cerini, M. E. D., Cumming, I. A. and Goding, J. R. (1972). The effect of prostaglandin $F_{2\alpha}$ on progesterone, oestradiol and luteinizing hormone secretion in sheep with ovarian transplants. *J. Endocrinol.*, 55, 253–263

Chamley, W. A. and Christie, M. (1973). Failure of prostaglandin $F_{2\alpha}$ to effect luteinizing hormone secretion in the ovariectomized ewe. *Prostaglandins*, 3, 405–412

Cleverley, J. D. and Folley, S. J. (1970). The blood levels of oxytocin during machine milking in cows with some observations on its half life in the circulation. *J. Endocrinol.*, 46, 347–361

Comline, R. S., Nathanielsz, P. W., Paisey, R. B. and Silver, M. (1970). Cortisol turnover in the sheep fetus immediately prior to parturition. *J. Physiol. (London)*, 210, 141–142P

Cook, B. and Taylor, T. (1973). Oestrogen binding activity in ovine corpora lutea. *Proc. Meeting of the Society for the Study of Fertility*, December 1973 (Abstr. 32)

Coudert, S. P., Phillips, G. D., Faiman, C., Chernecki, W. and Palmer, M. (1974a). Infusion of tritiated prostaglandin $F_{2\alpha}$ into the anterior uterine vein of the ewe. Absence of local venous arterial transfer. *J. Reprod. Fert.*, 36, 333–343

Coudert, S. P., Phillips, G. D., Faiman, C., Chernecki, W. and Palmer, M. (1974b). A study of the utero–ovarian circulation in sheep with reference to local transfer between venous and arterial blood. *J. Reprod. Fert.*, 36, 319–331

Coudert, S. P., Phillips, G. D., Palmer, M. and Faiman, C. (1972). Prostaglandin F concentration in the peripheral blood of the ewe during the oestrous cycle. *Prostaglandins*, 2, 501–509

Coudert, S. P. and Short, R. V. (1966). Prolongation of the functional life of the corpus luteum in sheep with experimental uterine infections. *J. Reprod. Fert.*, 12, 579–582

Cowie, A. T., Daniel, P. M., Prichard, M. M. L. and Tindal, J. S. (1963). Hypophysectomy in pregnant goats and section of the pituitary stalk in pregnant goats and sheep. *J. Endocrinol.*, 28, 93–102

Cox, R. I., Mattner, P. E. and Thorburn, G. D. (1971). Changes in ovarian secretion of estradiol-17β around oestrus in the sheep. *J. Endocrinol.*, 49, 345–346

Cox, R. I., Thorburn, G. D., Currie, W. B., Restall, B. J. and Schneider, W. (1972). Prostaglandin F group (PGF), progesterone and oestrogen concentrations in the utero–ovarian venous plasma of the conscious ewe during the oestrous cycle. *Adv. Biosciences*, 9, 625–630

Currie, W. B. and Thorburn, G. D. (1973). Induction of premature parturition in goats by prostaglandin F_α administered into the uterine vein. *Prostaglandins*, 4, 201–214

Currie, W. B., Wong, M. S. F., Cox, R. I. and Thorburn, G. D. (1973). Spontaneous or dexamethasone-induced parturition in the sheep and goat: changes in plasma concentrations of maternal prostaglandin F and fetal oestrogen sulphates. *Mem. Soc. Endocrinol.*, 20, 95–118

Debackere, M., Peeters, G. and Tuyttens, N. (1961). Reflex release of an oxytocic hormone by stimulation of genital organs in male and female sheep studied by a cross circulation technique. *J. Endocrinol.*, 22, 321–334

Denamur, R. (1968). Formation and maintenance of corpora lutea in domestic animals. *J. Anim. Sci.*, 27 (Suppl. 1), 163–169

Denamur, R. and Kann, G. (1973). Luteolytic effects of oestradiol after hypophysectomy or pituitary stalk section in cycling sheep. *Acta Endocrinol.*, 73, 635–642

Denamur, R. and Martinet, J. (1955). Effets de l'ovariectomie chez la Brebis pendant la gestation. *C.R. Seance, Soc. Biol.*, 149, 2105–2107

Denamur, R., Martinet, J. and Short, R. V. (1966). Secretion de la progesterone par les corps jaunes de la brebis après hypophysectomie, section de la tige pituitaire et hysterectomie. *Acta Endocrinol.*, 52, 72–90

Denamur, R., Martinet, J. and Short, R. V. (1970). Mode of action of oestrogen in maintaining the functional life of corpora lutea in sheep. *J. Reprod. Fert.*, 23, 109–116

Denamur, R. and Mauleon, P. (1963). Endocrine control of persistence of the corpus luteum in sheep. *C.R. Acad. Sci.*, 257, 527–530

Dingle, J. T., Hay, M. F. and Moor, R. M. (1968). Lysosomal function in the corpus luteum of the sheep. *J. Endocrinol.*, 40, 325–336

DuCharme, D. W. and Weeks, J. R. (1968). Cardiovascular pharmacology of prostaglandin $F_{2\alpha}$, a unique pressor agent. *Nobel Symposium*, 2, 173–181

Dutt, R. H. and Casida, L. E. (1948). Alteration of estrual cycle in sheep by use of progesterone and its effect upon subsequent ovulation and fertility. *Endocrinology*, **43**, 208–217

Findlay, J. K. and Seamark, R. F. (1973). The occurrence and metabolism of oestrogens in the sheep fetus and placenta. In: *The Endocrinology of Pregnancy and Parturition: Experimental studies in the Sheep*, 54–64 (C. G. Pierrepoint, editor) (Cardiff: Alpha-Omega-Alpha Press)

Fitzpatrick, R. J. and Walmsley, C. F. (1965). The release of oxytocin during parturition. In: *Advances in Oxytocin Research*, 57–71 (J. H. M. Pinkerton, editor) (London: Pergamon Press)

Flint, A. P. F., Anderson, A. B. M., Patten, P. T. and Turnbull, A. C. (1974a). Control of utero–ovarian venous prostaglandin F during labour in the sheep: acute effects of vaginal and cervical stimulation. *J. Endocrinol.*, **63**, 67–87

Flint, A. P. F., Forsling, M. L., Mitchell, M. D. and Turnbull, A. C. (1975). Temporal relationship between changes in oxytocin and prostaglandin F levels in response to vaginal distension in the pregnant and puerperal ewe. *J. Reprod. Fert.* **43**, 551–554

Flint, A. P. F., Grinwich, D. L. and Armstrong, D. T. (1973). Control of ovarian cholesterol ester biosynthesis. *Biochem. J.*, **132**, 313–321

Flint, A. P. F., Grinwich, D. L., Kennedy, T. G. and Armstrong, D. T. (1974b). Metabolism of the corpus luteum during luteolysis in the pseudopregnant rabbit. *Endocrinology*, **94**, 509–517

Folley, S. J. and Knaggs, G. S. (1966). Milk ejecting activity (oxytocin) in the external jugular vein blood of the cow, goat and sow in relation to the stimulus of milking or suckling. *J. Endocrinol.*, **34**, 197–214

Forsling, M., Jack, P. M. B. and Nathanielsz, P. W. (1974). Plasma oxytocin concentrations in the fetal sheep (In press)

Fuller, G. B. and Hansel, W. (1970). Regression of sheep corpora lutea after treatment with antibovine luteinizing hormone. *J. Anim. Sci.*, **31**, 99–103

Fylling, P. (1970). The effect of pregnancy, ovariectomy and parturition on plasma progesterone level in sheep. *Acta Endocrinol.*, **65**, 273–283

Ginther, O. J. (1968). Influence of exogenous progesterone and the uterus on ovarian activity in sheep. *Endocrinology*, **83**, 613–615

Ginther, O. J. (1970). Length of estrous cycle in sheep treated with estradiol. *Amer. J. Vet. Res.*, **31**, 973–975

Ginther, O. J. (1971). Response of corpora lutea to cauterisation of follicles in sheep. *Amer. J. Vet. Res.*, **32**, 59–62

Ginther, O. J. and Bisgard, G. E. (1972). Role of the main uterine vein in local action of an intrauterine device on the corpus luteum in sheep. *Amer. J. Vet. Res.*, **33**, 1583–1587

Ginther, O. J., Del Campo, C. H. and Rawlings, C. A. (1973). Vascular anatomy of the uterus and ovaries and the unilateral luteolytic effect of the uterus: a local venoarterial pathway between uterus and ovaries in sheep. *Amer. J. Vet. Res.*, **34**, 723–728

Ginther, O. J., Pope, A. L. and Cassida, L. E. (1966). Local effect of an intrauterine plastic coil on the corpus luteum of the ewe. *J. Anim. Sci.*, **25**, 472–475

Goding, J. R. (1974). The demonstration that prostaglandin $F_{2\alpha}$ is the uterine luteolysin in the ewe. *J. Reprod. Fert.*, **38**, 261–271

Goding, J. R., Baird, D. T., Cumming, I. A. and McCracken, J. A. (1972a). Functional assessment of autotransplanted endocrine organs. *Acta Endocrinol. (Copenhagen)*, **69, Suppl. 158**, 169–191

Goding, J. R., Blockley, M. A. de B., Brown, J. M., Catt, K. J. and Cumming, I. A. (1970). The role of oestrogen in the control of the oestrous cycle in the ewe. *J. Reprod. Fert.*, **21**, 368–369

Goding, J. R., Buckmaster, J. M., Cerini, J. C., Cerini, M. E. D., Chamley, W. A., Cumming, I. A., Fell, L. R., Findlay, J. K. and Jonas, H. (1973). Gonadotrophins in the ovine oestrous cycle. *J. Reprod. Fert.*, **Suppl. 18**, 31–37

Goding, J. R., Catt, F. J., Brown, J. M., Kaltenbach, C. C., Cumming, I. A. and Mole, B. J. (1969). Radioimmunoassay for ovine luteinizing hormone. Secretion of luteinizing hormone during estrus and following estrogen administration in the sheep. *Endocrinology*, **85**, 133–142

Goding, J. R., Cumming, I. A., Chamley, W. A., Brown, J. M., Cain, M. D., Cerini, J. C., Cerini, M. E. D., Findlay, J. K., O'Shea, T. D. and Pemberton, D. H. (1972b). *IVth Int. Seminar on Reprod. Physiol. and Sexual Endocrinol. Hormones and Antagonists* (P. Hubinont and S. Karger, editors) (Brussels)

Goding, J. R., Harrison, F. A., Heap, R. B. and Linzell, J. L. (1967b). Ovarian activity in the ewe after autotransplantation of the ovary or uterus to the neck. *J. Physiol. (London)*, **191**, 129–130P

Goding, J. R., McCracken, J. A. and Baird, D. T. (1967a). The study of ovarian function in the ewe by means of a vascular autotransplantation technique. *J. Endocrinol.*, **39**, 37–52

Goldberg, N. D., Haddox, M. K., Hartle, D. K. and Hadden, J. W. (1973). Cyclic GMP levels and PGF in uterine contractility. *Proc. 5th Int. Congr. Pharmacol., San Francisco 1972*, page 146

Grinwich, D. L., Kennedy, T. G. and Armstrong, D. T. (1972). Dissociation of ovulatory and steroidogenic actions of luteinizing hormone in rabbits with indomethacin, an inhibition of prostaglandin biosynthesis. *Prostaglandins*, **1**, 89–96

Hansel, W., Shemesh, M., Hixon, J. E. and Lukaszewska, J. (1975). Extraction, isolation and identification of a luteolytic substance from bovine endometrium. *Biol. Reprod.* (In press)

Harrison, F. A. and Heap, R. B. (1974). Prostaglandin secretion by the autotransplanted uterus in sheep. *J. Endocrinol.*, **64**, 13–14

Harrison, F. A., Heap, R. B., Horton, E. W. and Poyser, N. L. (1972). Identification of prostaglandin $F_{2\alpha}$ in uterine fluid from the non-pregnant sheep with an autotransplanted ovary. *J. Endocrinol.*, **53**, 215–222

Harrison, F. A., Heap, R. B. and Linzell, J. L. (1968). Ovarian function in the sheep after autotransplantation of the ovary and uterus to the neck. *J. Endocrinol.*, **40**, xiii

Hawk, H. W. (1967). Investigations into the antifertility effect of intrauterine devices in the ewe. *J. Reprod. Fert.*, **14**, 49–59

Hawk, H. W. and Bolt, D. J. (1970). Luteolytic effect of oestradiol-17β when administered after midcycle in the ewe. *Biol. Reprod.*, **2**, 275–278

Hearnshaw, H., Restall, B. J. and Gleeson, A. R. (1973). Observations on the luteolytic effects of prostaglandin $F_{2\alpha}$ during the oestrous cycle and early pregnancy in the ewe. *J. Reprod. Fert.*, **32**, 322–323

Hindson, J. C., Schofield, B. M. and Turner, C. B. (1967). The effect of a single dose of stilboestrol on cervical dilatation in pregnant sheep. *Res. Vet. Sci.*, **8**, 353–360

Hixon, J. E., Gengenbach, D. R. and Hansel, W. (1974). Failure of prostaglandin $F_{2\alpha}$ to cause luteal regression in ewes after destruction of ovarian follicles by x-irradiation. *Proc. 7th Meeting of the Soc. for the Study of Reproduction, Ottawa*

Hixon, J. E., Nadaraja, R., Schechter, R. J. and Hansel, W. (1973). Prostaglandin $F_{2\alpha}$ induced stimulation of estrone and estradiol-17β secretion in cattle. *Prostaglandins*, **4**, 679–687

Hunter, G. L. (1970). Life span of corpora lutea in ewes with one congenitally absent uterine horn. *J. Reprod. Fert.*, **23**, 131–133

Inskeep, E. K. (1973). Potential uses of prostaglandins in control of reproductive cycles of domestic animals. *J. Anim. Sci.*, **36**, 1149–1157

Inskeep, E. K. and Butcher, R. L. (1966). Local component of utero–ovarian relationships in the ewe. *J. Anim. Sci.*, **25**, 1164–1168

Irving, G., Jones, D. E. and Knifton, A. (1972). Progesterone concentrations in the peripheral plasma of pregnant goats. *J. Endocrinol.*, **53**, 447–452

Kaltenbach, C. C., Graber, J. W., Niswender, G. D. and Nalbandov, A. V. (1968). Luteotrophic properties of some pituitary hormones in non pregnant or pregnant hypophysectomized ewes. *Endocrinology*, **82**, 818–824

Kann, G. and Denamur, R. (1973). Changes in plasma levels of prolactin and LH induced by luteolytic or luteotrophic treatment in intact cycling sheep or in sheep after section of the pituitary stalk. *Acta. Endocrinol.*, **73**, 625–634

Karsch, F. J., Noveroske, J. W., Roche, J. F., Norton, H. W. and Nalbandov, A. V. (1970). Maintenance of ovine corpora lutea in the absence of ovarian follicles. *Endocrinol.*, **87**, 1228–1236

Keirse, M. J. N. C., Patten, P. T., Anderson, A. B. M., Turnbull, A. C., Johns, A., Wooster, M. J. and Pickles, V. R. (1973). Pregnant sheep myometrium responds to prostaglandins in *vitro* but not *in vivo*. *Int. Res. Commun. Syst.* (**73–4**), 8–5–1

Keirse, M. J. N. C. and Turnbull, A. C. (1975). *In vitro* metabolism of prostaglandins in tissues from the pregnant human uterus. *J. Endocrinol.*, **63**, 180

Keyes, P. L. and Bullock, D. W. (1974). Effects of prostaglandin $F_{2\alpha}$ on ectopic and ovarian corpora lutea of the rabbit. *Biol. Reprod.*, **10**, 519–525

Kimball, F. A. and Hansel, W. (1975). Estrogen cytosol binding proteins in bovine endometrium and corpora lutea. *Biol. Reprod.* (In press)

Kiracofe, G. H., Menzies, C. S., Gier, H. T. and Spies, H. G. (1966). Effect of uterine extracts and uterine or ovarian blood vessel ligation on ovarian function of ewes. *J. Anim. Sci.*, **25**, 1159–1163

Ladner, C., Brinkman, C. R., Weston, P. and Assali, N. S. (1970). Dynamics of uterine circulation in pregnant and non-pregnant sheep. *Amer. J. Physiology*, **218** (1), 257–263

Lamond, D. R. and Drost, M. (1973). The counter-current transfer of prostaglandin in the ewe. *Prostaglandins*, **3**, 691–695

LeMaire, W. J., Yang, N. J. T., Behrman, H. R. and Marsh, J. M. (1973). Preovulatory changes in the concentration of prostaglandins in rabbit Graafian follicles. *Prostaglandins*, **3**, 367–376

Liggins, G. C. (1968). Premature parturition after infusion of corticotrophin or cortisol into foetal lambs. *J. Endocrinol.*, **42**, 323–329

Liggins, G. C. (1973). Endocrine factors in labour. *Mem. Soc. Endocrinol.*, **20**, 119–139

Liggins, G. C., Fairclough, R. J., Grieves, S. A., Kendall, J. Z. and Knox, B. S. (1973). The mechanism of initiation of parturition in the ewe. *Rec. Progr. Hormone Res.*, **29**, 111–150

Liggins, G. C. and Grieves, S. A. (1971). Possible role for prostaglandin $F_{2\alpha}$ in parturition in sheep. *Nature (London)*, **232**, 629–631

Liggins, G. C., Grieves, S. A., Kendall, J. Z. and Knox, B. S. (1972). The physiological roles of progesterone, oestradiol-17β and prostaglandin $F_{2\alpha}$ in the control of ovine parturition. *J. Reprod. Fert.*, **Suppl. 16**, 85–103

Linzell, J. L. and Heap, R. B. (1968). A comparison of progesterone metabolism in the pregnant sheep and goat. Sources of production and an estimation of uptake by some target organs. *J. Endocrinol.*, **41**, 433–438

Lukaszewska, J. H. and Hansel, W. (1970). Extraction and partial purification of luteolytic activity from bovine endometrial tissue. *Endocrinology*, **86**, 261–270

Mattner, P. E. and Braden, A. W. H. (1972). Secretion of oestradiol-17β by the ovine ovary during the luteal phase of the oestrous cycle in relation to ovulation. *J. Reprod. Fert.*, **28**, 136–137

Mazer, R. S. and Wright, P. A. (1968). A hamster uterine luteolytic extract. *Endocrinology*, **83**, 1065–1070

McCracken, J. A. (1973). Comment. *Prostaglandins*, **3**, 696–701

McCracken, J. A., Baird, D. T. and Goding, J. R. (1971). Factors affecting the secretion of steroids from the transplanted ovary in the sheep. *Rec. Progr. Hormone Res.*, **27**, 537–582

McCracken, J. A., Barcikowski, B., Carlson, J. C., Green, F. and Samuelsson, B. (1973). The physiological role of prostaglandin $F_{2\alpha}$ in corpus luteum regression. *Adv. Biosciences*, **9**, 599–624

McCracken, J. A. and Caldwell, B. V. (1969). Corpus luteum maintenance in a ewe with one congenitally absent uterine horn. *J. Reprod. Fert.*, **20**, 139–141

McCracken, J. A., Carlson, J. C., Glew, M. E., Goding, J. R. Baird, D. T., Green, K. and Samuelsson, B. (1972). Prostaglandin $F_{2\alpha}$ identified as a luteolytic in sheep. *Nature New Biol.*, **238**, 129–134

McCracken, J. A., Glew, M. E. and Levy, L. K. (1970a). Regulation of corpus luteum function by gonadotrophins and related compounds. *Adv. Biosciences*, **4**, 377–397

McCracken, J. A., Glew, M. E. and Scaramuzzi, R. J. (1970b). Corpus luteum regression induced by prostaglandin $F_{2\alpha}$. *J. Clin. Endocrinol. Metab.*, **30**, 544–546

Meites, J., Webster, H. D., Young, F. W., Thorp, F. and Hatch, R. N. (1951). Effects of corpus luteum removal and replacement with progesterone on pregnancy in goats. *J. Anim. Sci.*, **10**, 411–416

Mitchell, M. D., Flint, A. P. F. and Turnbull, A. C. (1974) (Unpublished observations)

Mitchell, M. D., Flint, A. P. F. and Turnbull, A. C. (1975). Stimulation by oxytocin of prostaglandin F levels in utero–ovarian venous effluent in pregnant and puerperal sheep. *Prostaglandins*, **9**, 47–56

Moor, R. M. and Rowson, L. E. A. (1964). Influence of the embryo and uterus on luteal function in the sheep. *Nature (London)*, **201**, 522–523

Moor, R. M. and Rowson, L. E. A. (1966a). Local uterine mechanisms affecting luteal function in the sheep. *J. Reprod. Fert.*, **11**, 307–310

Moor, R. M. and Rowson, L. E. A. (1966b). Local maintenance of the corpus luteum in sheep with embryos transferred to various isolated portions of the uterus. *J. Reprod. Fert.*, **12**, 539–550

Moor, R. M. and Rowson, L. E. A. (1966c). The corpus luteum of the sheep: functional relationship between the embryo and the corpus luteum. *J. Endocrinol.*, **34**, 233–239

Moor, R. M. and Rowson, L. E. A. (1966d). The corpus luteum of the sheep. Effect of the removal of embryos on luteal function. *J. Endocrinol.*, **34**, 497–502

Moor, R. M., Rowson, L. E. A., Hay, M. F. and Caldwell, B. V. (1969). The corpus luteum of the sheep and effect of the conceptus on luteal function at several stages during pregnancy. *J. Endocrinol.*, **43**, 301–307

Moore, N. W., Barrett, S., Brown, J. B., Schindler, I., Smith, M. A. and Smyth, B. (1969). Oestrogen and progesterone content of ovarian vein blood of the ewe during the oestrous cycle. *J. Endocrinol.*, **44**, 55–62

Morris, B. and McIntosh, G. H. (1971). In: *Perfusion Techniques*, 145–168 (E. Diczfalusy, editor) (Stockholm: Karolinska Institutet for Reproductive Endocrinology)

Morris, B. and Sass, M. B. (1966). The formation of lymph in the ovary. *Proc. Roy. Soc. (Biol.)*, **164**, 577–591

Nalbandov, A. V. and Cook, B. (1968). Reproduction. *Ann. Rev. Physiol.*, **30**, 245–278

Nathanielsz, P. W., Comline, R. S. and Silver, M. (1973). Uterine activity following intravenous administration of oxytocin to the fetal sheep. *Nature (London)*, **243**, 471–472

Niswender, G. D., Dzuik, P. J., Graber, J. and Kaltenbach, C. C. (1970). Function of the corpus luteum in the ewe following relocation of the uterus or embryo. *J. Anim. Sci.*, **30**, 935–940

Oakes, G., Mofid, M., Brinkman, C. R. and Assali, N. S. (1973). Insensitivity of the sheep to prostaglandins. *Proc. Soc. Exp. Biol. Med.*, **142**, 194–197

Obst, J. M. and Seamark, R. F. (1972). Plasma oestrogen concentrations in ewes during parturition. *J. Reprod. Fert.*, **28**, 161–162

Obst, J. M., Seamark, R. F. and Brown, J. M. (1971). Application of a competitive protein binding assay for oestrogens to the study of ovarian functions in sheep. *J. Reprod. Fert.*, **24**, 140

O'Grady, J. P., Kohorn, E. I., Glass, R. H., Caldwell, B. V., Brock, W. A. and Speroff, L. (1972). Inhibition of progesterone synthesis *in vitro* by prostaglandin $F_{2\alpha}$. *J. Reprod. Fert.*, **30**, 153–156

Orczyk, G. P. and Behrman, H. R. (1972). Ovulation blockade by aspirin or indomethacin—*In vitro* evidence for a role of prostaglandin in gonadotrophin secretion. *Prostaglandins*, **1**, 3–20

O'Shea, J. D., Lee, C. S. and Cumming, I. A. (1974). Normal duration of the oestrous cycle in ewes with congenital absence of one uterine horn. *J. Reprod. Fert.*, **38**, 201–204

O'Shea, J. D. and Phillips, R. E. (1974). Contractility *in vitro* of ovarian follicles from sheep, and the effects of drugs. *Biol. Reprod.*, **10**, 370–379

Pexton, J. E., Ford, S. P., Wilson, L., Butcher, R. L. and Inskeep, E. K. (1973). Prostaglandin F (PGF) in I.U.D. treated ewes. *J. Anim. Sci.*, **37**, 324

Pharris, B. B. and Wyngarden, L. J. (1969). The effect of prostaglandin $F_{2\alpha}$ on the progestogen content of ovaries from pseudopregnant rats. *Proc. Soc. Exp. Biol. Med.*, **130**, 92–94

Pickles, V. R., Hall, W. J., Best, F. A. and Smith, G. N. (1965). Prostaglandins in endometrium and menstrual fluid from normal and dysmenorrhoeic subjects. *J. Obstet. Gynaecol. Brit. Cwlth.*, **72**, 185–192

Piper, E. L. and Foote, W. C. (1965). A luteotrophic effect of oestradiol in the ewe. *J. Anim. Sci.*, **24**, 927–928

Piper, E. L. and Foote, W. C. (1968). Ovulation and corpus luteum maintenance in ewes treated with 17β-oestradiol. *J. Reprod. Fert.*, **16**, 253–259

Piper, E. L. and Foote, W. C. (1970). The effect of 17β-oestradiol on corpus luteum function in sheep. *Biol. Reprod.*, **2**, 48–52

Radford, H. M., Wheatley, I. S. and Wallace, A. L. C. (1969). The effects of oestradiol benzoate and progesterone on secretion of luteinizing hormone in the ovariectomised ewe. *J. Endocrinol.*, **44**, 135–136

Ramsey, E. M. (1960). Placental circulation. In: *The Placenta and Fetal Membranes*, 36–62 (C. A. Villee, editor) (Baltimore: Williams and Wilkins)

Restall, B. J., Hearnshaw, H. R., Gleeson, A. R. and Thorburn, G. D. (1973). Observations on the luteolytic action of prostaglandin $F_{2\alpha}$ in the ewe. *J. Reprod. Fertil.*, **32**, 325–326

Roberts, J. S., Barcikowski, B., Wilson, L., Skarnes, R. C. and McCracken, J. A. (1974). Hormonal and related factors effecting the release of prostaglandin $F_{2\alpha}$ from the uterus. *Proc. IVth Int. Congr. on Hormonal Steroids, Mexico City*

Roberts, J. S. and Share, L. (1968). Oxytocin in plasma of pregnant lactating and cycling ewes during vaginal stimulation. *Endocrinology*, **83**, 272–278

Roberts, J. S. and Share, L. (1969). Effects of progesterone and estrogen on blood levels of oxytocin during vaginal distension. *Endocrinology*, **84**, 1076–1081

Rowson, L. E. A. and Moor, R. M. (1964). Effect of partial hysterectomy on the length of the dioestrous interval in sheep. *Proc. Vth Int. Congr. Anim. Reprod. and Artificial Insemination (Trento)*. **Vol. II**, 394

Scaramuzzi, R. J., Baird, D. T., Wheeler, A. G. and Land, R. B. (1973). The oestrous cycle of the ewe following active immunization against prostaglandin $F_{2\alpha}$. Acta Endocrinol. (*Copenhagen*), **Suppl. 177**, 318

Scaramuzzi, R. J., Boyle, H. P., Wheeler, A. G., Land, R. B. and Baird, D. T. (1974). Preliminary studies on the secretion of prostaglandin F from the autotransplanted uterus of the ewe after exogenous progesterone and oestradiol. *J. Endocrinol*, **61**, xxxv

Scaramuzzi, R. J., Caldwell, B. V. and Moor, R. M. (1970). Immunoassay of luteinizing hormone and estrogen during the estrous cycle of the ewe. *Biol. Reprod.*, **3**, 110–119

Scaramuzzi, R. J., Tillson, S. A., Thorneycroft, I. H. and Caldwell, B. V. (1971). Action of exogenous progesterone and estrogen on behavioural estrus and luteinizing hormone levels in the ovariectomized ewe. *Endocrinology*, **88**, 1184–1189

Sharma, S. C. and Fitzpatrick, R. J. (1974). Effect of oestradiol-17β and oxytocin treatment on $PGF_{2\alpha}$ release in the anoestrous ewe. *Prostaglandins*, **6**, 97–105

Short, R. V. (1964). Ovarian steroid synthesis and secretion *in vivo*. *Rec. Progr. Hormone Res.*, **20**, 303–333

Spilman, C. H. and Duby, R. T. (1972). Prostaglandin mediated luteolytic effect of intrauterine device in sheep. *Prostaglandins*, **2**, 159–168

Spilman, C. H., Howe, G. R. and Black, D. L. (1972). Alteration of uterine motility in the ewe by an intrauterine device. *J. Reprod. Fert.*, **28**, 269–272

Steele, P. A., Flint, A. P. F. and Turnbull, A. C. (1974). Evidence of steroid C-17, 20 lypase activity in ovine fetal placental tissue. *J. Endocrinol.*, **64**, 41p

Stormshak, F., Kelly, H. E. and Hawk, H. W. (1969). Suppression of the ovine luteal function by 17β-oestradiol. *J. Anim. Sci.*, **29**, 476–478

Stormshak, F., Lehman, R. D. and Hawk, H. W. (1967). Effect of intrauterine plastic spirals and HCG on the corpus luteum of the ewe. *J. Reprod. Fert.*, **14**, 373–378

Sykes, J. A. C., Williams, K. I. and Rogers, A. F. (1975). Prostaglandin production and metabolism by homogenates of pregnant human deciduum and myometrium. *J. Endocrinol.*, **64**, 18–19p

Thorburn, G. D., Cox, R. I., Currie, W. B., Restall, B. J. and Schneider, W. (1973). PGF and progesterone concentrations in the utero–ovarian venous plasma of the ewe during the oestrous cycle and early pregnancy. *J. Reprod. Fert.*, (**Suppl.**) **18**, 151–158

Thorburn, G. D. and Hales, J. R. S. (1972). Selective reduction in blood flow to the ovine corpus luteum after infusion of prostaglandin $F_{2\alpha}$ into a uterine vein. *Proc. Aust. Physiol. Pharmacol. Soc.*, **3**, 145

Thorburn, G. D. and Nicol, D. H. (1971). Regression of the ovine corpus luteum after infusion of prostaglandin $F_{2\alpha}$ into the ovarian artery and uterine vein. *J. Endocrinol*, **51**, 785–786

Thorburn, G. D., Nicol, D. H., Bassett, J. M., Shutt, D. A. and Cox, R. I. (1972). Parturition, in the goat and sheep: Changes in corticosteroids, progesterone, oestrogens and prostaglandin F. *J. Reprod. Fert.*, **Suppl. 16**, 61–84

Thorburn, G. D. and Schneider, W. (1972). The progesterone concentration in the plasma of the goat during the oestrous cycle and pregnancy. *J. Endocrinol*, **52**, 23–36

Virutamasen, P., Wright, K. H. and Wallach, E. E. (1972). Effects of prostaglandins E_2 and $F_{2\alpha}$ on ovarian contractility in the rabbit. *Fertility and Sterility*, **23**, 675–682

Waites, G. M. H. and Moule, G. R. (1961). Relation of vascular heat exchange to temperature regulation in the testis of the ram. *J. Reprod. Fertil.*, **2**, 213–224

Weiner, R. and Kaley, G. (1972). Lysosomal fragility induced by prostaglandin $F_{2\alpha}$. *Nature, New Biol.*, **236**, 46–47

Wilson, L., Butcher, R. L. and Inskeep, E. K. (1972b). Prostaglandin $F_{2\alpha}$ in the uterus of ewes during early pregnancy. *Prostaglandins*, **1**, 479–482

Wilson, L., Cenedella, R. J., Butcher, R. L. and Inskeep, E. K. (1971). Progesterone treatment on ovine endometrial prostaglandins. *J. Anim. Sci.*, **33**, Abstr. No. 298, 273

Wilson, L., Cenedella, R. J., Butcher, R. L. and Inskeep, E. K. (1972a). Levels of prostaglandins in the uterine endometrium during the ovine estrous cycle. *J. Anim. Sci.*, **34**, 93–99

Wiltbank, J. N. and Casida, L. E. (1956). Alteration of ovarian activity by hysterectomy. *J. Anim. Sci.*, **15**, 134–140

Wirz, H., Hargitay, B. and Kuhn, W. (1951). Lokalisation des Kunzentrierungsprozesses in der Niere durch direkte Kryoskopie. *Helv. Physiol. Acta*, **9**, 196–207

Woody, C. O., First, N. L. and Pope, A. L. (1967). Effect of exogenous progesterone on estrous cycle length. *J. Anim. Sci.*, **26**, 139–141

8
Practical Application of Prostaglandins in Animal Husbandry

M. J. COOPER and A. L. WALPOLE

8.1. INTRODUCTION

The use of natural prostaglandins (PGs) and their structural variants (analogues) in animal husbandry is a very recent development, still largely in an exploratory phase. Already, however, $PGF_{2\alpha}$ and a synthetic analogue, fluprostenol (ICI 81 008) under the trade marks, Prostin F2α Vet (Upjohn) and

Equimate (ICI) respectively, are commercially available in some countries for veterinary use. The results obtained with these and some related substances—notably ICI 79 939 and cloprostenol (ICI 80 996)—encourage the belief that products of this kind are destined to affect profoundly the management of breeding and the treatment of infertility in the larger domestic species within a very few years.

This article is concerned with past and current studies of the applications of prostanoids (natural PGs and PG analogues) in animal husbandry. Earlier reviews by Inskeep (1973) and Oxender, Noden, Louis and Hafs (1974) are restricted to studies with $PGF_{2\alpha}$ alone.

Most of the applications now being explored quite clearly depend on the capacity of $PGF_{2\alpha}$ and some of its analogues—including those mentioned above—to induce functional and morphological regression of corpora lutea (luteolysis). Prostaglandin $F_{2\alpha}$ has been found active in this respect, in appropriate circumstances, in all mammalian species studied (Pharriss, Tillson and Erickson, 1972), with the possible exception of man (Pharriss and Shaw, 1974) and dog (Jöchle, Tomlinson and Andersen, 1973). Its luteolytic activity was first demonstrated in laboratory animals in which active corpora lutea had been induced to persist for longer than is normal in unmated individuals of the species in question—as, for example, in pseudopregnant rats (Pharriss and Wyngarden, 1969), pregnant rats and rabbits (Gutknecht, Cornette and Pharriss, 1969) and hysterectomised guinea-pigs (Blatchley and Donovan, 1969). More recently these studies have been extended to normally cycling and pregnant animals of a variety of species in which luteal function is dominant during the greater part of the oestrous cycle. As a result it has been shown that $PGF_{2\alpha}$ has luteolytic activity in several of these, notably sheep (McCracken, Baird and Goding, 1971; Thorburn and Nicol, 1971; Douglas and Ginther, 1973), cattle (Rowson, Tervit and Brand, 1972a, b; Lauderdale, 1972), horses (Douglas and Ginther, 1972) and pigs (Diehl and Day, 1973; Diehl, Godke, Killian and Day, 1973). In all these species, the uterus is thought to be responsible for regression of the corpus luteum of the oestrous cycle, and these findings have implications for the vexed question of the identity of uterine 'luteolysin(s)'. More importantly, in the present context, the demonstration that $PGF_{2\alpha}$ can induce luteal regression in such species prompted studies of possible applications of this prostaglandin and its analogues in the breeding of livestock.

Some of the possibilities envisaged have already been realised, though not yet fully exploited; others are the subject of active exploration or as yet of speculation only. They fall into two categories. One comprises the 'regulatory' applications of luteolytic prostanoids—that is their use for the control of reproductive function in essentially normal animals. This includes the induction and synchronisation of oestrus in cycling animals, and the termination of pregnancy at any stage where this is still dependent, in the species in question, on luteal function. The second category embraces the therapeutic uses of induced luteolysis in aberrations or disorders of reproductive function.

The control and synchronisation of oestrus in farm animals has become a subject of major interest to stock breeders in recent years. In cattle and pigs, and in sheep during their breeding season, sexual activity in the unmated female is confined to rather brief periods, spaced at regular intervals, when she will accept the attentions of the male and is said to be in oestrus or heat. Thus coitus takes place at a time appropriate for conception, since it is during or shortly after oestrus that ovulation occurs. In these species the mean duration of oestrus ranges from about 1 to 3 days, and ovulation occurs, according to species, between about 24 hrs before and 12 hrs after the end of heat. The mean interval between the onset of oestrus in successive cycles—that is, the cycle length—is much longer, being about 17 days in sheep and about 21 in cattle and pigs. It follows that given a number of animals of a kind, cycling at random without reference to one another's behaviour, it is unlikely that at any one time, all, or even most of them, will be at the stage in the cycle when fertile mating can occur. It is desirable in some circumstances to control the day on which individual animals, or small numbers of them, come into oestrus. It may be even more desirable to manipulate the cycles in a whole group of animals so that most of them come into heat together and ovulate on the same, pre-ferably pre-set day. Such is the aim of oestrous synchronisation, and its advantages to the livestock industry are many. Not the least is that it facilitates the use of artificial insemination—which in turn is of value in the genetic improvement of stock, in the control of disease and potentially, if not yet actually, in terms of convenience and cost.

One approach to oestrous control and synchronisation is by way of induced luteolysis. In farm animals—as indeed in many species—oestrus and ovula-tion are suppressed during the greater part of the cycle (the luteal phase) by progesterone secreted by the corpus luteum (or corpora lutea). It is only after the corpus luteum has reached the end of its functional life span that the animal will again come into fertile heat. It is to be expected that the induction of luteal regression before the time when it would normally occur might be followed a few days later by the appearance of oestrus and ovulation. It might further be expected that any animal with a functional corpus luteum would respond in this way. Hence, by treating animals in the luteal phase of the cycle with a luteolytic agent, it might be possible to bring them into oestrus at will. Moreover, since on a statistical basis, a high proportion of randomly cycling animals will always be in the luteal phase, then by so treating a group at one time, without reference to the timing of their natural cycles, it should be possible to bring a high proportion of them into fertile oestrus at the same time.

How far these expectations have been realised with luteolytic prosta-glandins, first in cattle and then in some other species of commercial importance, will be reviewed below, and certain practical considerations will be discussed concerning the application of the results so far achieved to the management of livestock breeding in the field.

8.2 CATTLE

8.2.1 $PGF_{2\alpha}$: luteolysis and its sequelae

From the experience of several groups of workers it is now well established that when given at any time between days 5 and 16 inclusive of the cycle (onset of oestrus = day 0), prostaglandin $F_{2\alpha}$ will cause rapid luteal regression, followed by the onset of fertile oestrus 2–4 days after its administration.

Rowson *et al.* (1972a, b) showed that as little as 0.5 mg of racemic $PGF_{2\alpha}$ injected on two consecutive days via the cervix into the uterine horn ipsilateral to the corpus luteum was effective in 20 out of 21 heifers, 17 of them showing oestrus on the 3rd day after the first dose. Rowson *et al.* (1972a) were also among the first to observe the failure of the bovine corpus luteum to respond within the first few days of its formation. Lauderdale (1972) similarly found that a subcutaneous dose of 30 mg of $PGF_{2\alpha}$—THAM salt* would not induce oestrus when given to cows on days 2, 3 or 4 of the cycle, whereas it was fully effective in this respect between days 6 and 16.

Other workers (Inskeep, 1973; Liehr, Marion and Olson, 1972; Louis, Hafs and Morrow, 1972a, b; Hill, Dickey and Hendricks, 1973) obtained similar results with natural $PGF_{2\alpha}$ infused or injected *once* into the ipsilateral uterine horn, or into the body of the uterus, in a dose of about 2 mg upward. A dose of 5 mg (THAM salt) was effective in the contralateral uterine horn (Louis *et al.*, 1972b). Similar results have also been obtained by intramuscular injection of much larger doses (Stellflug, Louis, Seguin and Hafs, 1973; Lauderdale, Chenault, Seguin and Thatcher, 1973)—30 mg of the THAM salt has been commonly used and seems to be consistently effective.

For routine use on any scale, simple parenteral injection is clearly preferable to intrauterine administration: in particular, the procedure advocated by Rowson *et al.* (1972a, b) demands some technical expertise.

After an effective dose of $PGF_{2\alpha}$ the corpus luteum is reduced in size within 24 hrs and by 72 hrs is impalpable (Louis *et al.*, 1972a). Blood progesterone falls by about half within 4 to 6 hrs and within 48 hrs may be below the limit of detection (Inskeep, 1973; Liehr *et al.*, 1972) where it remains until after ovulation. The peak in plasma LH which follows this fall in progesterone commonly occurs at about the same time as the onset of oestrus (Inskeep, 1973; Louis *et al.*, 1972a, b) but may appear later (Stellflug *et al.*, 1973) and, as in natural heat, precedes ovulation. The induced oestrous cycle is normal in length: a mean duration of 21 ± 0.5 days has been reported (Louis *et al.*, 1972a). After ineffective doses the fall in progesterone is less profound and not so long sustained (Liehr *et al.*, 1972).

In the studies summarised by Oxender *et al.* (1974), plasma progesterone fell from 4.0 ± 0.4 ng ml^{-1} to 1.5 ± 0.2 ng ml^{-1} at 12 hrs and 0.8 ± 0.2 ng ml^{-1} at 48 hrs after an intramuscular injection of 30 mg of $PGF_{2\alpha}$-THAM salt into cows on day 11 of the oestrous cycle. Plasma LH peaked at 64 ± 4 hrs, oestrus began at 74 ± 3 hrs, and ovulation occurred at 104 ± 6 hrs after the injection. Oestradiol concentration more than doubled by 24 hrs after PGF_2: treatment and increased to 15.5 pg ml^{-1} by 72 hrs. The authors stressed the close similarity of this pattern of changes to that around spontaneous oestrus in the cow.

Fertility at oestrus induced with $PGF_{2\alpha}$ has been examined in several studies and seems to be within normal limits (Inskeep, 1973; Rowson *et al.*, 1972a, b; Roche, 1974; Lauderdale *et al.*, 1974). Some of the heifers used by Rowson *et al.* were given pregnant mares' serum gonadotrophin (PMSG) on the day before treatment with (racemic) $PGF_{2\alpha}$, to induce superovulation, and were inseminated at oestrus. Eggs recovered from them appeared to have been fertilised, and following surgical transfer, the pregnancy rate in the recipients

* Equivalent to 22.4 mg of the free acid.

was normal even though they had themselves been treated with the prostaglandin to initiate a new cycle.

In a much larger, collaborative study (Lauderdale *et al.*, 1974) a total of 392 cattle, including crossbred beef heifers and cows (some suckling calves) and Holstein, Jersey and Brown Swiss heifers were randomly assigned to one of three treatments (I, II or III) at each of four locations in such a manner that similar numbers were treated in each way. They were artificially inseminated, (I) about 12 hrs after the onset of natural oestrus detected during a period of 18 to 25 days, (II) about 12 hrs after the onset of oestrus detected during the 7 days following injection of 30 mg of $PGF_{2\alpha}$-THAM salt, or (III) without reference to oestrus but twice, at about 72 and 90 hrs after injection of the same dose of the prostaglandin as in II. (Cattle assigned to treatments II and III were given $PGF_{2\alpha}$ only if a corpus luteum was detectable by rectal palpation, or assumed to be present from previous palpation.) Pregnancy was diagnosed by rectal palpation 35–60 days after insemination. Conception rates were calculated on the basis of the numbers of cattle found pregnant and, for treatments I and II, the numbers inseminated or, for treatment III, the number that responded to $PGF_{2\alpha}$ and were inseminated. The conception rates and numbers inseminated were 53.3% of 122, 52.2% of 69 and 58.8% of 86 for treatments I, II and III respectively. Statistical analysis showed that fertility in the cattle inseminated at oestrus after $PGF_{2\alpha}$ or at fixed intervals after $PGF_{2\alpha}$ did not differ significantly from that in the controls.

It should be noted that fertility is here expressed as conception rate, which must not be confused with other measures of fertility, i.e. 'non-return' rate and calving rate. Confusion of these terms and their erroneous use over a number of years is probably responsible for the widespread belief that cattle are more fertile than they are in fact.

8.2.2 Synchronisation of oestrus

Some consideration may now be given to how the information derived from these studies may be utilised in practice to facilitate the use of artificial insemination. If, as in the example above, treatment with $PGF_{2\alpha}$ is limited to cattle in the responsive phase of the cycle (days 5–16) the proportion synchronised can be maximised and the animals artificially inseminated at the induced oestrus or at fixed intervals after dosing without oestrus detection. This, however, requires knowledge before dosing of the timing of the natural cycle of each animal, obtained by rectal palpation or, with greater precision, by oestrus detection. If, on the other hand, cattle are dosed indiscriminately, i.e. without reference to their natural cycles, the proportion responding will be lower and oestrus detection will then be needed to identify those to be inseminated, whether at oestrus or at fixed intervals after the dose. It would be most convenient, often, to be able both to dose and to inseminate animals without reference to oestrous behaviour and yet to be confident that a majority, at least, in any group are inseminated at the appropriate time(s).

This may be achieved by a procedure, sometimes referred to as the 'spaced (double) injection' technique. It is based on the knowledge that virtually all cattle given an appropriate dose of $PGF_{2\alpha}$ between days 5 and 16, inclusive, of the (21 day) cycle will come into fertile oestrus 2–4 days later, and on the assumptions, (a) that the oestrous cycles of animals not in the responsive phase at the time of injection will be unaffected by this treatment and (b) that the sequence of events following a second dose of $PGF_{2\alpha}$ will be determined by the same considerations and conform essentially to the same pattern as that following the first. The procedure consists in giving all the cattle in a group a luteolytic dose of $PGF_{2\alpha}$ on the same day and a second, similar dose, also on one day, not less than 9 nor more than 12 days after the first. By the time of the second dose, those animals which respond to the first should be in the responsive phase of the induced cycle, while those which fail to respond should be in the responsive phase of a natural cycle. Hence, theoretically at least, almost all the cattle in the group should respond to the second dose and come into oestrus together 2 to 4 days later.

A trial in which $PGF_{2\alpha}$ was used in this way has been reported by King and Robertson (1974). Thirty Holstein heifers, cycling at random, were each given two subcutaneous injections of 30 mg of the THAM salt, 10 days apart and were then artificially inseminated shortly after the detection of oestrus and again 12 hrs later. Ten of the 25 (40%) were found to be pregnant 60 days after insemination. Thirteen out of 15 control heifers (87%) were detected in oestrus during a 3-week period and were also inseminated twice during oestrus. Seven of the 13 (54%) were found pregnant 60 days later. Statistical analysis showed that the proportion of animals showing oestrus and subsequent pregnancy in the control and treated groups respectively were not significantly different.

The animals in this trial were dosed without reference to their oestrous cycles but were inseminated only when they were seen to come into heat. Trials in which cattle were similarly dosed but were inseminated at fixed intervals after the second of the two doses have been made using both $PGF_{2\alpha}$ (Hafs, Manns and Drew, 1975) and also some synthetic analogues related to it—in particular, cloprostenol (ICI 80 996).

8.2.3 Luteolytic analogues of $PGF_{2\alpha}$

Among the very numerous analogues of $PGF_{2\alpha}$ which have been synthesised for biological evaluation in recent years is a series of 16-aryloxyprostaglandins (Binder *et al.*, 1974). Several of these have proved to be many times as potent as $PGF_{2\alpha}$ in luteolytic activity without being correspondingly more toxic (Dukes, Russell and Walpole, 1974), thus having a wide margin of safety when used to indicate luteolysis in both laboratory and domestic animals. Three such compounds are shown on page 315.

Two of these, ICI 79 939 and ICI 80 996 (cloprostenol), have been studied in cattle. The former was shown by Tervit, Rowson and Brand (1973) to be luteolytic in heifers when given in a single intramuscular dose of 1 mg or less between days 5 and 16 inclusive of the oestrous cycle. Out of a group of 49 heifers, cycling at random, 43 returned to oestrus 2–4 days after the second of two doses of 750 µg of ICI 79 939, given 10 days apart (Cooper, M. J., personal observation). Dobson, Cooper and Furr (1975) have studied in detail the response to such treatment in 6 heifers to which the first of the two

R	ICI No	Free name	Trade mark*
p 604f	79 939	—	—
m Cl	80 996	cloprostenol	Estrumate
m CF$_3$	81 008	fluprostenol	Equimate

* The property of ICI Ltd.

doses was given between days 9 and 13 of their natural cycles. After both doses the sequence of changes in the reproductive tract and in plasma concentrations of progesterone, estradiol-17β and LH were closely similar to those occurring around natural oestrus. The animals returned to oestrus 48–96 hrs after the first, and 48–55 hrs after the second dose. A peak in LH was observed 62–103 hrs after the first, and 48–62 hrs after the second dose and was followed by ovulation in all animals. The corpora lutea formed were all functional as judged by plasma progesterone values and the cycles after the second dose were of normal length.

Cloprostenol (ICI 80 996) is of similar potency to ICI 79 939 but is less toxic. When given during the sensitive phase of the bovine oestrous cycle it is consistently effective as a luteolytic agent in an intramuscular dose of 500 μg (Cooper et al., in preparation). Luteolysis is followed by a return to oestrus 2–4 days later and ovulation at the usual time in relation to oestrus. The endocrine changes after injection of the compound have been described by Nancarrow, Radford, Connell and Mattner (1974), Cooper, Dobson and Furr (1974) and Cooper and Rowson (1975), and resemble closely those around spontaneous oestrus in the cow. No adverse reactions have been observed in any animal following treatment (Cooper, 1974) and the wide margin of safety of the compound is indicated by the fact that 200 times this dose (i.e. 100 mg) causes little more than mild and transient diarrhoea (Cooper and Furr, 1974).

In experiments by Cooper (1974) a total of 175 cycling Friesian heifers were given two intramuscular injections of 500 μg of cloprostenol, 11 days apart. The animals were at all stages of the cycle at the time of the first injection. No fewer than 171 were in oestrus between 48 and 96 hrs and 159 between 48 and 72 hrs after the second injection. In 45 of the heifers, rectal palpation was performed once or twice daily before and after each injection to monitor morphological changes in the uterus and ovaries. Cervical mucus samples were also taken and examined for spinnbarkeit and 'ferning'. By this means, luteal regression and the subsequent development of follicles was followed, ovulation being diagnosed by the disappearance of a follicle of pre-ovulatory size and the subsequent palpation of a well formed corpus luteum on the same ovary. Thus the conclusions from observations of oestrous behaviour were confirmed and extended. The results of this detailed study in 45 heifers is shown in Figure 8.1 and Table 8.1.

The subsequent behaviour of these animals was also carefully noted. After the synchronised heat, the 43 which responded showed cycles of normal length; they developed corpora lutea which had a normal lifespan and were presumably fully functional.

It is noteworthy (Figure 8.1) that the oestrus response following the second injection of cloprostenol was somewhat earlier and more closely synchronised than that following the first. This has been a consistent observation both with cloprostenol (Cooper, 1974) and with ICI 79 939 (Dobson, Cooper and Furr, 1975).

Of the remaining heifers, 119 were used to investigate fertility at the controlled heat. Thirty were inseminated twice, 72 and 96 hrs after the second

Table 8.1 Responses in 45 heifers (2 failures)

Hours after second injection	Number of heifers in oestrus	Number of heifers ovulating
48–72	39	4
72–96	4	34
96–120		5

injection of cloprostenol, without reference to heat, and of these 18 calved normal offspring after gestations of normal length. Eighty-nine were inseminated once only, towards the end of the controlled heat. The conception rate in these, based on rectal diagnosis of pregnancy at 8 weeks, was identical with that in a similar number of control heifers kept at the same time and inseminated once as they came into spontaneous heat. The animals that conceived following treatment produced normal calves after pregnancies of normal duration.

8.2.4 Tactical considerations

Any simple and successful method of controlling the bovine cycle will result in several well recognised benefits. Brief reference has already been made to the facilitation of the use of artificial insemination that can be thereby achieved—particularly where oestrus detection is inconvenient or impossible—enabling rapid genetic improvement of the herd to be made. This is valuable in groups of dairy heifers and even more so in single suckled beef herds, since weight-gain in young animals is a characteristic with a high degree of heritability.

Controlled breeding can also lead to a 'tighter' calving pattern, simplifying supervision and resulting in the rearing for sale of uniform groups of calves having similar growth rates. This not only overcomes many marketing difficulties but may also result in a saving of fodder during the growing period. Synchronised gestation may also facilitate the economical use of rations for the pregnant cow.

These and other benefits, like those obtained by greater control in any commercial situation, can be expected to make controlled breeding an attractive prospect. The method of using prostaglandins described above meets many of the criteria demanded of any such technique, but experience in the field indicates that the outcome is governed by a variety of practical considerations.

From what is already known about the luteolytic activity of these compounds in cattle it is clear that their use is only likely to be effective when ovarian cyclicity is normal. During the post-partum period in beef cows, the time of the first ovulation and of the re-establishment of normal oestrus cycles is extremely variable (Saiduddin, Queredo and Foote, 1968) and under many

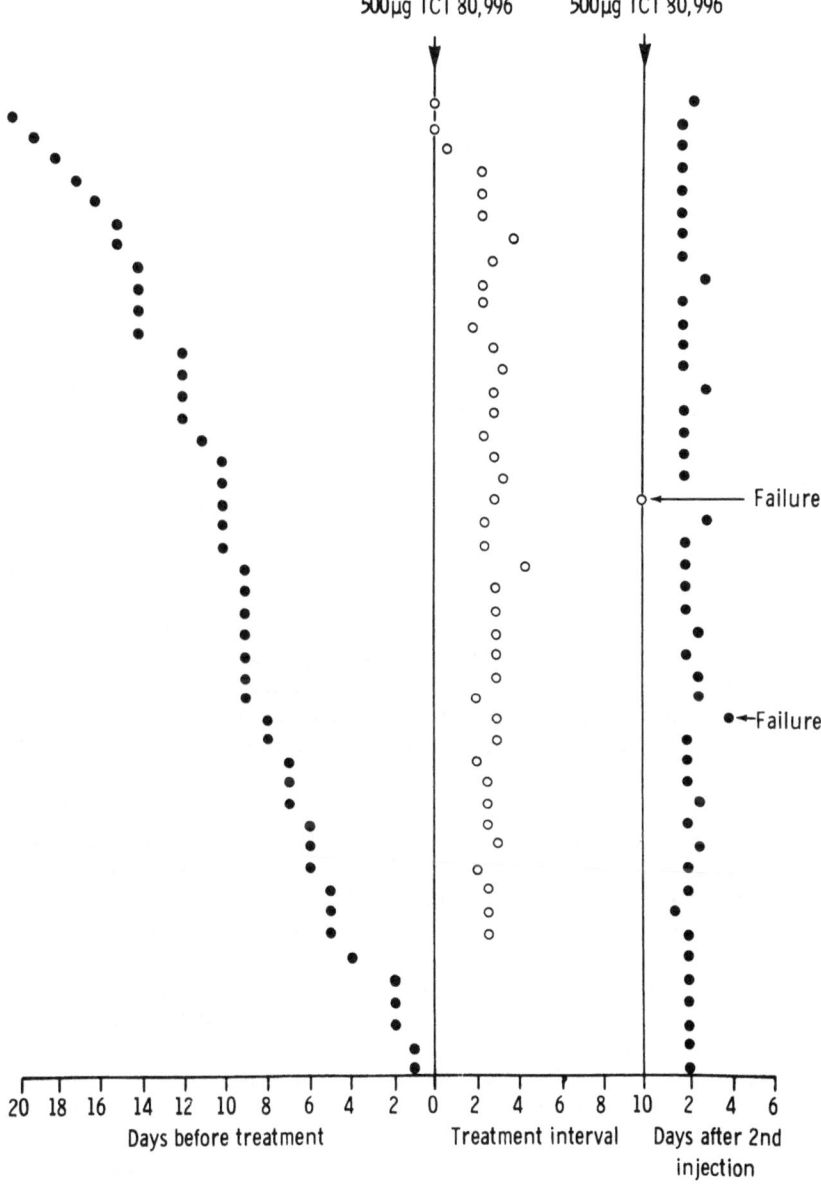

Figure 8.1   Synchronisation of oestrus in heifers with ICI 80 996. Key: • Oestrus before and after treatment; ○ Oestrus after first injection

conditions of management ovarian activity may be completely absent for some time after calving (Fielden, MacMillan and Watson, 1973). This condition can also occur in young heifers and is known to be related both to the season of the year and to the level of nutrition. From information currently available, there is no reason to suppose that luteolytic doses of prostaglandins will stimulate the inactive bovine ovary.

In cattle, as in other species of farm livestock, fertility is known to be influenced by nutrition and the best results from any system of controlled breeding can only be expected under optimal nutritional conditions.

The presence of unwanted or unsuspected pregnancy will also complicate the use of prostaglandins. This may occur both in heifers and in beef cows post partum, especially under poor conditions of management. Such pregnancies are not likely to be far advanced and will therefore be lost as a result of treatment, owing to the abortifacient effect of luteolytic prostaglandins during the earlier part of gestation in the bovine (see below). This complication can be avoided by routine examination of the cattle before treatment, but this will obviously increase the complexity and cost of the operation.

The work already cited suggests that, despite these complications, the informed use of prostaglandins can give results in a variety of field conditions which are very acceptable in terms both of the degree of synchronisation and fertility at the induced heat. This view is supported by the preliminary results of extensive field trials of $PGF_{2\alpha}$ (Hafs *et al.*, 1975, and Hafs, personal communication) and of cloprostenol (Cooper and Jackson, in preparation), used by the double-injection procedure.

It is pertinent at this point to enquire how far the use of prostaglandins is likely to satisfy all the criteria of an ideal synchronisation technique. The procedure must be simple and its outcome predictable and the agents used must be cheap. These requirements are certainly met with cloprostenol and perhaps other injectable analogues which are effective in very low doses. The controlled ovulation should be of normal fertility and should be synchronised to such a degree that oestrus detection is unnecessary and only a single insemination at a fixed time after treatment need be given. It is not yet clear how far this latter requirement can be met with prostaglandins. The preliminary results of the field trials mentioned above (Cooper and Jackson) in which more than 2000 cattle were treated with cloprostenol, suggest that optimum fertility can only be obtained by two inseminations given at, say, 72 and 96 hrs after the second injection of the prostaglandin. It is not yet known at what interval, precisely, after the prostaglandin a single insemination should be given or how far short of the optimum the conception rate may then fall.

It may be found that the degree of synchronisation of ovulation obtainable by the use of a prostaglandin alone is insufficient to yield a satisfactory conception rate from a single insemination at any fixed time. Already the possibility of improving the chances by additional treatment with other agents is being explored. It has been suggested, for example, that the carefully timed injection of a small dose of oestradiol benzoate (500 μg or less) following the second prostaglandin treatment may substantially improve synchronisation and allow a single insemination to be used (Nancarrow, personal communication). It seems possible that PMSG, and perhaps gonadotrophin releasing hormone (GnRH), might prove useful in this context. The use of a prostaglandin following pretreatment with a progestagen has also been tried with encouraging results (Wishart, 1974; Thimonier *et al.*, 1975).

The primary target of much endeavour is thus, very properly, a combination of treatment and insemination which avoids the need for oestrus detection. Nevertheless, the variation in the conditions met with in the management of herds is such that there are circumstances where other methods of using prostaglandins to control the oestrous cycle may be appropriate. For example, where large numbers of cattle are involved, and gathering and holding them is difficult, it may be preferable to give a single injection of prostaglandin followed by artificial insemination at a fixed time or on detection of oestrus. Although this cannot lead to the successful impregnation of more than a proportion of animals in the herd, it may yield the optimum benefit in the circumstances. Another technique which has been suggested for use in similar circumstances is to concentrate an artificial breeding programme into 10 days of persistent oestrus detection and insemination. A single luteolytic dose of a prostaglandin is given on the 5th of these days and by this procedure it is theoretically possible to inseminate the whole herd during oestrus, natural or induced. However, oestrus detection would need to be uncommonly efficient for this system to be successful.

There seems little doubt that luteolytic prostaglandins will have an important role in the future management of cattle breeding. It is clear, however, that the method of their use will vary considerably with the circumstances and that much development work remains to be done before the main variants become well defined.

8.2.5 Induction of abortion

It is well known that in cattle ovarian progesterone is required throughout the greater part of pregnancy to maintain the gravid uterus. Enucleation of the corpus luteum (McDonald, McNutt and Nichols, 1953) or ovariectomy (Erb, Estergreen, Gomes, Plotka and Frost, 1967) before about the 200th day of gestation leads to abortion, and prostaglandin-induced luteolysis would be expected to have the same result.

In cows 40–120 days pregnant, Lauderdale (1972) found that the injection of $PGF_{2\alpha}$-THAM salt in total doses of 150 or 45 mg invariably caused abortion; 30 or 15 mg aborted 3 out of 6 cows and 1 mg was ineffective. Abortion was preceded by luteal regression and ensued in 2 to 7 days after the higher doses and within a fortnight after 30 or 15 mg. Cloprostenol is effective at a similar stage of pregnancy in a single intramuscular dose of 500 μg (M. J. Cooper, unpublished).

Perhaps the most obvious situation in which it may be desirable to abort cattle is that following misalliance in young heifers. Under many conditions of management, the accidental impregnation of young animals by a straying bull or an improperly castrated steer is not uncommon and may lead to permanent damage to, or even death of the heifer. The use of a prostaglandin in this situation would seem to be a distinct improvement on the current practice of giving oestrogens which is unreliable. The early abortion of cattle may also be desirable where the sole object of pregnancy is to ensure lactation and here again luteolytic prostaglandins may prove useful. All in all, however, their potential use for the termination of pregnancy in the bovine is not likely ever to be more than one of the minor 'regulatory' applications of these agents.

8.2.6 Therapeutic applications

A preliminary report from Talbot and Hafs (1974) suggests that the removal of a mummified fetus, a less common but often more intractable problem than the induction of abortion in misalliance, may yield to a similar approach. A fetus dying fairly early in gestation may remain in the uterus, preventing luteal regression and thereby its own abortion.

Chronic endometritis in cattle which often follows the retention of the fetal membranes is in some respects a similar problem. The uterus becomes swollen and filled with pus, preventing normal luteal regression, and the situation is aggravated by the fact that while the corpus luteum is functional the uterus, being under the dominant influence of circulating progesterone, is unusually susceptible to infection (Rowson, Lamming and Fry, 1953). First attempts to treat this condition by inducing luteal regression with cloprostenol have given very promising results (Cooper and Jackson, unpublished), suggesting that this may be an important advance in veterinary therapeutics.

8.3 HORSES

A species in which prostaglandin-induced luteolysis has already proved to be of value in improving breeding performance is the horse. The mare is a seasonally polyestrous animal with a distinct breeding season during the spring and summer months. The average length of the oestrous cycle is 22 days: oestrus is variable in duration—from 3 to as many as 10 days—and ovulation occurs 24 to 48 hrs before it ends (Day, 1939).

Douglas and Ginther (1972) found that a subcutaneous dose of 1.25 mg or more of $PGF_{2\alpha}$ given (in aqueous ethanol) to pony mares on the 6th day of dioestrus—i.e. 6 days after ovulation—would shorten the cycle, oestrus appearing 3 or 4 days after treatment. They later reported (Douglas and Ginther, 1973) that treatment on day 4 of diestrus had less effect, and on day 1, little or none. Other workers have reported (Oxender et al., 1974) that, in larger mares, intrauterine deposition of 10 mg, or subcutaneous injection of 15 mg of $PGF_{2\alpha}$-THAM salt, 7 to 9 days after ovulation, resulted in a precipitous fall in blood progesterone concentration, a return to oestrus within about 2 days and the occurrence of ovulation about 2 days before the end of oestrus. Blood LH rose to a peak 2 days after ovulation, as is usual in the mare. Apart from a prolongation of oestrus by about 2 days, the cycles initiated by treatment closely resembled control cycles.

Studies with ICI 79 939 were started by Allen and Rowson (1973) in cycling Welsh pony mares during the breeding season of 1972. Treatment, given on 2 consecutive days, consisted of infusion of 100, 150 or 200 μg of the analogue (sodium salt in aqueous solution) into the body of the uterus, or intramuscular injection of 300 or 600 μg. Mares in which treatment started on days 4 to 12 of dioestrus returned to oestrus within 4 days of the first dose. Only 3 of the 5 dosed on days 3 and 4 responded and 4 treated on days 2 and 3 failed to respond. Most of the animals which responded (73%) returned to oestrus 3 days after the first dose and all ovulated normally during the induced oestrus. The interval between the first day of treatment and ovulation ranged from 7 to 12 days with a peak at 10 days.

In later studies Allen and various co-workers (Allen and Rossdale, 1973, Allen et al., 1974), demonstrated the efficacy of ICI 79 939 in causing luteal regression followed by fertile oestrus in thoroughbred mares, and its clinical value in mares in which the occurrence of spontaneous oestrus is delayed by persistent luteal function (see below).

Although controlled trials to determine the minimum luteolytic dose of ICI 79 939 in mares have not been undertaken, treatment of over 200 mares with the compound indicates that a single intramuscular dose of not less than 80 μg for Welsh pony mares and 100 μg for thoroughbreds consistently induces luteolysis and oestrus (Allen et al., 1974). In the course of this work it was noted, however, that in doses little above the luteolytic dose, this analogue produces side-effects which, although apparently innocuous, are undesirable. In pony mares given very high doses—1 mg or more by intrauterine instillation or intramuscular injection—these are severe and take the form of (a) profuse sweating of the head, chest and lower abdominal regions of the body, (b) increased cardiac and respiratory rates, (c) gastrointestinal hypermotility accompanied by colic of variable severity, (d) watery diarrhoea, and (e) mild depression and reduced appetite. Most of these effects are transient, but diarrhoea and depression persist for up to 24 hrs. Sweating, gastrointestinal hypermotility and increased heart and respiration rates were seen in all ponies given 500 μg of ICI 79 939 and in some given as little as 250 μg.

Frank (1972) and others have observed similar side-effects in thoroughbred mares given the normal luteolytic dose of 5 mg of natural $PGF_{2\alpha}$. Although this prostaglandin, as the THAM salt, is now on sale for use in mares, no reports have yet appeared in the literature describing its value in clinical practice.

In laboratory species, as noted above, fluprostenol (ICI 81 008; Equimate), though rather less potent than ICI 79 939 as a luteolytic agent, is very much less toxic in several respects (Dukes, Russell and Walpole, 1974). The minimum effective luteolytic dose of this analogue by the intramuscular route is 125 μg for ponies and 250 μg for thoroughbred mares. In pony mares, 6 to 8 times this dose, i.e. 750–1000 μg, is required for detectable side-effects and after a dose as high as 32 times that needed to effect luteolysis, sweating and diarrhoea are comparatively mild and pass off quickly (Allen et al., 1974). It appears to be a preferred analogue for use in mares.

8.3.1 Regulatory applications

Demonstration of the luteolytic activity of $PGF_{2\alpha}$ and ICI 79 939 in mares prompted Allen and Rowson (1973) to suggest that these substances might be of value in horse breeding, particularly where the artificial insemination of mares is practised, and that even in thoroughbred mares, where artificial insemination is not permitted, they might be useful for controlling and short-ening the cycle of individual animals. By appropriately timed treatment it might be possible to avoid the awkward situation which often arises in large studs when many mares booked to be covered by the same stallion come into oestrus at the same time. Moreover, the covering season for thoroughbreds is arbitrarily restricted in length and, for various reasons, many mares come to the end of the season after having been in oestrus only once or twice. In this situation luteolysis might be used to reduce valuable time lost by brood-mares as they pass through dioestrus.

These 'regulatory' applications of prostaglandins in horse breeding have not yet been fully explored. However, some evidence is available (Palmer and Jousset, 1975) that behavioural oestrus and ovulation can be synchronised in groups of mares by the strategic use of fluprostenol and human chorionic gonadotrophin (HCG). This may well prove, in certain circumstances, to be an important aid to the management of breeding mares.

8.3.2 Therapeutic applications

One of the main reasons for the comparatively poor reproductive performance of thoroughbred mares is the failure of many of them to exhibit regular and normal oestrous cycles within the limits of the covering season. Allen and Rossdale (1973), Hughes, Stabenfeldt and Evans (1973) and Allen *et al.* (1974) have shown that by far the most common cause of this is the abnormal per-sistence of luteal function ('prolonged dioestrus'). This may occur (a) with-out apparent cause—as, for example, in barren and maiden mares—and in the following circumstances.

(b) After early fetal death. In as many as 8 to 10% of mares that conceive, the fetus dies during the first 100 days of gestation and the conceptus is resorbed or aborts. Such animals may not return to oestrus for many weeks.

(c) In 'pseudopregnancy'. Some mares which have not returned to oestrus after being served and show other clinical signs of pregnancy are found to be empty when examined manually between 19 and 45 days after service.

(d) In 'lactational anoestrous'. Some mares while suckling a foal and after exhibiting a 'foal heat' a few days after parturition, fail to come into oestrus during the next 2 to 3 months.

Both ICI 79 939 (Allen and Rossdale, 1973, Allen *et al.*, 1974) and flu-prostenol (Allen *et al.*, 1974; Allen, 1974; Berwyn-Jones and Irvine, 1974) have been shown to be effective in the treatment of infertility in mares in the circumstances (a–d) outlined above. All the thoroughbred mares treated by Allen *et al.* (1974) had failed to exhibit oestrus during the previous 28 days and had persistent luteal activity on the evidence of plasma progestin levels (typically around 3–5 ng ml^{-1}). A total of 144 were given a single intra-muscular injection of 100 or 200 μg of ICI 79 939 and 63 received fluprostenol, 52 being given a single dose of 250 μg and the remainder 100 or 200 μg on two consecutive days. (The response was similar in both these latter groups.) The mares were teased daily after treatment and examined frequently *per rectum* and *per vaginam* to monitor follicular development and ovulation. Samples of peripheral blood were taken regularly and assayed for progestin by a competitive protein binding method.

Of the 144 mares treated with ICI 79 939, 134 returned to oestrus within 4 days and subsequently ovulated: 119 were covered during the induced oestrus and of the 110 for which the results were known, 51 (46%) were later found to be in foal to this service. Of the 63 mares treated with fluprostenol, 55 came into oestrus within 4 days and ovulated: 52 were covered and of the 45 whose subsequent history was known, 18 (40%) were found to be pregnant to this mating. In mares which responded to treatment with either compound, the plasma progestin concentration fell rapidly to and remained at basal values until after ovulation.

The conception rate to mating during the induced oestrus in these mares was considered to be entirely satisfactory, especially as many of them had very bad breeding histories. It supported the view that oestrus induced in mares with prostaglandins is no less fertile than a naturally occurring oestrus.

One situation in which a mare in prolonged dioestrus will not respond satisfactorily to treatment with prostaglandins is that where the animal has active endometrial cup tissue in the uterus and, in consequence, has a high concentration of gonadotrophin (PMSG) in the blood. This situation arises in some mares which have lost their conceptus after 40 days of gestation and in all mares from which twin conceptuses have been washed from the uterus after day 40. Allen (1974) examined 12 mares in which twin conceptuses had been removed from the uterus after 42 days of gestation and 3 which had resorbed spontaneously but continued to show high levels of PMSG in their serum. Treatment of all these animals with ICI 79 939 or fluprostenol on one or more occasions induced luteolysis as judged by plasma progestin determinations. However, in all cases the ovaries became progressively smaller and less active after treatment and, although some animals exhibited intermittent oestrous behaviour when teased, none showed normal follicular development or ovulated until PMSG had disappeared from the blood. In contrast, a mare treated with fluprostenol after removal of twins at 35 days of gestation—i.e. before the development of endometrial cups—returned to oestrus 3 days after oestrus ovulated normally.

There is now extensive evidence from international clinical trials (Cooper et al. in preparation) that fluprostenol can play an important part in equine veterinary practice. Detailed case records are available on nearly 1000 mares, of which about 80% responded to treatment with this agent as judged by the appearance of behavioural oestrus within a few days. The mares were served during this estrus and out of 504 that were subsequently examined for pregnancy, no less than 49% were found to be in foal. Most equine stud practitioners would regard this figure as being in the middle of the normal range for mares.

In clinical practice, situations can arise (other than those already referred to) where a mare which fails to come into oestrus during the breeding season does not respond to routine treatment with prostaglandins. There are several possible reasons for this.

(a) The mare may be in anoestrus rather than dioestrus, having completely inactive ovaries with no luteal tissue present. As with cattle, such animals are unlikely to respond and (in contrast to cattle) are difficult to diagnose by rectal palpation alone.

(b) In a mare which is cycling 'silently' or where supervision has been poor and oestrus has passed unobserved, treatment may be given at the wrong stage of the cycle. As with cattle, there is a period following luteal regression and lasting until the establishment of the next corpus luteum (about day 4 of dioestrus in mares) when luteolytic doses of prostaglandins have no apparent effect.

(c) The mare may have ovulated during dioestrus. This occasionally happens and if prostaglandin treatment is given shortly after such an occurrence it may be ineffective in inducing oestrus. The original corpus luteum of the cycle will regress but the new one may still be insensitive.

It is not known how often such ovulations occur but they will obviously contribute to the number of animals which fail to respond.

(d) The mare may be pregnant. Douglas and Ginther (1973) have reported that in mares estimated to be 40–120 days pregnant, subcutaneous injection of $PGF_{2\alpha}$ in doses of 1.25 and 2.5 mg caused abortion in 3 of 7 and 4 of 8 animals. The effects of prostaglandins in pregnant mares needs more extensive investigation.

In spite of these apparent difficulties, veterinary surgeons who have experience of these compounds regard their use as a major advance over existing methods—i.e. various types of uterine irrigation—for the treatment of temporary infertility in the mare.

8.4 PIGS

8.4.1 Oestrous synchronisation

In the domestic pig, the period after ovulation during which the corpora lutea are insensitive to luteolytic prostaglandins is considerably longer than in the cow or mare. Diehl and Day (1973) found that a dose of 2 or 5 mg of $PGF_{2\alpha}$, injected into the uterine horns of gilts on day 10 of the oestrous cycle, or given as a single intramuscular injection on day 12, had no effect upon plasma progesterone levels or cycle length. On the other hand, a sufficient dose of a prostaglandin given between days 12 and 15 of the cycle has been found to induce premature luteal regression and shorten the cycle (Polge, 1975).

This prolonged insensitivity of the corpus luteum makes it impracticable to use prostaglandins alone to synchronise oestrus in randomly cycling pigs. Polge (1975), using ICI 79 939, has overcome the difficulty by procedures based on the following observations.

(a) Corpora lutea maintained beyond day 12 by giving oestrogen regress synchronously after injection of the prostaglandin.

(b) Accessory corpora lutea induced by administration of PMSG and HCG (human chorionic gonadotrophin) at any stage of the cycle persist, and can be caused to regress by injecting the prostaglandin 12 days after HCG.

(c) Corpora lutea of pregnancy are highly sensitive to the prostaglandin after the 12th day of gestation.

About 80% of animals treated as in (b) or (c) showed oestrus 4 to 7 days after injection of the prostaglandin, and fertility and embryonic survival following insemination at the induced oestrus were normal. Although these results are of theoretical interest, the procedures involved are probably too cumbersome for use in commercial pig-breeding.

8.4.2 Induction and synchronisation of parturition

In pregnant pigs, luteolysis can be induced by means of prostaglandins from about the 12th day of gestation onward and, since in this species pregnancy depends throughout on the presence of the ovaries (Du Buisson and Dauzier, 1957), it is not surprising that effective doses cause abortion or premature parturition.

In 4 out of 7 gelts given an intramuscular injection of 5 mg of $PGF_{2\alpha}$ at 23 to 30 days of gestation, Diehl and Day (1973) observed a fall in peripheral progesterone levels followed by abortion 28 ± 2.3 hrs after treatment. Similarly, a total of 2.1 mg of this prostaglandin infused over 10 hrs into 5 pregnant gelts 5 to 7 days before the expected time of parturition caused premature delivery in all of them (Diehl et al., 1973). The average time from the start of infusion to the birth of the first piglet was 28.9 ± 1.9 hrs as compared with 78.9 ± 18.4 hrs in 4 saline-infused controls. The mean gestation lengths were 109 ± 0.03 and 111.5 ± 0.02 days respectively. All the treated pigs had abundant colostrum before the onset of parturition and 94.1% of the piglets were born alive as compared with 95.8% for the controls.

The response of sows to an intramuscular injection of $PGF_{2\alpha}$ late in pregnancy has been examined by Henricks and Handlin (1974). A dose of 5 to 25 mg of the THAM salt was given 2 to 6 days before the expected date of parturition to 14 sows. In 9 of these, parturition began within 48 hrs of the injection (mean, 25 hrs; range 28–48 hrs) at least 20 hrs before the expected time. In one other it began within 60 hrs, while the remaining 4 started to farrow only one day before, or on the expected day. At all doses given $PGF_{2\alpha}$ seemed equally effective, but it was most effective in those sows in which plasma progesterone decreased rapidly. The response was not affected by the gestational age at treatment.

More precise control of parturition was achieved by Ash and Heap (1973) in a study with ICI 79 939 in 7 gilts and 3 sows. The analogue was given by intramuscular injection of 50–150 μg, repeated at about 8 hr intervals, in total doses up to 750 μg (mean, 530 ± 32 μg). Treatment started on days 109 to 110 of gestation induced parturition after 26.4 ± 0.9 hrs. The length of gestation which was 114 ± 0.2 days in 147 untreated pigs in this herd, was reduced to 111 ± 0.2 days (P<0.01) in the treated pigs. In this trial no side-effects of treatment were detected, the average birth and 3-week weights of piglets were within the normal range, and sows usually returned to normal oestrus within a week after weaning.

Ash and Heap draw attention to the practical advantages of induced synchronous parturition and especially the prospect of inducing farrowing during the daylight hours of a 5-day week. At the same time they point out that early induction of parturition is not without its hazards, particularly in gilts. In their trial, there seemed to be an appreciable secretion of colostrum at the time of parturition in all the treated animals. However, mammary secretion was depressed in some gilts for a period of about 24 hrs starting 12–18 hrs after the induction of delivery and a number of piglets succumbed, including 15 from two gilts that showed this lactational insufficiency. They suggest that the induction of parturition too early may curtail the final stages of mammary development prior to the onset of lactogenesis with subsequent effects on mammary secretion. Thus in the practical application of this technique for the induction of parturition, optimum results in terms of live piglets may well depend on precise timing of treatment in relation to known service dates.

References

Allen, W. R. (1974). Prostaglandins in equine stud management. *Vet. Ann.*, 15, 168–174

Allen, W. R. and Rossdale, P. D. (1973). A preliminary study upon the use of prostaglandins for inducing oestrus in non-cycling thoroughbred mares. *Equine Vet. J.*, 5, 137–140

Allen, W. R. and Rowson, L. E. A. (1973). Control of the mare's oestrous cycle by prostaglandins. *J. Reprod. Fert.*, 33, 539–543

Allen, W. R., Stewart, F., Cooper, M. J., Crowhurst, R. C., Simpson, D. J., McEnery, R. J., Greenwood, R. E. S., Rossdale, P. D. and Ricketts, S. W. (1974). Further studies on the use of synthetic prostaglandin analogues for inducing luteolysis in mares. *Equine Vet. J.*, 6, 31–35

Ash, R. W. and Heap, R. B. (1973). The induction and synchronisation of parturition in sows treated with ICI 79, 939, an analogue of prostaglandin $F_{2\alpha}$. *J. Agric. Sci., Cambridge*, 81, 365–368

Berwyn-Jones, M. D. and Irvine, C. H. G. (1974). Induction of luteolysis and oestrus in mares with a synthetic prostaglandin analogue (ICI 81,008). *N.Z. Vet. J.*, 22, 107–110

Binder, D., Bowler, J., Brown, E. D., Crossley, N. S., Hutton, J., Senior, J., Slater, L., Wilkinson, P. and Wright, N. C. A. (1974). 16-Aryloxyprostaglandins: a new class of potent luteolytic agent. *Prostaglandins*, 6, 87–90

Blatchley, F. R. and Donovan, B. T. (1969). Luteolytic effect of prostaglandin in the guinea-pig. *Nature, Lond.*, 221, 1065–1066

Cooper, M. J. (1974). Control of oestrous cycles of heifers with a synthetic prostaglandin analogue. *Vet. Rec.*, 95, 200–203

Cooper, M. J., Dobson, H. and Furr, B. J. A. (1974). Endocrine changes in Friesian heifers during luteolysis and oestrous synchronization with ICI 80, 996, a synthetic analogue of prostaglandin $F_{2\alpha}$. *J. Steroid. Biochem.*, 5, 403 (abstr.)

Cooper, M. J. and Furr, B. J. A. (1974). The role of prostaglandins in animal breeding. *Vet. Rec.*, 94, 161 (abstr.)

Cooper, M. J. and Rowson, L. E. A. (1975). Control of the oestrous cycle in Friesian heifers with ICI 80 996. *Ann. Biol. Anim. Bioch. Biophys.*, 15 (in press)

Day, F. T. (1939). Sterility in the mare associated with irregularities of the oestrous cycle. *Vet. Rec.*, 51, 1113

Diehl, J. R. and Day, B. N. (1973). Effect of prostaglandin $F_{2\alpha}$ on luteal function in swine. *J. Anim. Sci.*, 37, 307–308 (abstr.)

Diehl, J. R., Godke, R. A., Killian, D. B. and Day, B. N. (1973). The induction of parturition in swine with prostaglandin. *Biol. Reprod.*, 9, 104 (abstr.)

Dobson, H., Cooper, M. J. and Furr, B. J. A. (1975). Synchronization of oestrus with ICI 79, 939, an analogue of $PGF_{2\alpha}$ and associated changes in plasma progesterone, oestradiol 17-β and LH in heifers. *J. Reprod. Fert.*, 42, 141–144

Douglas, R. H. and Ginther, O. J. (1972). Effect of prostaglandin $F_{2\alpha}$ on length of diestrus in mares. *Prostaglandins*, 2, 265–268

Douglas, R. H. and Ginther, O. J. (1973). Effect of prostaglandin $F_{2\alpha}$ in ewes and pony mares. *J. Anim. Sci.*, 37, 308 (abstr.)

Du Buisson, F. de M. and Dauzier, L. (1957). Influence de l'ovariectomie chez la truie pendant la gestation. *C.R. Soc. Biol., Paris*, 151, 311–313

Dukes, M., Russell, W. and Walpole, A. L. (1974). Potent luteolytic agents related to prostaglandin $F_{2\alpha}$. *Nature, Lond.*, 250, 330–331

Erb, R. E., Estergreen, V. L., Gomes, W. R., Plotka, E. D. and Frost, O. L. (1967). Progestin levels in corpora lutea and progesterone in ovarian venous and jugular vein blood plasma of the pregnant bovine. *J. Dairy Sci.*, 51, 401–410

Fielden, E. D., Macmillan, K. L. and Watson, J. D. (1973). The anoestrous syndrome in New Zealand dairy cattle. *N.Z. Vet. J.*, 21, 77–81

Frank, C. J. (1972). Personal communication to W. R. Allen

Gutknecht, G. D., Cornette, J. C. and Pharriss, B. B. (1969). Antifertility properties of prostaglandin $F_{2\alpha}$. *Biol. Reprod.*, 1, 367–371

Hafs, H. D., Manns, J. G. and Drew, B. (1975). Onset of oestrus after $F_{2\alpha}$ in cattle. *Vet. Rec.*, 96, 134–135

Henricks, D. M. and Handlin, D. L. (1974). Induction of parturition in the sow with prostaglandin $F_{2\alpha}$. *Theriogenology*, 1, 7–14

Hill, J. R., Dickey, J. F. and Henricks, D. M. (1973). Estrus and ovulation in $PGF_{2\alpha}$/PMS treated heifers. *J. Anim. Sci.*, 37, 315 (abstr.)

Hughes, J. P., Stabenfeldt, G. H. and Evans, J. W. (1973). Clinical and endocrine aspects of the estrus cycle of the mare. *Proc. 18th Am. Ass. Equine Practit.*, p. 119

Inskeep, E. K. (1973). Potential uses of prostaglandins in control of reproductive cycles of domestic animals. *J. Anim. Sci.*, 36, 1149–115

Jöchle, W., Tomlinson, R. V. and Andersen, A. C. (1973). Prostaglandin effects on plasma progesterone levels in the pregnant and cycling dog (beagle). *Prostaglandins*, 3, 209–217

King, G. J. and Robertson, H. A. (1974). A two injection schedule with prostaglandin $F_{2\alpha}$ for the regulation of the ovulatory cycle of cattle. *Theriogenology*, 1, 123–128

Lauderdale, J. W. (1972). Effects of $PGF_{2\alpha}$ on pregnancy and the estrous cycle of cattle. *J. Anim. Sci.*, 35, 246 (abstr.)

Lauderdale, J. W., Chenault, J. R., Seguin, B. E. and Thatcher, W. W. (1973). Fertility in cattle after $PGF_{2\alpha}$ treatment. *J. Anim. Sci.*, 37, 319 (abstr.)

Lauderdale, J. W., Seguin, B. E., Stellflug, J. N., Chenault, J. R., Thatcher, W. W., Vincent, C. K. and Loyancano, A. F. (1974). Fertility in cattle following $PGF_{2\alpha}$ injection. *J. Anim. Sci.*, 38, 964–967

Liehr, R. A., Marion, G. B. and Olson, H. H. (1972). Effects of prostaglandin on cattle estrous cycles. *J. Anim. Sci.*, 35, 247 (abstr.)

Louis, T. M., Hafs, H. D. and Morrow, D. A. (1972a). Estrus and ovulation after uterine $PGF_{2\alpha}$ in cows. *J. Anim. Sci.*, 35, 247–248 (abstr.)

Louis, T. M., Hafs, H. D. and Morrow, D. A. (1972b). Estrus and ovulation after $PGF_{2\alpha}$ in cows. *J. Anim. Sci.*, 35, 1121 (abstr.)

McCracken, J. A., Baird, D. T. and Goding, J. R. (1971). Factors affecting the secretion of steroids from the transplanted ovary in the sheep. *Rec. Prog. Horm. Res.*, 27, 537–582

McDonald, L. E., McNutt, S. H. and Nichols, R. E. (1953). On the essentiality of the bovine corpus luteum of pregnancy. *Amer. J. Vet. Res.*, 14, 539–541

Nancarrow, C. D., Radford, H. M., Connell, P. J. and Mattner, P. E. (1974). Hormonal changes occurring in cattle around normal oestrus and following administration of several luteolytic prostaglandins. *J. Steroid. Biochem.*, 5, 402 (abstr.)

Oxender, W. D., Noden, P. A., Louis, T. M. and Hafs, H. D. (1974). A review of prostaglandin $F_{2\alpha}$ for ovulation control in cows and mares. *Amer. J. Vet. Res.*, 35, 997–1001

Palmer, E. and Jousset, B. (1975). A two PG-HCG sequential treatment for synchronisation of oestrus and ovulation in the mare. *Ann. Biol. Anim. Bioch. Biophys.*, 15 (in press)

Pharriss, B. B. and Shaw, J. E. (1974). Prostaglandins in reproduction. *Ann. Rev. Biochem.*, 36, 391–412

Pharriss, B. B., Tillson, S. A. and Erickson, R. R. (1972). Prostaglandins in luteal Function. *Rec. Prog. Horm. Res.*, 28, 51–89

Pharriss, B. B. and Wyngarden, L. J. (1969). The effect of prostaglandin $F_{2\alpha}$ on the progestogen content of ovaries from pseudopregnant rats. *Proc. Soc. Exp. Biol. Med.*, 130, 92–94

Polge, C. (1975). The use of prostaglandins for the control of the sexual cycle in pigs. *Ann. Biol. Anim. Bioch. Biophys.*, 15 (in press)

Roche, J. R. (1974). Synchronization of oestrus and fertility following artificial insemination in heifers given prostaglandin $F_{2\alpha}$. *J. Reprod. Fert.*, 37, 135–138

Rowson, L. E. A., Lamming, G. E. and Fry, R. M. (1953). The relationship between ovarian hormones and uterine infection. *Vet. Rec.*, 65, 335–340

Rowson, L. E. A., Tervit, R. and Brand, A. (1972a). The use of prostaglandins for synchronization of Oestrus in cattle. *J. Reprod. Fert.*, 29, 145 (abstr.)

Rowson, L. E. A., Tervit, R. and Brand, A. (1972b). Synchronization of oestrus in cattle by means of prostaglandin $F_{2\alpha}$. *Proc. 7th Int. Cong. Anim. Reprod. Munich*, (ii), 866–869

Saiduddin, S., Quevedo, M. M. and Foote, W. D. (1968). Response of beef cows to exogenous progesterone and estradiol at various stages postpartum. *J. Anim. Sci.*, **27**, 1015–1020

Stellflug, J. N., Louis, T. M., Seguin, B. E. and Hafs, H. D. (1973). Luteolysis after 30 or 60 mg $PGF_{2\alpha}$ in heifers. *J. Anim. Sci.*, **37**, 330 (abstr.)

Talbot, A. C. and Hafs, H. D. (1974). Termination of a bovine pregnancy complicated by mummified foetus. *Vet. Rec.*, **95**, 512

Tervit, H. R., Rowson, L. E. A. and Brand, A. (1973). Synchronization of oestrus in cattle using a prostaglandin $F_{2\alpha}$ analogue (ICI 79939). *J. Reprod. Fert.*, **34**, 179–181

Thimonier, J., Chupin, D. and Pelot, J. (1975). Synchronisation of oestrus in heifers and cyclic cows. *Ann. Biol. Anim. Bioch. Biophys.* **15**, (in press)

Thorburn, G. D. and Nicol, D. H. (1971). Regression of the ovine corpus luteum after infusion of prostaglandin $F_{2\alpha}$ into the ovarian artery and uterine vein. *J. Endocrinol*, **51**, 785–786

Wishart, D. F. (1974). Synchronisation of oestrus in cattle using a potent progestin (SC21009) and $PGF_{2\alpha}$. *Theriogenology*, **1**, 87–90

Index